The Radiance of Being
Complexity, Chaos and the
Evolution of Consciousness

by

Allan Combs

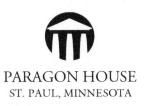

PARAGON HOUSE
ST. PAUL, MINNESOTA

First U.S. edition, 1996

Published in the United States by

Paragon House
2700 University Avenue West
St. Paul, Minnesota 55114

First Published in 1995 by Floris Books, Great Britain

The Omega Books series from Paragon House is dedicated to classic and contemporary works about human development and the nature of ultimate reality.

Library of Congress Catalog-in-Publication Data

Combs, Allan, 1942-
    The radiance of being: complexity, chaos and the evolution of consciousness / by Allan Combs
        p. cm.—
    Includes bibliographical references and index.
    ISBN 1-55778-755-7
    1. Consciousness. 2. Evolution. 3. Brain.   I. Title
BF311.C575   1996
150.19'8—dc20   96-41972
                                                                      CIP

It is evident, however, that the primary function of theories is as a lure for feeling, thereby providing immediacy of enjoyment and purpose ... Consider a Christian meditating on a saying in the gospels. He is not judging 'true or false'; he is eliciting their value as elements in feeling. In fact he may ground his judgment of truth upon the realization of value ...

Independent of the atmosphere of feeling all systems are equal, and equally uninteresting.
Alfred North Whitehead, *Process and Reality*

As webs come out of spiders, or breath forms in frozen air, worlds come out of us.
William Irwin Thompson, *Imaginary Landscape*

A contribution of The General Evolution Research Group

OMEGA BOOKS

The OMEGA BOOKS series from Paragon House is dedicated to classic and contemporary works about human development and the nature of ultimate reality, encompassing the fields of mysticism and spirituality, psychic research and paranormal phenomena, the evolution of consciousness, and the human potential for self-directed growth in body, mind and spirit.

John White, M.A.T., Series Editor of OMEGA BOOKS, is an internationally known author, editor, and educator in the fields of consciousness research, and higher human development.

MORE TITLES IN OMEGA BOOKS

KUNDALINI EVOLUTION AND ENLIGHTENMENT
Edited by John White

LIFECYCLES: Reincarnation and the Web of Life
Christopher M. Bache

THE SOUL: AN OWNER'S MANUAL
Self Discovery and the Life of Fullness, George Jaidar

THE MEANING OF SCIENCE AND SPIRIT
Guidelines for a New Age, John White

WHAT IS ENLIGHTENMENT?
Exploring the Goal of the Spiritual Path, Edited by John White

KUNDALINI EMPOWERING HUMAN EVOLUTION
Selected Writings of Gopi Krishna, Edited by Gene Kieffer

Contents

Dedicated to

Ed Mulligan and David Loye

Mentors

With appreciation to Ervin Laszlo, Stanley Krippner, Christopher Moore, Georg Feuerstein, Sally Goerner, Charles Tart, Guy Burneko, Marnie Muller, David Smith, and to my wife, Julie, for reasons they well know.

And to Herbert Guenther for his support, friendship and the sharing of his wealth of thought throughout the writing of this book.

Permissions

All the chaotic attractors were produced on a PC using the program supplied with Julien C. Sprott's *Chaotic Attractors: Creating Patterns in Chaos,* and reproduced with his permission.

The attractor figures from the olfactory bulb of the rabbit were supplied courtesy of Leslie Kay and Walter J. Freeman, Department of Molecular and Cell Biology, University of California, Berkeley.

Other drawings are reproduced with permission of the artist, Brent Garren.

The nonlinear limerick in Chapter 2, note 16, is quoted with permission from Ted Melnechuk of the Institute of Neuropoetics.

The poem by Sodo in Chapter 11, from *A Net of Fireflies,* is reproduced with permission of Charles E. Tuttle, Co.

The poem, *The Sheikh Who Played with Children,* quoted in part in Chapter 11, is reproduced from *The Longing: Poetry, Teaching Stories, and Letters of Rumi,* with permission of Threshold Books.

All Tibetan poems were translated by Herbert Guenther and are reproduced with his permission.

Foreword

In this eminently readable book Allan Combs sets himself the formidable task of providing not only an up-to-date overview but also a critical assessment of the various attempts to resolve the age-old tension between process and structure. He weaves the welter of models that evolved since before the common era to the present into a coherent tapestry in which each thread appears in new patterns and ever fascinating combinations.

For the most part Western and Eastern intellectual history has been of a structured type, with process, the dynamic quality, more or less subordinated — 'quality is nothing but poor quantification' on one side of the spectrum, and the behavioral fashion, 'beyond freedom and dignity,' on the other. Only in recent years has this worldview begun to crumble. This occurred at the microscopic level, precisely where it was least expected, and at a moment when the materialist worldview, having grown out of a reductionist science and led *ad absurdum* by its own momentum had to re-introduce the human individual as a creative participant. This collapse of the old order ushered in new ideas of a non-material field, of harmony beyond music, of co-ordination, inspiration, and wholeness, and above all of evolution as the unfolding of a self-directed theme — not as a kind of Darwinian adaptation but as dynamic, the foremost example of which is still inadequately and restrictively called 'consciousness.'

Evolutionary ideas are not new. In rudimentary form they occurred already in the Upanishads, apart from the Vedas the earliest Indian literary documents, where what is called *Brahman*[1] either transforms itself into the multiplicity of the phenomenal world or unfolds through different, usually three, levels in a hierarchical order.[2] Leaving Buddhism and Vedanta aside for the moment because of their complexity, the tension between reductionist and evolutionary trends in early Indian thought was already patent in the grouping of various philosophical systems.[3] The reductionist trend so deeply ingrained in human nature was represented by the Nyaya-Vaishesika systems, the atomists (Vaishesikas), and the adherents of logic (Nyaya).[4] The evolutionary trend was represented by the Samkhya Yoga systems, which found their modern revival in the writings of Sri Aurobindo.[5] The high esteem in which Sri Aurobindo held Darwin was due to a familiarity with the Samkhya system on to which his Yoga was grafted.

Samkhya viewed mind as a subtle but essentially material process.[6] The idea that mind or what we call knowledge is matter was not abhorrent to the early Indians. Still they felt uneasy about it and claimed that the *purusha,* Atman or Self, was like some light without which all cognitions would be blind. In order to resolve the many inherent difficulties, Indians long before Sri Aurobindo noted that unless they wanted to embark on an infinite regress, they had to come up with a super-Atman or God — this magic word that effectively prevents any further questioning. This ruse was not unknown to the Upanishadic thinkers, though in a less piously evocative form, for when, in the Brhadaranyaka Upanishad, Gargi continued asking questions about the Ultimate, Yajnavalkya, running out of answers, told her to stop asking or her head would burst!

Yoga, of which many varieties were to evolve, had already at the time of Panini (sixth or fifth century BC) acquired the meaning of control of the senses and was used by Patanjali (second century AD) in the sense of a partial or full restraint and steadying of the states of mind as inner experiences — of which some are positive and some negative in terms of the overall movement of the mind toward emancipation. It was this emphasis on control that endeared the yoga disciplines to the Westerner's dominance psychology, so much the more so as it leaves intact, indeed reinforces, a narrow and restricted ego-logical 'vision.'

Specific to the yoga discipline is the idea of a human being presenting a hierarchically organized multilevel system, its levels — seven in Hinduism, Buddhism being less dogmatic as to numbers — referred to by the technical term *cakra,* each one forming a focal point of experience or energy flow pattern interacting with the other focal points and with the human system's environment. The hierarchical arrangement is teleologically oriented and, while the ascent from a lower level to a higher one may be seen as an emphasis on process rather than on structure, it is not evolutionary in the strict sense of the word as an unfolding and reaching-out into a non-predetermined future. This 'dead end' feature of an older teleological evolution (a straightforward goal-seeking) and of a newer, contemporary, teleonomic evolution (a goal-seeking by way of possible processes involving detours) is not overcome by adding new levels or by speaking of maximum ascension,[7] but actually contradicts the open-ended self-organization of dynamic systems.

It is not without significance that before presenting his many innovative and illumining ideas the author examines the very meaning of the word 'evolution.' It is used, according to him, in the sense of being a biological notion, in the sense of a general theory, and in the sense of psychological or spiritual growth to which there can be no limits. This re-examination releases it from the hold of the outdated Darwinian model of mere adaptation and paves the way for a deepening understanding of the self-organization and self-determination of all that is alive. This fresh vision makes the author not only aware of the dangers that lie in any model-building that as a creative activity always tends to end in some artefact and prompts us to forget that it is a human artefact, but even more so makes him avoid the 'narcissistic' trap into which this model-building likes to lead and then hold us captive. It may not be out of place to quote the words of the late Erich Jantsch:

> So desperate is our dependence on viable models and myths
> that we subconsciously try to elevate them from the muddy
> world of human emotions and interests to the crisp, clear
> heights of absolute truth. Physical models are set absolute,
> and the myth of science is created. Social models are set
> absolute and their corresponding myths, or ideologies,
> subsequently imposed by social habits and taboos, or also
> by intimidation and force. Spiritual or cultural models are
> set absolute and their imperialism is defended on the
> grounds of belief in the form of religion or other
> evolutionary or pseudoevolutionary myths.

In assessing and weaving together the various models the author emphasizes their positive points without, however, concealing their negative aspects. He is one of the rare individuals who can listen rather than simply coming up with 'definite' statements that, in spite of the high esteem in which they are held by professionals and lay-people, are the ultimate in reductionist insipidity. He invites the reader to cultivate the rare gift of thinking. His book will be required reading for any serious student of the mystery that we are.

Herbert Guenther

Introduction

The roots of consciousness

Rather than discrete things and independent events, there are but ripples upon ripples upon waves upon waves in this universe, propagating in a seamless sea.

Ervin Laszlo

Finally the neural network people had succeeded in building a computer as intelligent as a human being. It not only was as smart as a human, but was able to report out the secret and invisible workings behind its own intellect. Scientists rubbed their hands in anticipation. They asked the first question.

'What is the nature of human knowledge?'

Lights momentarily flickered and a soft resonant voice replied, 'Let me tell you a story ...'[1]

This book is a story of a search for the truth of human nature and its possibilities, my possibilities and your possibilities. It is a search that takes place in this world where truth itself is woven from the clear chronicles of science and the profound tales of mystics. It is my own search, but I do not quest alone. Not since late antiquity with its myriad religions, philosophical crosscurrents, and mystery schools, have people in such numbers looked beyond the limits of tradition for the deep narratives of their own souls. In those days, as today, ideas from as far away as India and China were discussed side by side over meals with the religious, scientific, and philosophical thought of Greece and Rome. Egypt's Alexandria was the scientific and wisdom center of a civilization. Today the world has spiralled back around, but at a different octave. Once more we have access to knowledge of the past, some rediscovered and some returned to us from Eastern sources where all along it has been growing. We now have the added benefit and wisdom of a science finally outgrowing its adolescence and turning to matters of essence.

My intent in this book is to serve as part guide and part fellow traveler on a quest into the labyrinthine realms of science and traditional wisdom in search of the roots of consciousness. My hope is to seek a thread of truth and follow it to its end. This requires more than data and hard logic, and even more than intuition. It requires a balancing act that at once clings to the best that science has to offer while all the time holding a reverence for traditional wisdom, knowing that the truths of science change daily while traditional wisdom is so deeply steeped in metaphor that its foundations are often obscure. More than anything else, however, it requires an honesty that is relentless and penetrates to the bone, an honesty that calls upon us to reject even our most cherished beliefs and biases when facts, common sense, and intuition rebel against them. No one is a perfect pilot in this domain, but we must hold to all that can guide us in navigating the web of possibilities that will follow. You, the reader, may well come to different conclusions than my own, but let us proceed together as companions.

The thread of truth to which I will cling is a process view of human consciousness, one that honors its fluid and evolving complexity in each moment as well as the historical unfolding of its evolutionary roots. This thread is consistent with my own background in chaos theory and the sciences of complexity. It views human experience as a process in flux rather than a fixed event, more of the nature of rippling water than of the rocks over which it flows. The ideas in this book present a radically revised understanding of what it is to be human. We will begin to see ourselves, not as static organisms, but as living processes evolving into the future in a continuous dynamic event of self-creation.

As a psychologist I have considerable respect for those 'transpersonal' psychologists such as William James, Carl Jung, Abraham Maslow, Charles Tart, Ken Wilber, Stanislav Grof, Michael Washburn, and others, who have fought for the importance and legitimacy of recognizing the larger possibilities of human nature. Several of these will play important roles in the pages to come, as will the contributions of Eastern wisdom traditions. Indeed, the contemporary Tibetan wisdom master, Chögyam Trungpa, observed that the language and terms of modern psychology 'often come closer to those of Buddhism than to those of Western philosophy or religion.'[2] Thus, we are today better suited to seek a fusion of Eastern ideas with Western thought than ever before.

The book is arranged into three major sections. The first introduces ideas that will fuel the later sections. Beginning with a discussion of the nature of consciousness and the mind, it includes a basic description of chaos theory and self-creating systems as well as some observations on the brain. I also explain a process view of consciousness that will be useful throughout the book. The second section reviews important theories of the evolution of consciousness from that of the eighteenth-century philosopher Giambattista Vico, through the Indian sage philosopher Sri Aurobindo Ghose, and on to contemporary thinkers such as Jean Gebser and Ken Wilber. The third section begins with a critical evaluation of previous theories and proceeds to an examination of consciousness and the higher reaches of human nature.

Appendix I is a technical glossary that presents for convenience a list of terms, mostly from chaos and general systems theory. It also includes a second glossary of terms from Eastern philosophies, explaining more about their origins and meaning than is found in the main body of the book.

It seems that many theorists interested in the nature of consciousness, both in the East and West, have also been interested in its historical evolution. For this reason the review in the middle section of the book, which summarizes the thought of Henri Bergson, Teilhard de Chardin, Sri Aurobindo, Jean Gebser, and Ken Wilber, among others, turns out to cover much of the basic theoretical ground of transpersonal psychology itself. With this in mind, I thought it useful to include an *Appendix II* which summarizes the two major contemporary views of transpersonal psychology not touched on elsewhere. These are the theories of psychiatrist Stanislav Grof and philosopher Michael Washburn.

PART ONE

Complexity

1. Minding Consciousness

Consciousness and mind

This book is about consciousness, but it is also about the mind, as the two are not easily separated. So let's start by giving form to these concepts here at the beginning.

Consciousness: the very essence of it

There are few words that have been used as many different ways as the word *consciousness*.[1] If I were to review all of them we would still be at it till well after dinner. Here I will simply give my own idea of consciousness as plainly and directly as possible. It represents a practical and intuitive synthesis of many years of reading, thinking, and simply sitting with the topic. It seems to me to minimize conflicts with other views, while at the same time getting us down the road to understanding the richness and mystery of human nature.

Consciousness is the essence of experience. Its touch is the bearer of meaning. It is pointed neither inward nor outward; I mean it is neither introverted nor extroverted. It is not simple nor is it complex. It has no structure of its own but only essence. It is not static nor is it in motion. Consciousness is the perfect transparent *subjectivity* through which the phenomenal world shines. Without it, knowledge is only information. Without it the cosmos is dead.

Consciousness, however, is always *about* something. For instance, we can think about a tree — be conscious of it — but the tree itself is not *about* anything. Likewise, we can dream about a lake, but the lake is not about anything either. Thus consciousness is always in the business of bringing objects into awareness, whether through thoughts, dreams, memories, feelings, or sensory impressions such as tastes, sounds, and visual images. In other words, consciousness always has a point. In formal terms it is said to be *intentional*.[2] Something is

intended by it. There may be exceptions, for example in certain meditative and mystical states that we will explore later in the book,[3] but
for practical purposes these are rare and unusual.

Intentionality is dynamic. Like a polarizing magnetic field that
draws iron filings into formations of multiple ellipses, consciousness
aligns the processes of the mind into patterns with direction and
purpose. For example, even now as I sit writing in a local coffee shop
an old man enters my field of vision, makes his way across the street,
and steps through the door. He is hunched over with age and wears a
heavy brown coat against a cold wind. He wears a beret on his head
that gives him the appearance of an aged artist or scholar. Without
meaning to take my mind from my work I find myself the object of
a series of fantasies about this old man's life — his years of writing
or painting, or teaching at some college or university — and I also
become aware of memories of other such men whom I have met or
seen in photographs or paintings. I notice in myself a feeling of fond-
ness for this man out of all proportion to what I actually know of him,
perhaps because I might one day be such an old man myself. The
point of all this is that the old man's entry into my consciousness had
a dramatic effect on me, not only activating my visual sense — as I
watched him — but triggering a whole set of feelings, reflections,
thoughts and memories. All this was brought about by the effortless
touch of consciousness. In a word, the old man caught my *attention*.
It is the polarizing touch of consciousness in the form of attention that
activates the senses, awakens memories, quickens the emotions,
kindles desire, and animates the imagination.[4]

Attention can apparently be trained by the practice of virtually any
task that requires its unbroken concentration. A hundred years ago
William James commented on the importance of cultivating attention,
remarking that:

> The faculty of voluntarily bringing back a wandering
> attention, over and over again, is the very root of judgment,
> character, and will. No one is *compos sui* if he have it not.
> An education which should improve this faculty would be
> *the* education *par excellence.*

Though James could not have known it a century ago, the rigorous training of attention is an essential aspect of the required training in virtually all wisdom traditions, whether Indian yoga, Zen Buddhism, Taoist meditation, or the forms of Western esotericism such as alchemy, magic, and the Kabbalah.

None of this is to suggest that consciousness is any kind of *entity,* or *substance,* such as René Descartes' *res cogitans.*[5] During his philosophical period William James once argued that consciousness of itself 'is the name of a nonentity, and has no right to a place among first principles.'[6] He went on to state that consciousness is a relation between two terms in which one *knows* the other. In other words, the essential nature of consciousness is simple awareness; one thing (a person or animal) is aware of another. I would be inclined to agree with James were it not for the dynamic aspects of consciousness mentioned above. These suggest something more active than the sparse relationship of one thing knowing another.[7]

To make myself even more disagreeable, I do not feel it sufficient to say, as do many current theorists, that consciousness is explained as an emergent or higher order property of the brain.[8] The single fact of the subjectivity of consciousness, in other words that it is *like* something to be a human being but apparently not like anything to be a brick, a baseball bat, or even a computer, sets consciousness so far apart from matter that, to my mind, it makes no sense at all to conclude that it is any kind of *property* of it.[9]

Personally, I am inclined to think of consciousness as a subjective *presence.* This feels good to me and honors the experience we all have toward other persons and animals as well that 'something is there,' something that most palpably departs at death. But here we approach metaphysics, and, for me, it is a relief to realize that my opinions about the final nature of consciousness are not at all critical to most of the ideas in this book. Few of the notions presented in the following pages would be lost if consciousness turned out to be entirely comprehensible as some miraculous outgrowth of the living brain.

Having said all the above, I now plan to make myself entirely objectionable by being perfectly libertine in my use of the word *consciousness,* promising only to return to the above carefully considered limitations by the end of the book. This is because otherwise I would drive myself, and you dear reader, crazy with constant updates, corrections, harangues about how others use the word and how I ought to be more careful about it myself. I ought not to say, for example, 'states of consciousness,' but rather 'patterns of mind or brain activity that structure regimens of experience in a certain way,' and pedantically on like that. But I will try to use the word *consciousness* with the democratic pragmatism of reality itself, so that if one pays attention things will usually make sense. Then, in the final chapters, I will begin to pull in the reins again to bring us to a safe and ordered philological landing.

Mind, on the other hand

The word *mind* has been used almost in as many ways as the word *consciousness.* In the largest sense it is often taken to mean the entire inner life of an individual. Thus it is said, 'she is healthy in both body and mind.' Here the word *mind* points to her thoughts, attitudes, dreams, desires, and so on.

Throughout history, however, there has been a tendency to put a spin on the concept of mind in favor particularly of the intellectual aspects of the inner life. Thus, to 'live the life of the mind' means to live an intellectual life. This spin is found in the West and East as well.[10] It is found, for instance, near the very beginnings of Western thought in Plato's reflections on the soul. In the *Phaedo* he has Socrates discuss the ideal situation of the soul after death. Here the soul is presented entirely as a thinking being, reasoning toward truth and virtue. Plato's student, Aristotle, took a more holistic view, seeing the soul as infusing the physical body with life. In *De Anima* he named several distinctly different functions of the soul, but even so only rational thought and the search for truth were given uniquely human status, and thus seen to be eternal. Following along this line the philosophers and writers of the Middle Ages celebrated the rational, reasoning, side of human nature while condemning the irrational side as base and animal-like. At the beginning of the modern era, when René Descartes formulated his remarkably influential concept of mind as distinct from the body, he proposed a thinking mind that was very much like Plato's soul.

Consistent with the above, modern thinking about the mind is largely dominated by the cognitive or mental sciences. These include computer design and artificial intelligence, the neurosciences and cognitive psychology, as well as certain strains of philosophy, linguistics, and anthropology. They form a loosely knit community of disciplines which share an interest in computers, information processing, symbolic logic, and the like. As a group they view mind in terms of computation, symbol manipulation, and information exchange, all of which emphasize the mind's rational operations.[11]

In this book I will not limit the idea of mind to the cognitive or intellectual side of the inner life alone. Rather, I will take *mind* to be all those inner processes and conditions that shape and color consciousness, producing the unique landscapes of experience that characterize each moment of our lives.[12] A person's thoughts, feelings, desires, dreams, memories, and aspirations are all mental events, all productions of the mind.[13] They are all, as well, objects of conscious experience if one attends to them.

Though consciousness tends to exhibit wholeness, the mind does not. It is the unity of consciousness and the integrity of its field that collects the various elements of the mind into a coherent fabric. Penetrating deconstructions of the mind by Western philosophers from David Hume to Daniel Dennett, and centuries of Buddhist analysis, have failed to find unity in it, though the observing consciousness is rarely without wholeness. This is to say that under hard scrutiny the processes of the mind are seen to be fragmented and surprisingly separate.[14] If consciousness weakens, as when we become drowsy, these disparate processes drift into disarray, and fragmented thoughts, memories, and feelings float aimlessly through awareness.[15]

From the point of view of consciousness, looking down at the mind discloses many interesting features but its essential operations are mostly hidden from view. Indeed, the prominent psychologist Karl Lashley once commented, 'no activity of mind is ever conscious'! For instance, where do memories reside, and what are the mechanisms that call them on to the stage of awareness? Where, in fact, do thoughts come from, and what is the studio that produces the imagination?

What faculties organize perception, to present to consciousness, *fait accompli,* an entire visible world built from the rippling shades of retinal light? How is the perfect stride chosen to take us smoothly up a flight of stairs or around a corner? Indeed, honest assessment leads to the conclusion that we understand little and experience less of the ground level activities of the mind.[16]

With these thoughts I conclude our brief introduction to consciousness and the mind, though we will return to them often in the pages to come. In Chapter 2, however, we will stop to explore briefly some ideas about evolution and chaos. These will be useful for coming to a new and deeper understanding of consciousness and the mind.

2. The Fire and the Rose

Beauty in chaos

And all shall be well and
All manner of thing shall be well
When the tongues of flame are in-folded
Into the crowned knot of fire
And the fire and the rose are one.
                    T.S. Eliot, *Little Gidding*

The image of stillness in chaotic motion is powerfully suggestive of a deeper mystical awareness. Here is tension between impermanence and eternal pattern, a tension experienced in the heart of the whirl-wind, and in the rainbow at the waterfall. This chapter is one story of how science has come to recognize this tension. The ideas introduced here will be useful throughout the rest of the book.

All the world is made up of the two dimensions of flux and stasis, of process and structure. Whether through historical accident or evolutionary intention, however, we lean toward structural, even static conceptions of the cosmos and of ourselves. This is the case in the East as well as the West. It is a tendency that has blinded us in part to the chaotic and fluid nature of the cardinal events of our lives; of thought, of emotion, of growth and transformation in all their myriad aspects, and of human relationships and everything they entail.

Centuries ago the Enlightenment legacy of Descartes, Newton, and the other architects of modern mechanistic science, left us with a notion of reality that centered almost exclusively on material objects. In this view processes were reduced to by-products of motion. Consciousness had no place at all in such a cosmos, and was in fact evicted from it by Descartes' influential dualism.[1] As a consequence, evolution still is usually explained as the lone result of the random play of physical elements. Meanwhile it is far from clear how complex organisms such as human beings could ever have come into existence in such a haphazard fashion. Process thinking is a major alternative to this perspective.

Process thinking is not new. In the West it was found in ancient Greece, where the philosopher Heraclitus, recognizing the ever-changing nature of reality, shrewdly observed that it is not possible to step into the same river twice. In the East, process thinking was also apparent in the ancient philosophy of Taoism, according to which the visible world is undergirded by an organic growth principle, or *tao*.[2] Certain Buddhist thinkers as long ago as the sixth century AD, developed a detailed and penetrating process understanding of human experience.[3] More recently, the twentieth-century British philosopher Alfred North Whitehead constructed an influential process. For the most part, however, all these approaches have either been purely subjective,[4] as in the Buddhist traditions, or metaphysical, as with Whitehead. What was missing was a way to translate the process perspective into diverse practical and theoretical applications, in other words a theoretical approach interesting as well as fertile in the everyday world.

Self-creation

A breakthrough came in the sixties and seventies when general systems theory, already developing in the writings of Ludwig van Bertalanffy and others, came under the influence of cybernetics, created by mathematicians such as Norbert Wiener.[5] Systems ranging from computers to living organisms, and on to entire ecologies, in time came to be seen as self-regulating processes that utilize cybernetic feedback loops for growth and stabilization. Theorists such as Erich Jantsch and Ervin Laszlo systematically explored the implications of these ideas for a wide range of issues in both philosophy and science.[6]

An important contribution to this developing line of thought was the introduction, in the mid-seventies, of the notion of self-creation, or *autopoiesis,* suggested by South American biologists Humberto Maturana and Francisco Varela.[7] The idea is that certain systems, including living organisms, are in a business, the primary object of which is no less than to constantly create themselves. For example, the net result of the metabolic activity of a living cell is the cell itself. Much the same can be said of more complex organisms such as plants and animals, and indeed entire ecologies and even human societies.[8] Autopoietic systems do not simply maintain stasis in the face of changing external conditions; they dynamically recreate themselves. Maturana and Varela originally defined such systems as networks of interconnected component-producing processes that, interacting, re-create these very networks. Such systems are best thought of in terms of patterns of processes rather than as material structures, the substance of which may be left behind. The human body, like a living cell, continuously recreates itself out of new molecular material, while patterns of hormonal, metabolic, and neural activity remain more or less constant.

The notion of autopoiesis is steeped in process thought because in it we see what is essential to an organism, ecology, or society, is not its physical composition or momentary structure, which constantly changes, but the continuing processes by which it re-creates itself. These processes sustain its identity, whether it be a simple amoeba wriggling through the waters of a farm pond, a knobby caterpillar transforming into an exquisitely mottled butterfly, a child maturing into an adult, or an evolving star. We will later see that the mind itself is an autopoietic process.

Putting turbulence in order

Simultaneous with the above developments, changes in the field of mathematics lead to new and more effective ways to conceptualize process aspects of complex systems.[9] These new ways, now collectively called *chaos theory,* form a loosely knit fabric of theory that includes René Thom's catastrophe theory, Edward Lorenz's discovery of the first of an unlimited variety of chaotic *attractors* — of which we will have more to say shortly — and Benoit Mandelbrot's unveiling of a strange and irregular *fractal* geometry.[10] An important but often understated aspect of these new approaches is that they use intuitively appealing topological, or graphic, representations, beautiful in themselves and more readily grasped than abstract algebraic formalisms. These innovations in mathematics provide powerful tools for understanding complex systems. They have already been applied to an ever growing variety of physical and biological systems ranging from pendulums to entire ecologies. They have also been used in medical research on the human heart and the electrical activity of the brain, and have even been used to describe entire social and economic systems.[11]

One of the richest ideas in chaos theory, and one that will be very useful to us in understanding the nature of consciousness, is the above-mentioned *attractor*. This is a state or pattern of activity toward which a system tends to slide of its own accord.[12] Several types of attractors have been identified. The simplest is demonstrated by a pendulum that, set into motion, swings in decreasing arcs until it comes to rest. This rest state is termed a *static attractor* because it represents the stationary configuration to which the pendulum system is drawn after friction brings it to a full stop. Another example is an empty coffee cup which, placed roughly on a table spirals round and round, circling till it comes to a stop — again in the rest state. It is as if the pendulum and the cup are drawn or 'attracted' to their final stationary positions. In these instances we see an important feature of all attractors, namely that they represent the *final* disposition of a system, often after it passes through an initial period of change. In our study of consciousness we will not often find uses for static attractors. Other, more interesting types of attractors, however, will be of much value.

Some systems do not arrive at a static configuration at all, but remain in continuous motion. For instance, if a small energy source were connected to the pendulum to offset the drag of friction, as is the case with a grandfather clock, the pendulum could continue swinging. In this case we would refer to its pattern of motion as a *fixed cycle* or *periodic attractor*. A more complete description of this pattern might involve the mapping of its motion as seen on the left in Figure 1, in which the moment-to-moment velocity of the pendulum is plotted on the vertical axis against its instant-to-instant position on the horizontal axis. The result is a closed loop indicating cyclic motion.[13] If the clock were to run down, allowing the swing of the pendulum to decrease

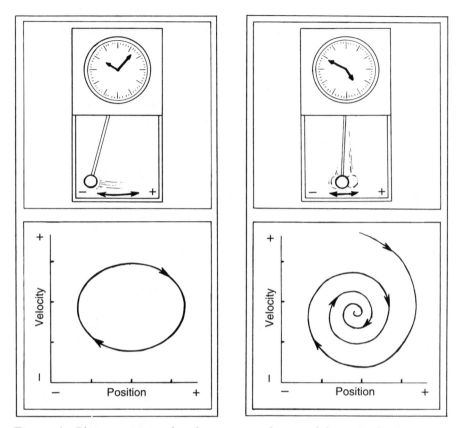

Figure 1. Phase portraits for the motion of a pendulum. Each shows its simultaneous change in position and velocity with the passage of time. In the portrait on the left its motion continues normally, describing a fixed cycle attractor, while in the portrait on the right it gradually comes to a stop, or point attractor, as the clock's spring runs down.

until it stopped, the figure produced would be a spiral, indicating a smooth decrease of displacement and velocity toward the original point attractor, as seen on the right.

The basic human circadian rhythm of sleep and wakefulness approximates the behavior of a fixed cycle attractor. Here, however, variations occur in the larger cycle with the appearance of dreams at roughly ninety minute intervals during the night as well as cycles of alertness and drowsiness during the day.[14] More important, the rhythm is not smooth, but reflects normal day to day irregularities in patterns of sleep and wakefulness. Thus, our circadian rhythms are far from smooth or perfect cycles. Indeed, they might be better characterized as chaotic, or at least chaotic-like.

Resembling our own circadian rhythms, many complex systems oscillate in a more or less periodic fashion which, unlike the pendulum, does not come to rest and does not ever quite repeat itself. This is the case, for instance, with weather patterns, animal population cycles, and stock market fluctuations. It would also appear to be the case with the ebb and flow of moods and emotions.[15] Such processes are unpredictable in the strictest sense, though their overall patterns can be recognized and identified and short term projections of rough accuracy can be drawn of their future progress, as is the case with weather. Such irregular rhythms have often been termed *chaotic,* and plotting the course of such a rhythm is said to yield a *chaotic attractor* (also called a *strange attractor).* As seen in Figure 2, such attractors may appear to be made up of sets of lobes or wings of varying complexity. Here we see the famous Lorenz attractor, sometimes called the 'Lorenz mask,' discovered in 1963 by MIT meteorologist Edward Lorenz. It is produced by a simple set of equations that he used to model weather.

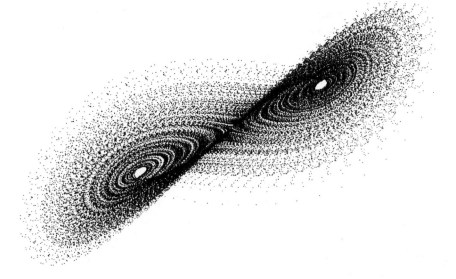

Figure 2. The Lorenz 'mask,' a three-dimensional attractor discovered by Edward Lorenz in 1963 while modeling weather patterns. It was the first known instance of a chaotic attractor.

Strictly speaking, the behavior of a system must meet certain mathematical criteria to qualify as chaotic.[16] The Lorenz attractor does so easily, while moods and emotions may only partially qualify.[17] At the time of this writing it is unknown for sure whether circadian rhythms qualify at all. For these and other reasons, in this book I will use a somewhat relaxed definition of chaos, referring to circadian rhythms and similarly irregular but globally patterned processes as *chaotic* or *chaotic-like,* without holding them to the fire for the formal criteria.[18] Other writers and researchers are following a similar course as it becomes increasingly apparent that many systems of interest, ranging from simple single cell organisms to entire ecosystems, are broadly chaotic, but either do not precisely fit the mathematical criteria or cannot for practical reasons be shown to do so.[19]

Tottering on the edge of chaos

Some complex systems, apparently including those that undergird conscious experience, appear to exist *on the edge of chaos.* For them, ordinary stability is punctuated by periods of chaos. This notion was first introduced to describe processes such as the intricate metabolic cycles of living cells, or the exquisitely complex neural events of the human brain.[20] Systems on the edge of chaos shift back and forth between predictable behavior and chaotic activity. In doing so, they may undergo important transformations that can produce growth. This is a notion that we will return to in the next chapter where we examine it in the context of psychological maturation. Periods of chaotic activity can throw a system out beyond its ordinary grooves, affording it an opportunity to come down in a different path, a new attractor. Complex systems can relax out of their habitual patterns of behavior. Were they, on the other hand, to remain in chaotic states all the time they would risk losing their identity and descending into absolute disorder.

It is helpful to visualize the behavior of complex systems in terms of attractors. Mathematically speaking, an attractor is always located in a *basin.* This can be thought of as an indentation carved into the surface of a table top, one into which, for example, a marble might be rolled. This indentation includes along its slopes all the initial states of the system that could lead it down to the attractor at the bottom. For instance, if the indentation is simply a round bowl-shaped cavity, the marble will roll around in it, eventually finding its way to the bottom. Here, the final condition of the marble represents the static attractor of the marble-in-the-bowl system.

The analogy between the real system and the mathematical one need not be so literal. For example, a super-saturated solution of sugar dissolved in water will form rock candy if a string is dropped down into it. To picture this system we could construct a diagram, or topological surface, representing sugar concentration on one axis and water temperature on the other. Across a particular region of this surface the dissolved sugar will begin to crystalize into rock candy. This region is the basin for the static rock candy attractor. Making rock candy, however, involves more than a simple increase in the concentration of the sugar. It also requires the formation of a crystal, a dramatic shift in the structural organization of the sugar molecules away from their dissolved state. Such a basic change in a system is often called a *bifurcation.* We will see many instances of psychological bifurcations as we go along, for example, when consciousness slips from wakefulness to sleep, or when a child becomes an adolescent. Interestingly, both transitions involve temporary periods of chaos, pleasant in the first instance, but not always so pleasant in the second.

More complex than the sugar solution example, the metabolism of a living cell is best described not as a static attractor, but as a cyclic attractor that moves through a variety of states as part of its ordinary activity. If it is destabilized by some novel situation, however, it might shift, or bifurcate, into a new chaotic or chaotic-like pattern of activity. This would launch it into a complex trajectory leading through a series of divergent states that never quite repeat themselves. In the course of these travels the system might find itself sliding into a new groove, a new cyclic attractor. Such processes may well underlie certain kinds of growth or transformation in the cell. We will explore later the idea that the turbulence which often accompanies periods of personal transformation may be of a like nature.

An interesting situation occurs when two equally compelling attractors are available to the system. Then it might choose either one at random. But if there is chaos in the system it may seesaw between

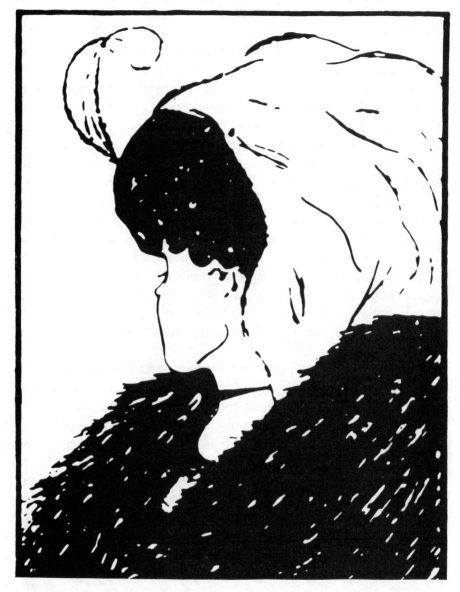

Figure 3. The curious drawing of the young girl and the old woman.

them, unable to settle conclusively into one or the other. For instance, when one views certain ambiguous pictures one of two possible images can be seen, but rarely both at once. Such pictures are called *multi-stable images,* because they present the eye with more than one temporarily stable perception. Figure 3 demonstrates this curious situation with the famous drawing of the 'young girl and the old woman.'[21]

The visual brain embraces either the perceptual attractor of the young girl, or that of the old woman, but not both at once. This is another way of saying that the patterns of neural activity in the visual brain settle into either of the two possible attractors after a short initial chaotic search for form. But notice that neither attractor is deep enough to hold the perceptual system for long, and inescapable flips between images occur from time to time. An analogous process might well underlie the unstable oscillations experienced in multiple personality disorders.[22]

Such seeming instability may protect a system from getting stuck in a rut. In the instance of multistable visual images, it keeps perception from settling on a single view and missing all other possibilities. Often we are confronted with a situation in which we are not entirely certain what we are seeing. Is this someone we know? Is there an animal on the dark road, or simply the play of light on leaves waving in the wind? Is the last digit of a scrawled handwritten phone number a five or a three?

In the case of memory, the mind likewise benefits from agile uncertainty. As we try to recall a nearly forgotten name, a series of prospects are paraded by the mind's eye for inspection, each a small attractor for memory. Each candidate temporarily holds our attention till one name takes hold of the mind as a powerful singularity and we know we have what we are looking for. The unstable situation seen in the case of multiple personalities seems pathological, but even here we may be seeing the extreme form of a desirable process. The natural tendency of systems on the edge of chaos toward supple flexibility is certainly a desirable trait in a healthy personality. The ability to easily change states from mother to lover, from teacher to student, and from work to play, and anger to joy, is unhealthy only if out of control.

Complexity and the grand evolutionary synthesis

Systems thinking and chaos theory are only part of a larger shift seen in many fields, and indeed in society as a whole. This is a shift toward increasing *complexity*.[23]

For example, my auto mechanic recently explained to me that in order to repair cars these days he practically needs degrees in electrical engineering and computer technology, as well as the traditional mechanical skills! This is because advanced cars today are controlled by on-board computers which in turn utilize complex electrical circuitry to regulate the gas flow, timing of the spark, engine temperature, and so on. Such cars have forced many a back-yard mechanic to seek other hobbies.

But why do such complex and difficult to repair cars survive in the marketplace? Mihaly Csikszentmihalyi, the gifted psychologist who a few years ago coined the notion of psychological *flow*,[24] discusses a similar situation with cameras. Suppose you are about to buy a camera, he proposes. You go to the camera store and examine the variety of models on display. Some are easier to use than others, performing operations such as setting time exposures and lens adjustments by themselves, so you can concentrate on the picture and not on the camera. These same models are likely also to offer additional features such as a built-in zoom lens for portraits, or automatic film rewinding. These, of course, are the most complex cameras in the store, and if you can afford them they are very likely the ones you will select. Thus, like the complex cars, they tend to survive in a complex and competitive marketplace.

Csikszentmihalyi believes the growth of complexity to be the hallmark of evolution.[25] This holds for all sorts of evolution, for example the evolution of biological organisms, the evolution of ecologies, and the subtle evolution of the inner self. Exactly why this might be the case is not entirely apparent, and Csikszentmihalyi does not explain it. At least part of the answer, however, can be found in a new understanding of evolution itself, one that comes from the process perspective as well as from systems theory. It reveals why physical, biological, and social systems all complexify as they evolve. Its ideas will also be useful to us in gaining a richer understanding of the nature of consciousness.

In the 1970s Nobel laureate chemist Ilya Prigogine and his associates discovered how systems such as living organisms utilize energy available in their environments to reorganize themselves to increasingly higher orders of complexity. In doing so such systems create disorder, or entropy, as a by-product. The latter takes the form of dissipated heat, for example, and its associated random or Brownian motion. It is essential that these systems be located in an energy flow such as light or heat, and that it be capable of capturing and using some of this energy before releasing it into the environment.[26] The Earth itself is such a system. It absorbs energy from the sun, releasing it again in the form of radiant heat. Before its release, however, the captured energy fuels the living biosystems of the Earth. This feature of the Earth more than any other has made possible the evolution of complex life.

An example of this kind of energetic process is seen when water is placed in the energy flow created by a burner on the stove. As the water absorbs heat the Brownian movement of its molecules increases, forming whorls and eddies. This is a turbulent phase in which the individual molecules thrash about with increasing independence. It is the unstable moment just prior to transformation. If the heat continues to increase, the entire system undergoes a change, or bifurcation, and distinct well-organized vertical convection currents appear. These are called *Bénard cells.* They are hexagonally shaped and can be seen not only in heated water, but also in oceanic as well as atmospheric currents, occasionally producing hexagonal imprints on ocean floors and desert sands.

The appearance of Bénard cells is an example of the emergence of a new, more complex organization from the turbulent and energy driven motion of the heated water. Notice that here we also see the appearance of a primitive tiered or hierarchical organization. The individual water molecules continue their independent random movement, but now are carried about in the larger complex system of Bénard cells. While I know of no instance in which the Bénard cells, in their turn, form the foundation stones for some even higher formation, instances of the spontaneous appearance of multilevel structures seem to be a common feature in evolution. For instance, the early phases of the creation of the physical universe appear to have involved the spontaneous formation of a variety of very small particles which in their turn formed the basis of more elaborate arrangements. Eventually, complex atoms self-organized from sub-atomic particles. Such atoms in turn came to comprise the building blocks for a virtually infinite variety of molecules, some of which form the elements of organic matter.

The appearance of hierarchical organization is just as apparent in biological evolution. According to biologist Lynn Margulis, for example, eucaryotic cells such as those that form the human body originally evolved from a cooperative relationship between at least two earlier types of cells, one of which was probably a parasite nested in the other.[27] The two eventually developed a cooperative or symbiotic relationship. Today the eucaryotic cell carries within it small cell-like structures termed *mitochondria,* the vestiges of the original parasite cells and an important component of the eucaryote's energy metabolism. Mitochondria, however, still retain a significant degree of individual integrity, including the possession of their own genetic material. Thus, the modern eucaryotic cell is a hierarchical structure, 'built up from other cells ... [in] a community of interacting microbes.'

An important feature of hierarchical systems is that each level exhibits its own characteristics, experiences its own domain of freedom, and operates by its own set of rules. The eucaryotic cell was originally formed of more elemental cells. Of these the mitochondria retain a certain independence, including the management of their own cell division. The entire symbiotic system of the eucaryote with its mitochondria, however, is the product of more elemental chemical processes, best understood at the molecular level where the laws of chemistry that govern them have dominion. Chemical processes, in turn, are woven together of events at the atomic level. Like Chinese boxes, each level is undergirded by another, and is itself the foundation for a higher tier. Eucaryotic cells exhibit characteristics of their own, independent of the smaller cells that comprise them. On the upward scale they in turn form the organs of the human body. These interact in a cooperative fashion to create the body itself. At each level a new system emerges, with its own autonomy, its own patterns of interaction, and its own unique environment.

Apparently, each new level of organization offers an energy gain over the previous one. The appearance of Bénard cells yields an increase in the efficiency with which heat is transmitted through the hot water.[28] Eucaryotic cells gather energy in the form of food more efficiently than their constituent predecessors. The grouping of eucaryotic cells into organs and human bodies allows even more effectiveness in food gathering. When human beings form social groups they further increase their food gathering capacities and their energy managing capacity in general, whether it be heat in the form of fire, electricity, or even atomic energy. Thus, societies, cultures, and civilizations are formed.

All the above suggests a new general model for understanding evolution. This new model recognizes a broad tendency for evolution to move in the direction of increasingly complex and cooperative interactions between subsystems, leading to the formation of emergent higher-order systems of the autopoietic type. This tendency is witnessed in the physical universe as well as in the evolution of life. It is a tendency that also characterizes the evolution of ecological, social, economic, and political systems. Hungarian systems philosopher Ervin Laszlo has termed this new model the *grand evolutionary synthesis,* writing:

> In the penultimate decade of the twentieth century science is sufficiently advanced to resolve the puzzles that stymied scientists in the last century and demonstrate, without metaphysical speculation, the consistency of evolution in all realms of experience. It is now possible to advance a grand evolutionary synthesis based on unitary and mutually consistent concepts derived from the empirical sciences.

Laszlo provides a readily accessible overview of the grand evolutionary synthesis in his book, *Evolution: the Grand Synthesis.* A more technical introduction is found in Vilmos Csányi's *Evolutionary Systems and Society: a General Theory of Life, Mind, and Culture.*[29]

Considering the breadth of this conception of evolution, it is not surprising that it would also have implications for the evolution of consciousness. This is indeed the case, as we shall soon see.[30]

3. Like a City Built across the Ages

Consciousness and the brain

In fact, the brain is a complex matrix of superimposed and interwoven systems corresponding to the various stages of evolution, and the self that arises from it is something like a city built across the ages ... Each of us carries within his own nervous system the whole history of biological life on the planet, at least that belonging to the animal kingdom.

Danah Zohar, 1990

In the previous chapter I introduced a variety of notions about process thinking, complex systems, and evolution. This chapter introduces ideas about the brain and consciousness. The ideas in both chapters are intended to put us on the path to a new vision of consciousness and its evolution, one which will unfold as we go along.

The unity of the brain

It seems that from the beginning the brain has followed a now familiar formula. It has been a cooperative effort between separate and relatively autonomous subsystems which have come together to support a very special unity. That unity is conscious awareness. In this respect the brain represents, in microcosm, the basic pattern for the entire human body, itself a cooperative venture between the living cells that make up its various organs, and the organs, in turn, which form its whole living structure.

Biologist Lynn Margulis believes that the very nerve cells (or *neurons*) that form the brain, like all nucleated cells, represent symbiotic partnerships between several types of bacteria whose ancestors once lived quite independent lives.[1] One of these, the *spirochetes,* seems to have been a predator on another, the *archaebacteria*. She writes:

> Our nerve cells are the outcome of an ancient, nearly
> immortal marriage of two arch enemies who have managed
> to coexist: the former spirochetes and former archaebacteria
> that now comprise our brains ... These former free-living
> bacteria are inextricably united. They probably have been
> united for more than one thousand million years.

She goes on to note that the complex operations of the brain itself arise from the interactions of such nerve cells, quite literally forming a nervous system ecology. That ecology is the support of our mental lives. 'If we feel possessed of several minds, if we feel overwhelmed by complexity, it is because we are inhabited by and comprised of complexities.'

When we consider the complexity of the human brain we are confronted with the now familiar motif of levels within levels — the Chinese boxes which, when opened, are found to contain a whole series of smaller replicas of themselves. What we are discussing here is a hierarchical system. The level of the nervous system that will most interest us is that of the large subsystems which comprise the most evident functional units of the brain. These have appeared over a vast span of evolutionary time. Some are exceedingly ancient, while others came into existence only yesterday on the evolutionary time scale. The result, as Danah Zohar writes above, is that the modern human brain, and the mind that is supported by it, is like a city built across the ages.[2]

An inner bestiary

We can see the above themes begin to take form in a fascinating and well-articulated model of the human brain, one that is rooted in evolutionary thought from its inception, namely, Paul MacLean's theory of the *triune brain*.[3] According to this view the brain is an ancient structure comprised of three major strata, or subsystems. Each represents a separate evolutionary layer.

From years of research into the primate brain, MacLean concludes that this brain, which is also our own, is composed of three major subsystems, which he terms the *reptilian brain,* the *paleomammalian brain,* and the *neomammalian brain.* Anatomically these correspond to the evolutionarily ancient reticular activating system of the brain stem, the limbic system of the central forebrain, and the most recent evolutionary acquisition, the neocortex. The reptilian brain is the oldest major subsystem of the human brain. It was essentially the brain of the reptile, the mammal's evolutionary predecessor. Today it is the control center for basic states of brain activation such as sleep and wakefulness, and dream and nondream sleep. The paleomammalian brain, which appeared first in early mammals, gives rise to emotion and represents a major advance of the mammalian nervous system over that of the reptile. The neomammalian brain, however, embodies the most recent phase of evolution, expanded to the greatest extent in primates as well as in whales and dolphins. It is the thinking brain.

In the evolution of the nervous system old structures rarely disappear. Rather, they are over-topped by newer ones. In primates — humans included — all three of MacLean's major systems are active simultaneously, meaning that *we* inherit the tendencies of all of them. In this sense the brain conserves its history, and the influence of these structures represents three ancient attractor basins that still influence our mental life and behavior.

The foremost quality of the reptilian brain is its stubbornness and extreme inability to learn anything new. According to MacLean, it 'programs stereotyped behaviors according to instinctual and ancestral memories.' This brain plays a dominant role in genetically programmed activities such as defending territory, hunting, mating, and forming social pecking orders. It is prone to repeat old behaviors endlessly, as seen in the routine migrations of sea turtles, learning new ones only with great difficulty.

The paleomammalian brain, on the other hand, is 'nature's attempt to provide the reptilian brain with a thinking cap, and to emancipate it from stereotyped behaviors.' This thinking cap, however, is an emotional one, for the unique quality of the mammal is its ability to experience emotion, and through it to benefit from personal experiences, retained as emotional reactions to predators, friendly members of the same species, and so on. It also allows close emotional bonding between mating partners, parents and infants, members of families, and larger extended groups.

Finally, the neomammalian brain is more flexible than the paleo-mammalian one, providing the capacity for language and other intellectual skills. MacLean refers to the neocortex as the brain of 'reading, writing, and arithmetic.' It is widely recognized as the foundation for the higher intellectual functions. Many neuroscientists also feel that conscious experience is exclusively associated with the neocortex.

These three major brain subsystems, acquired at different legs in our long evolutionary journey, still retain, even in the modern brain, a surprising degree of identity and independence. Their chemical signatures are recognizably different, they are each anatomically unique, and they exhibit individual electrical patterns. MacLean refers to this state of affairs as a 'schizophysiology,' by which he refers to the tendency of the modern brain, and thus the mind that it supports, to be pulled in several directions at once.[4]

Brain modules

The idea of multiplicity, both of mind and brain, is all but universal, and paradoxically has existed side by side with another nearly universal theme, that of unity. We will meet these again and again in the following pages. They mirror the more fundamental dichotomy of complexity and simplicity. Human experience is rich in both.

In the mid-nineteenth century newspaper advertisements for professional positions such as accounting were frequently accompanied by a requirement that the applicant bring a report from a certified phrenologist to the job interview. The popular idea of phrenology, though never fully accepted by the medical community, was that the cerebral cortex could be physically divided into functions, or 'faculties' as they were often called in psychology, such as logic, memory, ability, poetic ability, computation, and so on. Phrenologists' skulls could be easily purchased. These were curious items, usually bone white and marked off with thin black lines into a fine grid with the names of faculties written in tiny print in the squares.

Eventually phrenology fell from favor, but in the fields of psychology as well as neurology the idea that intelligence can be divided into a collection of separate operations continued in a much more prestigious history. It has recently returned to the brain sciences in the guise of the modular brain.[5] This notion is suggestive of the familiar picture of a working community of subsystems that ultimately form a single fabric. It is an idea that has been explored in depth by neuro-psychologist Michael Gazzaniga, who believes that the brain contains a large number of more or less independent subsystems which he terms *modules*.[6] He writes:

> I argue that the human brain has a modular-type organiza-
> tion. By modularity I mean that the brain is organized into
> relatively independently functioning units that work in
> parallel. We seem only to have access to the product of
> these brain modules and not to the process itself.

The last sentence above refers to a fact we have already noted, that a substantial portion of the processes that undergird intelligence goes on behind the scenes. Gazzaniga asserts not only that the brain is composed of modules, but that at the level of consciousness we are aware only of the final product or read-out of these modules, not of what actually goes on in them. We will return to the latter point, as it has profound implications for the nature of ordinary consciousness. Let us first note, however, that unlike the triune brain of Paul MacLean, which reduces the entire brain to three major conceptual units, Gazzaniga speaks in terms of a considerable number of modules. This is not a conflict, as each of MacLean's major units can itself be analyzed into a variety of subsystems. MacLean is interested in broad evolutionary divisions, while Gazzaniga is captured by the richness of the brain's many subsystems.

The fact that many brain subsystems act independently of one another, and that they often do not report their activities to conscious awareness, is demonstrated by a wealth of experimental findings in the field of cognitive psychology.[7] It is shown most dramatically, however, in the clinic, where we see cases in which one system badly malfunctions while others continue as if nothing were the matter. The resulting behavior can be bizarre. For example, Gazzaniga tells the story of a woman hospitalized at the Memorial Sloan-Kettering hospital in New York City because of damage to her right parietal lobe. She seemed intelligent, charming, and in good humor, except for one thing; she insisted that she was still at her home in Freeport Maine. Nothing could convince her otherwise. In desperation, Gazzaniga pointed to the big hospital elevators just outside her room; he asked, 'And what are those things over there?' She answered, 'Those are elevators. Do you have any idea what it cost to have those put in my house?!'[8] Gazzaniga interprets this strange behavior as due to the malfunction of a single subsystem responsible for keeping track of one's physical location. Even though this subsystem's output was dramatically distorted, the other subsystems continued to function as usual, oblivious to this gaping error.

One of the obvious and compelling arguments in favor of the modular brain is the common experience of a thought or emotion that pops into the mind with no obvious conscious antecedent whatsoever. This can be anything from a sudden desire for pizza, to a stroke of creative genius for which one can give no accounting. Some time ago, while breakfasting in a café, I experienced an event which strikingly demonstrated the fact that we have little direct understanding of the sources of the ideas that often pop into our minds. An old acquaintance walked in and, saying hello, sat down at the table with me. I have always had a bad memory for names, and this time it let me down completely. I sat racking my brain for a clue as to his name. As the waitress delivered his order, however, it popped forcefully into my mind; he was Burnie Frisbee. 'Burnie Frisbee,' said the waitress, and walked away!

With a puzzled expression on his face he called her back to the table, asking: 'How did you know my name?'

'Your name?' she said.

'Burnie Frisbee.'

'Oh, no. It was just a joke,' she said. 'I meant your toast is burned like a frisbee!' And again she departed.

The matter received no more discussion at the time. And I was too befuddled to sort out my own thoughts till later. One thing that seems clear to me, however, is that the waitress had no idea in the world why she said 'Burnie Frisbee,' and even when asked for an accounting of it, was quick to provide a wrong answer. Such barely sensible but manifestly wrong answers are well known in the neurological clinic, where they are termed 'confabulations.' In the latter case they seem to be a desperate attempt to put a good light on one's own muddled state of mind, particularly in certain deteriorated brain conditions such as Korsakoff's Syndrome. The above events would seem to suggest, however, that this kind of behavior, reflecting a total absence of conscious understanding of what is going on in our own mind, may be more common than we have imagined.

Why be conscious?

After all the above comments concerning the extent to which conscious experience is excluded from the nuts-and-bolts operations of the brain one might be inclined to ask, just what *is* the role of consciousness in the brain?

A person who has spent a great deal of time thinking about such matters is the psychologist Bernard Baars, of the Wright Institute in Berkeley, California.[9] He believes that consciousness plays an essential role in distributing vital information broadly throughout the many modules or systems of the brain. In his own words, 'conscious experience involves a *global workspace,* a central information exchange that allows many different specialized processors [read systems] to interact ... "Global" in this context simply refers to information that is usable across many different subsystems.' Information of broad interest to many systems could include anything of real significance to the person, from the sight of a loved one or the appearance of something dangerous, to an item of interest in a newspaper or a book. In other words, *whatever captures our conscious attention becomes available to many if not all the subsystems of the brain.*

Michael Gazzaniga's conclusions about the role of consciousness run on the same track as Baars', but in the opposite direction. As already noted, Gazzaniga views consciousness as a single read-out of information from the many separate subsystems or modules. Presumably such a read-out would be available to the other subsystems, so that in reality it ends up performing precisely the same information distributing function suggested by Baars. For Gazzaniga, however, what is most interesting about consciousness is that it represents our ability to report out to others, and to ourselves, what seems to be going on inside of us. It does this through its close association with one unique brain module located in the left hemisphere, which he terms the *interpreter.*

It is not only the responsibility of the interpreter to report on the output of other brain modules, but more importantly to make some kind of sense out of the big picture of what is going on in the brain as a whole. In doing so, it must find a single interpretation of the information it gets from the entire set of modules it is in touch with. In other words, it must monitor the sensory modules which provide vision, hearing, and the other senses, observe internal emotional states and desires, check for reports from the memory systems, and so on, and produce a running interpretation of what it finds. It might conclude, for example: 'My memory tells me that I have not eaten for several hours, my stomach feels hollow, my mouth is watering, and I am experiencing fantasies of food. I interpret all this to mean I am hungry.' This example is a bit too literal, as if the interpreter were conscious of its own process, and apparently it is not, but captures the basic idea well enough.

The interpreter module has very practical implications for understanding human behavior. These turn on the fact that the interpreter must perform its interpretative function no matter how sparse, or even flawed, the input it receives might be. It seems to be the hardest thing in the world for us humans to simply say we don't know something, or we have no opinion about it. Data or not, we are stuffed full of beliefs and opinions about everything under the sun, and if others disagree with us then let them be damned! This is the interpreter at work.

It appears that the interpreter is most tenacious, however, when it comes to making sense out of what goes on in our own nervous system. Here it will brook no criticism, even when faulty information from malfunctioning modules provide it with data that is absolutely preposterous. A good example is the lady described above, who insisted that she was not in a hospital but at home, despite the reports of her senses and what she was told by everyone who walked in her room.

The archives of clinical neurology are full of bizarre behavioral symptoms apparently brought about by the interpreter's failure to compensate for the distortions of one or more malfunction modules. For fascinating reading along these lines see neurologist Oliver Sacks' *The Man who Mistook his Wife for a Hat: and other Clinical Tales.*

Gazzaniga tells a story, for instance, of a young man who had undergone an operation to disconnect his two cerebral hemispheres, apparently creating a condition in which each hemisphere supports its own independent stream of conscious experience. With cleverly conceived procedures it was possible to send messages to one hemisphere while withholding them from the other. This is done by flashing a word on to a screen to either the right or the left of the young man's direction of gaze. The word registers only in the opposite hemisphere — the left side of the visual field is registered by the right hemisphere, and vice versa.[10] Gazzaniga flashed a message on to the left half of the screen that asked the man to leave the room. Only the right hemisphere received it, but nonetheless he got out of his chair and proceeded immediately to walk toward the door. Keep in mind that the left hemisphere, which contains the interpreter module, did not have privy to the message and was forced to interpret the situation entirely from its own resources. This is exactly what it did. Midway across the room the young man was asked just where he thought he was going. He replied that he was on his way to get a coke and would be back shortly!

Now this young man, like the lady in the New York hospital, was not entirely naive to his own situation. He knew he had been through brain surgery, and he knew his behavior was interesting enough to be the subject of an extended program of psychological testing. He also had heard his operation explained many times to his mother and others. Nevertheless he did not respond to Gazzaniga's question by stating the obvious, that he frequently and understandably was disoriented because his brain was not normal! Rather, his interpreter functioned in what is evidently a perfectly normal way, trying to make sense, right or wrong, out of the concrete facts of the situation. That situation was that he was unaccountably walking toward the door, that he may have been thirsty, and that his memory system told him there was a coke machine nearby.[11]

But let us return to the problem of consciousness and the brain. Both neuropsychologist Gazzaniga and cognitive psychologist Baar view consciousness as playing an important role in distributing information. This is typical of *functionalist* explanations of consciousness. They ask what role, or 'function,' consciousness plays in the life of the organism. This is at root a Darwinian approach, in which it is assumed that consciousness adds something extra to the survival capacity of an organism or it would not have come along in the first place.

A related but somewhat different tilt on this basic idea is that consciousness emerged as a 'higher order' process when, through evolution, the brain reached some critical level of complexity. It then, presumably, made itself useful. This view, with its many variations, is common among artificial intelligence theorists, especially those who believe that sufficiently complex computers will also acquire consciousness. The idea, however, is not sound. It is one thing to speculate that the primate hand, which evolved in part while primates were living in trees, could, with a few modifications, later became useful for manipulating tools. It is quite another to assert that the elaborate structure of the brain evolved without consciousness, only then to later discover itself to be perfectly suited to support the exquisite varieties of awareness that each of us experiences every day.[12] Aware of this problem, many biologists, physicists, and philosophers have come to the opinion that some form of consciousness, or at least the potential for consciousness, exists in all forms of life, no matter how simple or primitive, and indeed perhaps in all matter, right down to elementary particles.[13]

Perhaps the most elegant advocate of the notion that consciousness emerges from complexity is the Nobel laureate neurologist Roger Sperry. He stresses the role of consciousness as a dynamic and emergent property of the uppermost level of the hierarchy of brain organization. He writes:

> The causal power attributed to the [conscious mind] is nothing mystical. It is seen to reside in the hierarchical organization of the nervous system combined with the universal power of any whole over its parts ... The whole

has properties as a system that are not reducible to the
properties of the parts.

For Sperry, consciousness exhibits its own unique properties. Moreover, it exerts 'downward' control over the subsystems, or modules,
that comprise the lower orders of the brain. This view of consciousness is the most inclusive of those we have seen in connection with
the study of the brain. It allows for consciousness to fulfil both Baars'
and Gazzaniga's informational roles, while including the dynamic
aspect of it typical of our own experience of consciousness as an
active agent. It is also broadly consistent with the grand evolutionary
synthesis, discussed previously.

We might well ask, however, if Sperry's theory does not run
aground for the same evolutionary reasons, above, that rebel against
the simple theory that consciousness is a product of sheer complexity?
Indeed, it would seem to be the case. Let us remind ourselves, as well,
that consciousness is more than the cognitive scientists have usually
been willing to recognize. It is more than a flow of information, or a
decision function, or any other function. It is a subjective reality that
stands at right angles to any description that limits it to a function or
role in the brain process, though it may well serve such functions or
roles.[14] Whatever its relation to the brain, the subjective dimension of
consciousness is so radically different from any objective property of
matter that to my way of thinking it makes no sense whatsoever to
think that it simply popped up, full blown, from an evolutionary progression that previously had nothing to do with it. We could hedge on
this problem by suggesting that consciousness gradually developed as
the nervous systems evolved. This is of no help to Sperry, though, because if consciousness is a higher-order function of the brain, then it
could not have come about until the hierarchy of systems in the brain
became sufficiently advanced through evolution to give birth to it.

Fortunately, we are in a better position to consider this problem
than is Sperry, because we are not dedicated to a philosophy which,
if not patently materialistic, at least ties consciousness inextricably to
the material brain. To my way of thinking the problem here reduces
to a confusion between association and identity. Clearly consciousness
is ordinarily associated with the brain, and in particular with certain

of the higher-order operations of the brain such as memory and decision-making. From all the above, and much more, there can be no argument about this. But to conclude that it arises from and is rooted in the brain in an *ontological* sense, in the sense that its very essence or being has no possibility except as a function of the brain is quite a different matter.

I do not propose to solve the enigma of the relationship of consciousness to the brain, *the mind-body problem,* here. It is arguably the greatest conundrum in human experience. Arthur Schopenhauer called it the 'world knot.' My own view, the one expressed in this book, however, places consciousness in a considerably larger context, while at the same time not denying its involvement at the level of the brain.

Chaos in the head

One of the most exciting recent developments in the neurosciences is the discovery that chaos may play a significant role in the operation of the brain.[15] In the previous chapter we noted that the brain may support chaotic activity, and that such activity might express itself in the form of chaotic attractors. From this it seems likely that mental states such as moods, desires, intentions, and even entire states of consciousness such as sleep and wakefulness, are undergirded by similar brain processes, themselves on the edge of chaos. Dream sleep, for example, might be seen as a self-organizing pattern of brain activity with its own global structure and its own deep attractor basin. Indeed, if dreaming is viewed as a biological need, as surely it must be,[16] then much if not all the very power of the state to draw us to it is contained in the brain attractor itself.

Some of the best known work on chaos in the brain was done by the Berkeley neurologist Walter Freeman, who studied the perception of odors by rabbits.[17] He found that when a rabbit is inactive the cells

Figure 4. Activity from the olfactory brain of the rabbit. The first figure represents the loose chaotic pattern of inactivity. When an odor such as that of a carrot is presented, the pattern is transformed through an 'explosive' bifurcation to the second, more defined but still chaotic attractor. These diagrams are from Walter Freeman's laboratory.

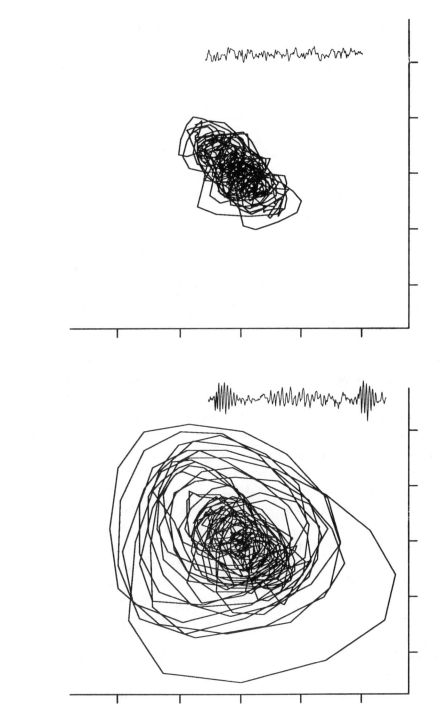

of its smell brain follow a loose-knit chaotic pattern, as shown on the top in Figure 4. When the rabbit is exposed to a stimulus such as the odor of a carrot, however, this gnarled attractor suddenly undergoes a rapid, 'explosive,' bifurcation to a much larger and better defined structure, as seen at the bottom of the figure. It is this sudden transition to this new but still chaotic pattern that seems to be the basis for the animal's odor recognition.

A fascinating feature of the smell brain is that if the rabbit learns to recognize the scent of, say, a carrot, then learns a new odor such as the smell of a mango, then upon returning to the original carrot its response will have changed. The carrot attractor has modestly but noticeably changed. In other words, the experience of the new learning has modified the brain so that, though it still recognizes the carrot, its response has been transformed by experience. The important implication here is that brain activity is constantly modified by new experiences. This is a principle that apparently is not limited to the smell brain of rabbits, but in fact applies broadly to higher order functions including consciousness.[18]

Freeman speculates that chaotic activity of the type described above, 'underlies the ability of the brain to respond flexibly to the outside world and to generate novel activity patterns, including those that are experienced as fresh ideas.' It would seem that in some subtle way each new experience has its impact on all of our later experiences. In Freeman's words, you can go and see Shakespeare's *Hamlet,* and then you can go and see *Rosencrantz and Guildenstern are Dead,* but if you come back to *Hamlet* again it will not be the same. Thus, consciousness is both the lens and focal point of all our past experience, and is ever informed by the accumulated wealth of living.

The roughly circular attractor produced by the rabbit's brain when smelling a carrot might be thought of alternatively as not a single attractor at all, but as a small portion of a vast unseen attractor of multidimensional complexity, one in which each odor represents activity in a particular zone or lobe. This is an important idea. Let us follow it further.

Imagine a grand chaotic attractor in which individual perceptions, even entire experiences and states of consciousness, are represented as unique locations or perhaps lobes, each a mini attractor in its own right. Examples of something like this are seen in Figures 5, 6, and 7. The first represents a complex three-dimensional attractor space in which distinct regions of activity can be seen. Depending on our level of discussion these could represent perceptual responses such as the recognition of particular odors, or they could be states of conscious-ness such as ordinary wakefulness, dream sleep, and non-dream sleep. In the second figure we find three epicenters of activity connected by weak or low density regions, while the third depicts a swarm of epicenters, each loosely connected to the others. Such chaotic-like figures are richly suggestive. In Chapter 10, for instance, we will use them to illustrate different kinds of personality organizations.

In this vein, a young chaos mathematician, Ben Goertzel, at the University of Western Australia, has developed an amazingly complex and extensive model of the mind that he calls the *cognitive equation*.[19] This equation, which can only be broadly characterized but not written in detail, specifies a grand attractor for an individual's entire mental life. Subpatterns, or lobes, within this attractor represent habits of thought and even entire belief systems. Goertzel writes:

> The brain, like other extremely complex systems, is
> unpredictable in the level of detail but roughly predictable
> on the level of structure. This means that the dynamics of
> its physical variables [and the mental processes they
> support] display a strange attractor with a complex structure
> of 'wings' or 'compartments.'

The whole story of Goertzel's work is rich, occupying three books and numerous articles.[20] He views the mind as a dynamically self-organizing autopoietic system. This is very similar to my own idea of it, as we will see below. The similarity was made strikingly apparent in my first introduction to Ben Goertzel at the Toronto meeting of the Society for Chaos Theory in Psychology in the summer of 1993. I was presenting my idea of the mind as a self-organizing process, and had come to the point of emphasizing the notion that mental events such as thoughts, memories, and dreams can interact to give birth to new and original ideas, when Ben stood up and exclaimed: 'These are not just abstract speculations. They can be demonstrated mathematically

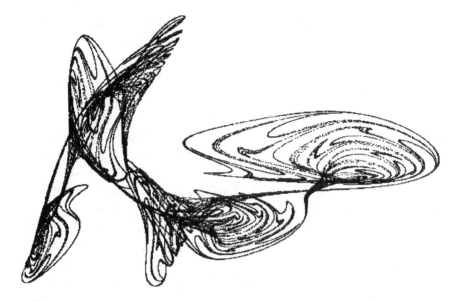

Figures 5, 6. 7. Large encompassing attractors in which individual perceptions or even entire experiences are represented as unique locations, or lobes, each a mini attractor in its own right.

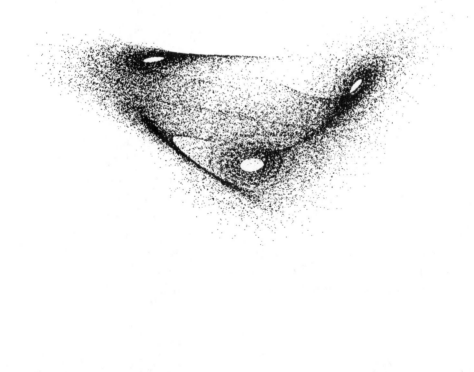

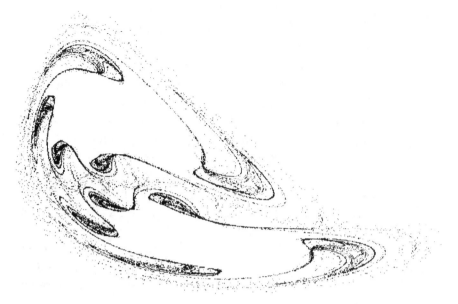

and are in fact the subject of my next book.'[21] I was stunned. I felt like Woody Allen in the film *Annie Hall,* where in the midst of a heated discussion over Marshall McLuhan, out steps McLuhan himself from behind a billboard and declares, 'This man is perfectly right!'

In later conversations we discovered many similarities in our thinking, though our ideas had developed quite independently. Ben had come to his conclusions through long and creative work on computational models of intelligence and the brain, whereas my own thoughts were the product of years of study of psychology and the neurosciences applied intuitively to chaos theory. Interestingly, however, both of us had been influenced by the ideas of a European systems theorist by the name of George Kampis, a one-time student of the Hungarian ethologist and evolutionary theorist Vilmos Csányi — one of the architects, along with Ervin Laszlo, of the grand evolutionary synthesis mentioned in the previous chapter.[22]

Kampis had pondered a great deal about self-creating or autopoietic systems, which he terms 'component systems' to emphasize they are made of up of many elements, or more accurately, processes, that interact in such a fashion as to re-create the entire event of which they are parts. Kampis' thinking, however, went beyond previous notions of autopoietic systems. First, it relies more on formal logic than on biological concepts, as did Varela and Maturana's concept of auto-poietic systems, or Goertzel's mathematical model of the mind. More important, it stresses the creation of new and emergent properties, components, or processes, entirely original and which cannot be predicted by logic or computation even in principle.

It works like this. The interaction of the processes that form a complex system such as the mind — thoughts, images, memories, and so on — give rise to new processes. For example a novel idea or feeling might appear. So far so good, and one might argue at least up to this point that the system, in principle at least, ought to be predictable with something, for example, like Goertzel's cognitive equation. But things get worse. These new processes now interact with the original ones to create yet other novel processes, second order emergent events, and these are in principle entirely free and unpredictable.[23] Thus, according to Kampis, the mind, and indeed many complex processes in nature such as the evolution of organisms and the growth of ecologies, is capable of fundamentally original productions that cannot even in principle be predicted or foreseen. One thinks of original creative ideas or inspirations, but the idea here is not limited to thought in the usual sense, but applies to dreams, feelings, and probably even to memories, which are famously unreliable![24]

Kampis' idea of the production of fundamental novelty is reminiscent of the French turn-of-the-century philosopher Henri Bergson's idea of original events, or *emergents*, he believed to be created in the process of evolution. We will have more to say about Bergson in Chapter 4. In the meantime, I note for interest's sake that in personal communications with Kampis he expressed both familiarity and affection for Bergson's thought.

With the ideas of Kampis, and Goertzel as well, we find our thoughts shifting away from the brain and moving in the direction of the mind and consciousness. It would seem that the creative complexity of the brain is reflected in the creativity of mind and conscious experience. Let us, then, turn our attention fully in this direction, examining consciousness itself.

States of consciousness

I have frequently spoken of states of consciousness. Let us begin here by examining them a bit more closely.

Charles Tart

In 1975 a University of California psychologist Charles Tart published a book titled *States of Consciousness,* in which he outlined a theory of the nature of consciousness based on then-current ideas about systems. Here I will make an effort to extend his seminal work by taking advantage of newer ideas drawn from chaos theory and evolutionary thought.

Charles Tart considered *states of consciousness* to be formed by coherent patterns of psychological processes such as emotion, memory, cognition, sense of identity, body sense, and so on. He thought of the latter as subsystems of the mind. In each state they form a working regimen, different than in other states. According to Tart, a state of consciousness is 'a unique, dynamic pattern or configuration of psychological structures, an active system of psychological subsystems.'

The subsystems undergo changes from state to state. For example, the quality of thought might be quite different during marijuana intoxication than in ordinary consciousness or in a dream state. Similarly, memory is sensitive to one's overall emotional situation. When we are depressed we tend to entertain oppressive recollections. When we are angry, on the other hand, we recall annoying events, and when we are feeling good we tend to have pleasant memories.[25] Tart emphasized the importance of the mutual fit of the various subsystems. In each state of consciousness they work together smoothly, making a unique and stable configuration.

In Tart's theory a state of consciousness is secured or sustained by four stabilizing processes. He designated these by terms drawn from cybernetics. The first, *loading stabilization,* involves keeping busy with activities that tend to anchor the person in the desired state. Hard goal-directed work, for instance, is a product of ordinary everyday consciousness. If I am engaged in such work I will usually remain in ordinary consciousness. If a child can be kept busy doing homework, he or she will not float off into a state of daydreaming.

The second, *negative feedback stabilization,* involves making adjustments to bring back to a desired state of consciousness if a person begins to slip out of it. For instance, if I begin to drowse off while driving my car I might toss my head, take a few deep breaths, or even slap myself on the leg, all providing negative feedback to the process of drowsing off. I might also utilize *positive feedback stabilization* by finding something to do that enhances my wakefulness in a positive way, such as listening to a story on tape, or picking a more interesting highway on which to drive. The fourth, *limiting stabilization,* simply denies access to other states of consciousness. I might, for instance, drink so much coffee that I can't go to sleep!

States of consciousness do change, however, and in Tart's theory the transitions are governed by two types of agents, *disrupting forces* and *patterning forces,* both of which will take on considerable importance later. These forces can be psychological, behavioral, biological, or environmental. In each case they tend to move us out of one state of consciousness and into another. Consider, for example, falling asleep. When we want to go to sleep we usually engage in a ritual preparation that includes washing and changing into light comfortable night clothes, then laying down and closing our eyes. An important environmental patterning force for going to sleep is the presence of the familiar bedroom. People who frequently travel may take along a small pillow from home, like a security blanket, to have, as it were, a piece of their bedroom with them. Going to bed at the same hour every night aligns one with powerful biological patterning forces connected to physiological circadian rhythms. At the same time, by removing ourselves from loud noises and conversation, turning off the lights, and closing our eyes, we disrupt those forces that confine consciousness to the waking state.

Tart makes the assumption that consciousness comes in discrete states rather than as a continuous spectrum. According to this view, states such as ordinary wakefulness, dreaming, deep meditation, various forms of drug intoxication, and so on, do not manifest by graded transitions from previous states, but by more or less complete transitions. At first glance this may seem questionable, but it turns out to be a very useful assumption for discussions of similarities and differences between states of consciousness. Moreover, there is reason to suspect that transitions between states are more abrupt than we might suspect from the evidence of casual introspection. Sleep research, for example, demonstrates that falling asleep involves an abrupt loss of awareness of the outer world at the moment the eyes begin a slow vertical roll.[26] If, at this instant, a strobe light flashes in a person's eyes, they will not see it. The onset of dream sleep, as well, seems to be abrupt. States of drug intoxication brought about by alcohol or marijuana often involve a particular moment when one becomes aware of being intoxicated and suddenly begins to act the part.

States and structures: all strangely attractive

Rather than viewing a state of consciousness simply as a system, let us also view it as an attractor. This is natural, as an attractor is a pattern to which a system is drawn according to its own nature. The basin for a state of consciousness would include all the situations from which one is likely to slide back into that state. For ordinary consciousness, for instance, these include brief periods of drowsiness, episodes of day dreaming, and the momentary dizziness when one stands up too fast. If the conditions that support ordinary consciousness are altered past some critical point, however, the system will slide into a new pattern, represented by a different attractor with its own basin. If we drowse off too far we slip out of the attractor basin of ordinary consciousness and begin to slide down into the basin of sleep. The slope of this basin is steep, especially if we are fatigued, and once into it considerable energy may be needed to escape it before we are rested. The dream state, incidentally, can be a particularly powerful attractor. It seems the brain protects this state by blocking sensory messages from reaching the higher brain centers.

Viewing each state of consciousness as an attractor allows us to square the fact that each state is unique with the everyday observation that transitions between them are often not entirely abrupt. Like a marble rolling on an uneven surface, we cross the ridge between states slowly, then accelerate down into the neighboring basin.

Now I want to extend our discussion to include the idea of *structures.* I will use the term to refer to relatively large configurations, ones within which particular states occur. For instance, a bugle with its hollow air-filled interior is a structure in which a number of resonant sound frequencies, or states, can be produced as the bugler varies the tension of his lips. In chaotic systems terms, the tension is called a *control variable,* because it regulates the state of the system. To take another example, in the last chapter we noted that the metabolic structure of a living cell can support more than a single state. As a system on the edge of chaos, for instance, it can support both cyclic and chaotic activity depending on its own control variables, which might include internal conditions such as genetic instructions from the nucleus, or external changes such as alterations in the chemistry of the surrounding tissues. Perhaps the most complex structure known, however, is the human brain. It is apparently capable of assuming a virtually infinite variety of states.[27]

Now, we might think of a state as a process, while the structure that supports it appears static and unchanging. The difference is relative, though, because the structure itself may cloak a process underneath. For instance, certain theories in physics would view the metallic matter of the bugle as made up, in the final analysis, of particle interactions, or even of the complex interplay of wave action at the subatomic level. In the case of the living cell it is easy to see its metabolic structure as a chemical process. Indeed, in the last chapter we noted that the idea of *autopoiesis* came originally from the observation that cells are matrices of processes that as a group are geared toward self-creation. The living brain is a static structure only in photographs. In reality it is a dynamic edifice fashioned of living cells, each formed of chemical processes undergirded, in turn, by atomic events, and so on down to the limits of speculation.

The concept of structures is like that of states in the sense that both carry the implication of coherency. The elements form a working whole. A psychological structure, for instance, is an entire agenda in which a variety of states may occur. For years psychologists have studied mental structures as they unfold developmentally in the individual. Here they are typically spoken of as developmental *stages.* Some stage theorists, such as Swiss psychologist Jean Piaget, have examined the growth of cognitive abilities from infancy through maturity.[28] Others, such as Harvard's Lawrence Kohlberg, and Carol Gilligan, have concentrated on moral development.[29] Many psychologists, such as Abraham Maslow and Erik Erikson, have studied the development of the personality.[30] A few, such as philosopher Michael Washburn, independent theorist and psychologist Ken Wilber, and Esalen scholar and psychiatrist Stanislav Grof, have studied spiritual growth and development.[31] Of course, these categories are somewhat artificial, and a complete understanding of any one of them would require some knowledge of the others as well.

A number of years ago, the European student of consciousness, Jean Gebser, introduced the notion of *structures of consciousness,* meaning entire styles or regimes in which reality presents itself to the viewer.[32] He identified a number of such regimes, about which we will have much more to say in Chapter 5, where we will examine Gebser's theory in detail. At this point I just want to introduce the idea that a structure, especially a structure of consciousness, like a state, is a pattern of processes that can be understood as an attractor.

Since it seems unlikely that any unique moment of conscious experience ever repeats itself exactly, we might also conclude that structures and states of consciousness are strange (chaotic) or chaotic-like attractors.[33] We already have seen that states of consciousness can be transformed if changes in their control variables bring about sufficient alterations in them, and we will later find the same to be true of structures of consciousness. All this suggests that if a large enough portion of the elements which form either a state or structure of consciousness are altered, the entire system can be up-ended and sent looking for a new attractor — a new stable pattern. Here in a nutshell is the process that underlies many techniques for personal and spiritual growth. In them old structures are dismantled and new ones substituted. We will continue to examine these ideas as we go along.

Personal bifurcations

Transformations are the very stuff and substance of psychological growth and development. When, through maturation or experience, a person's physical and mental systems cross critical thresholds of complexity, that person is thrown out of his or her comfortable previous state into a temporary but fertile period of chaos which heralds the appearance of a new stage of development. For instance, the hormonal control variables that change during adolescence combine with a young person's expanding life experience to produce widely felt effects which complexify both the biological and the psychological dimensions of life. The natural response to this situation is confusion and disorientation, that is, chaos. Eventually, however, the young person settles into new, more complex and mature patterns of life. Stage theories in psychology see maturation as proceeding through a series of such bifurcations, each heralding a quantal jump in complexity. This is especially apparent in structural theories such as Jean Piaget's model of cognitive growth, or Lawrence Kohlberg's model of moral maturation.

In the developmental history of a system, bifurcations are decision points, junctures at which it must 'choose' between future configurations or attractors. In the case of psychological development, if correct choices are not made the individual may be drawn into the basin of regressive or even pathological attractors. Erik Erikson's model of personality development and contemporary psychodynamic theory both emphasize this idea.[34] According to Erikson, the growth of personality is characterized by a series of 'crises,' chaotic episodes in which a life issue must be successfully resolved if one is to continue to grow in a healthy way. During the first year of life, for instance, the infant must acquire a trusting attitude toward the world or face the alternative possibility of going through life with negative and hostile expectations. Needless to say, the parents play a very important role in providing the infant with this attitude of trust, for if they fail to meet the infant's emotional or physical needs, he or she may take away a permanent feeling that the world is hostile and not to be trusted. Another instance from Erikson's theory is the adolescent identity crisis in which the young person is forced to seek a sense of personal identity beyond that of the child. Failing at this, one may go through life without a firm sense of who one really is.

Ken Wilber has articulated a major model of psychological growth and pathology in which maturation from birth through several transpersonal levels of development is viewed as a series of bifurcations, the outcomes of which lead either to growth or pathology.[35]

Cascading complexity

The evolution of complexity often involves the weaving together of simple motifs to produce a whole fabric which, when finished, exhibits complex features of its own, in no way evident from its constituents. This fabric in turn may become part of a larger garment. This is the story of the grand evolutionary synthesis, seen in the previous chapter. Subatomic processes weave atomic level events, which in turn undergird molecular processes that are the foundations of chemistry. Chemistry yields the worlds of life, of living cells that behave according to their own rules and dominion, but are only the building blocks for multi-cellular organisms ranging all the way up to cats, dolphins, and human beings. Humans form societies, the characteristics of which cannot be predicted from the study of individuals, as any sociologist would be quick to tell us. And so on, in a grand tiered hierarchy of reality.

The human mind is likewise structured in such a tiered fashion. Its development from the simplicity of infancy to the exquisite complexity of full maturity parallels the general pattern for the evolution of complexity seen above. In Jean Piaget's theory of the growth of the child's intellect, simple patterns of thought and behavior, termed *schemata* (the singular form is *schema)*, interact to create more complex patterns which, in turn, weave into still larger structures that are the bases for the major stages of development.

A visible form of this progression is the growth of children's art. Psychologist Rhonda Kellogg found that young children from virtually all cultures first begin to draw by scribbling basic solid shapes such as circles and squares.[36] In time, they are drawing only the outlines of these forms, and they later combine these into more complex patterns. Such a pattern might represent a human figure — let's say Daddy! — as a single circle with smaller circles for eyes and a mouth, and straight lines to represent arms and legs. A house might be drawn in the form of a square with smaller squares for doors and windows. In time children begin to combine these basic patterns, along with others such as spirals, triangles, grids, and so on, to construct drawings of houses, trees, cars, people, and animals. The fascinating thing about this progression is that the forms created at each stage of development are not lost, but integrated as components into the next stage.

Transitions from stage to stage, bifurcations in systems terms, can occur gradually or swiftly. In stage theories such as Piaget's, one thinks of gradual change, although transitions sometimes occur with surprising speed. For example, a young child quickly acquires the schema for using the suffix -*ed* to convert a verb to its past tense. Within just a few weeks he or she might be using it in almost every possible instance, including the 'irregular' exceptions where it is inappropriate. We hear three-year-olds say, 'I runned all the way home!' or 'She sitted on the little stool.' At this point the rule, or schema, has been over-generalized, meaning that the child now uses it in all instances, even when not appropriate. Here, as often is the case in language learning, it will take the child much longer to learn the exceptions than it did to acquire the rule.

Transpersonal or spiritual growth would seem to follow the same pattern as in ordinary psychological development. Transitions from stage to stage usually occur gradually, as patterning forces in the form of life experiences or spiritual practices are introduced and maintained over substantial periods of time. Exceptions occur, however, and may be dramatic. States of liberation, for example, can arise suddenly. In chaos theory, the abrupt appearance (or disappearance) of an attractor 'out of the blue' is called a *catastrophic bifurcation.* In this event the system may suddenly find itself in the basin of a major new attractor. An example was the illumination of the great Indian sage Ramana Maharshi, which swept over him suddenly and permanently at the age of sixteen.[37] The Rinzai school of Zen Buddhism is famous for stories of 'lightning realization,' though it is clear that considerable preparation has usually taken place before the student is made ready for it.[38]

Interestingly, the Rinzai school makes extensive use of koan practice, or the contemplation of paradox. The student is forced to confront reality at a level beyond the constructs of the rational mind. Such practice destabilizes the attractor of 'everyman's consciousness.' The final realization comes when a catastrophic bifurcation takes over and hurtles consciousness directly out into the state of realization.

The brain-mind reality kit

From much of the above it seems apparent that the mind, and the brain that supports it, are not passive bystanders to everyday reality, but actively participant in its creation. First, consider the brain.

It is not unduly idealistic to say that we have no real estimate of the true native capacity of the human brain. In a fascinating reassessment of the entire problem of the brain and mind, neuropsychologist Larry Vandervert argues that the brain is the source of a much higher order of intelligence than is the mind, which for him is made up of mentation and particularly of mental models and beliefs.[39] Vandervert's ideas are based on an analysis of the evolution and energy ecology of the brain, but also contain some highly original notions of a more general nature. To begin with, he argues that the brain is self-similar to the world, that is, its circuitry, or more accurately its inherent routines (algorithms), represent an exact microcosm of the macrocosm of the world. This is a modern restatement of the ancient Hermetic dictum, 'as above, so below.' In his view it becomes possible for the brain to find within its own structure many of the 'secrets' of the outer world. For instance, it suggests an answer to the enigma of why mathematics, created solely by the human mind, provides such an 'unreasonable' fit to systems studied in the physical sciences.

For Vandervert mind, in its turn, is self-similar to the brain, a derivative of it, and a less efficient subset of the brain's total computational capacity. The appearance of the mind through evolution came about because of its usefulness to the brain, roughly like the computer came about because of its usefulness to the mind. The first instances of mind were the appearance of mental maps, examples of which were projected as paleolithic cave paintings. These maps played important social roles such as increasing group cohesion and transmitting information from generation to generation. As time passed, the information embodied in mental maps became more abstract and efficient, giving rise to pictorial and nonrepresentational writing. As history continued, thought forms and their various outward expressions became more and more efficient, though still not as efficient as the brain that originally produced them. The mind is not up to the quality of the brain, just as the computer is not up to the quality of the mind. Thus, we find ourselves players in a paradoxical drama in which the evolution of thought and knowledge struggle to catch up with the already superb original brain that gave birth to them in the first place. This is a strange idea. But as has been said of scientific theories, if they are not sufficiently strange they don't stand a chance of being true.

Vandervert's distinction between mind and consciousness is similar to my own. Mind is made up of mental events while consciousness is the open ground across which these play.[40] Beyond this, however, Vandervert sees consciousness as an evolutionarily ancient production of the brain by which we as organisms place ourselves in a world of space and time. In his own words, 'consciousness continuously constructs this model of space-time in the brain.' The idea here is that survival in the very complex universe in which we live requires that we frame reality in terms we can deal with.

This way of thinking is reminiscent of the theory that quantum physicist David Bohm developed during the past two decades, namely that the world we experience is only the surface of a deeper reality, one in which space and time are mutually enfolded into a dynamic 'implicate order.' From this point of view space and time are simply the ways we experience the 'unfolding' of the implicate order. Bohm's student and colleague, the prominent neuroscientist Karl Pribram, spent decades developing a detailed understanding of how the brain accomplishes this feat.[41] To proceed into his work at this point, however, would take us far afield.

In Bohm's cosmos the prize question, as asked by Alex Comfort's delightful multi-dimensional demon Gezumpstein, is:

> How far experience and reality are explicates demanded by evolution in response to the inability of organisms to react appropriately to large lumps of the implicate *Brahman.*

Just how far must reality be modified to make it possible for us to live in it?

The basic notion that we don't see reality directly is as ancient as Plato's *Allegory of the Cave,* and has played a role in Western metaphysics ever since. It is a central theme in Kant's philosophy, which argued that space and time are categories of the mind and not of the world. Similar ideas are found widely in Eastern thought. But the notion of the *brain* as the weaver of reality, at least in a non-trivial sense that we might have some hope of understanding, is much more recent. In 1973, after years of studying the evolution of the nervous system, paleo-neurologist Jerison wrote:

> The simplest intuitive description of the brain's work (for me) is that it creates a 'real' world. Within that real world all the events of a lifetime take place.

It is unlikely, however, that Jerison would have gone as far as does Ben Goertzel, who recently observed that:

> The belief system which we call external reality is a collection of processes for constructing three-dimensional space, linear time and coherent objects out of noise- and chaos-infused sense-data.

Here there is a hint of flexibility. Indeed, Goertzel's whole notion of the cognitive equation, when examined in depth, carries the clear and intended implication that the brain is not simply a blind transducer of reality but, at least for human beings, this transduction is flexible, based on belief systems or habits of the mind.

Just how flexible, however, can reality be? Is it just putty to be molded into any shape whatsoever? Few would argue for this position, though certain postmodern constructionist thinkers seem to flirt with it. A more likely position is that reality is only incompletely defined in terms readily understood by nervous systems. In this case the principal occupation of science and philosophy is to sharpen up its corners for us, grinding the right set of lenses through which to see it truly. This is the most common opinion of philosophers these days. Unfortunately such questions cannot be answered with any finality.[42]

My own ideas on this matter follow from my view of consciousness and how it is molded. For example, states of consciousness are unique configurations of experience, particular worlds if you like. There are potentially a rich variety of them, but each is defined and constrained by its own unique structure. In other words, states of consciousness are not arbitrary. They represent working patterns of activity among functions such as memory, perception, and feelings, which in turn are supported by complex brain activity. Thus, an individual can experience many states of consciousness during a lifetime, but none of them are random productions. Beyond this, the notion of structures of consciousness represents an even larger vessel for human experience, each supporting a variety of states. The intertwining of these states and structures yields a rich horizon of potential worlds of experience.

Boot-strapping reality

Psychological productions such as Tart's states of consciousness, Piaget's or Erikson's stages of development, and, as we will see later, Gebser's structures of consciousness, can all be viewed as self-creating or autopoietic in their own right. As we know, this is a property of many complex systems. Their elements cling together in a particular fashion. They have self-resonant properties in which their subsystems — Piaget's schemata, Tart's psychological subsystems — conspire to create an overall unity which, in turn, forms the context for the subsystems themselves. For instance, we have seen that the state of depression tends to support itself by selecting memories such that we tend to recall oppressive episodes from our past.[43] These memories in turn feed our mood of depression, and so perpetuate a continuous cycle of memory and mood. If we want to break this cycle, we must disrupt the circuit and apply new patterning forces, or control variables, compelling the system to seek a new attractor. A good belly-laugh, a rousing piece of music, a brisk walk in the forest, and the atmosphere of depression has evaporated, overthrown completely.

A similar situation is found with the cognitive processes described by psychologists such as Piaget. For the latter, the complex hierarchical networks of schemata that ultimately come together to form adult intelligence are not static like information stored on a magnetic disk. They represent active processes by which we interpret reality. These processes act in a dynamic coordinated fashion to form hierarchical structures, each element of which supports the others. For example, the schema or concept of *conservation,* by which we know that matter does not appear or disappear out of nowhere, is supported by the schema of *reversibility*. The latter is simply an ability to run a mental operation in reverse. For instance, when a young child sees a tall narrow glass of water poured into a short wide glass he or she will report that there now is less water in the wide glass than was previously seen in the tall narrow one. This mistake is made because the child judges the amount of water solely on the basis of its height in the glass, which is lower in the instance of the wide glass. Having acquired the schema of reversibility, however, an older child will run the operation backward in his own imagination. He will then reply that the amount of water remains the same because, if you poured it back into the tall glass it would fill the glass to its original height. My point here is that such schemata form complex structures or networks which conspire to mutually support and create each other, and thus to create the network itself.

Speaking experientially, each combination of state and structure, or schemata and stage, constitutes an entire world. As such, it in turn supports the elements, the subsystems, of which it is formed. Seen in terms of conscious experience, this cyclic, self-resonant, aspect of reality could not be otherwise, for it is this tendency of the whole experience to support its constituents, and for them in turn to create the whole, that gives consciousness its stability. The child lives in a child's world, made of a child's dreams, perceptions, and fantasies. But these together are the very fabric of the child's world. When one or more of these is altered beyond some critical threshold, however, the entire construction is upended. The child loses the childhood world for adolescence, never to gain it back again.

PART TWO

Evolution

4. Here and Elsewhere

Historical tales of evolution

*Here and elsewhere we shall not obtain the best insight into
things until we actually see them growing from the
beginning.*

Aristotle

Here and in the following three chapters we will explore several
theories of the evolution of what might be called consciousness, mind,
or the spirit. A few of these are quite old. Most are Western, where
the concept of evolution is tied to much older notions of linear as
opposed to cyclic time, and of history as progress. The latter idea has
roots in the ancient Hebrew conception of history as a record of God's
hand in the affairs of men. Fully conceived linear time as a physicist
would think of it, however, waited till the Renaissance and paved the
way for the concept that nature advances in a forward direction.

These pages, however, will not simply be a tour through a museum
of Western antiquities. The next two chapters will bring us face to
face with two very contemporary views of the nature of consciousness, and of its evolution, namely those of Jean Gebser and Ken
Wilber. And Chapter 7 explores a leading Eastern view, namely the
ideas of the great Indian yogi and philosopher, Sri Aurobindo.

Ovid and Giambattista Vico

If evolution is taken in the broad sense as simply a temporal progression of forms, then it is quite an old notion in East and West as well.
Eastern and especially Indian conceptions emphasize the evolution of
spirit toward increasingly subtle forms of expression even today. We
will return to this perspective in the following chapters. Here we begin
with Western notions, which address not only the evolution of the

spirit but the evolution of biological organisms and also the maturation of societies. The essential idea dates back at least to the world of antiquity. Matthew Arnold's comment on first learning of Darwin's theory more than a hundred years ago was: 'It's all in Lucretius!'[1] The notion that the long span of human history has included several distinct periods of psychological development is also quite old.

In the *Metamorphoses,* for example, the Roman poet Ovid described four ages in human history. The first, the Golden Age, was said to be an age of paradise, a time when humankind lived completely in the bounty of nature. It was a period when 'Earth, untroubled, unhurried by hoe or plowshare, brought forth all that men had need for, and those men were happy, gathering berries from the mountain sides, cherries, or blackcaps, and the edible acorns.' The second of Ovid's ages, the Age of Silver, was also much like a paradise, but the human's distance from nature had increased. Farming became a way of life. Winter and autumn were added to the previous seasons of spring and summer, and people lived in 'bark-bound' shelters.

Ovid's third age, the Age of Bronze, brought with it aggression and distrust. Men became quick to take up arms at the least offense, though Ovid states that people as yet were 'not entirely evil.' Finally, with the Iron Age 'came trickery and slyness, plotting, swindling, violence and the damned desire of having.'

Ovid's mythical history describes a slow and incremental decline of the human spirit from a paradisiacal state somewhere in antiquity. This was a common notion in Ovid's day, and is widely found among ancient myths all around the world.[2] Confucius, for instance, saw his own era as a period of decline from a perfect society long past. For Ovid, the description of the last age may well have been intended as a commentary on his own times. He was born shortly after turmoil in the old Roman Republic had resulted in the rise and subsequent assassination of Julius Caesar. His light-hearted and irreverent attitude toward the austere traditional Roman virtues eventually got him banished by the emperor Octavian (Augustus) to life in an obscure town on the coast of the Black Sea.

In the eighteenth century the Italian social philosopher Giambattista Vico proposed a strikingly similar theory of human history, one that involved three ages which he called the Age of Gods, the Age of

Heroes, and the Age of Men.[3] The first of these, the Age of Gods, was much like Ovid's Ages of Gold and Silver, though Vico stressed an intimate relationship between humankind and the Divine during this period. It was said to be a time when the gods spoke directly to humans, and government was conducted by priests who received communications directly from them. The language was that of hieroglyphics or high symbolism. Vico's Age of Heroes was a period when human society was controlled by warrior heroes such as Odysseus and Achilles, many of whom were demigods remembered in mythology as born of the coupling of a god or goddess with a human. Such men spoke the language of poetry. Armed conflict was frequent, but motivations were still largely noble. Clearly this age corresponds to Ovid's Age of Bronze. Vico's final period, the Age of Men, finds government in the hands of ordinary people speaking ordinary language. They may not be evil to begin with, but they are subject to all the weaknesses of the human temperament. These ages, according to Vico, repeat themselves over large spans of time so that history is in fact cyclic.

Interestingly, William Irwin Thompson has recently added a fourth age to Vico's original three. This is an Age of Chaos, said to be transitional between the Age of Men and the next Age of Gods. He believes the world to be in such a period at the moment:

> Because our culture is in a transitional stage there now
> exists a great polarization between the mystics and the
> mechanists. One section of the culture is caught up in
> visions of total control, in space colonies and genetic
> engineering; the other is caught up in the spiritual visions of
> a Doris Lessing, a Karlheinz Stockhausen, a David
> Spangler. The age of chaos and the new age of gods
> overlap.

Vico's theory is not truly evolutionary because it views history as cyclic rather than as a progression. In this respect it has more in common with very ancient notions of history. Beyond this, we see in Vico as in Ovid the idea that history runs downhill; things get worse, and so do people.[4]

Georg Wilhelm Friedrich Hegel

While not without antecedents, the German philosopher Georg Wilhelm Friedrich Hegel was the first to argue eloquently for the idea that human consciousness develops through a historical progression leading to increasingly *higher* forms of expression. In *The Phenomenology of the Spirit,* published in 1807, Hegel asserted that the human being contains, infolded and shrouded within, the spirit of the absolute. This indwelling spirit, emanating as consciousness, comes to know itself as infinite only by assuming the limitations of finite existence and triumphing over them. In other words, the human is the vehicle by which God, the infinite spirit, comes to self-recognition.

As the spirit struggles to know its true essence it passes through a sequence of epochs representing different expressions of the spirit in human life. These can be understood as stages in the evolution of consciousness. In the first, the world is experienced in terms of sense perception. Hegel speaks of this most basic expression of consciousness as Nature, meaning that this form of experience was the least abstracted from the elemental experience of the natural world. The second stage emphasized society, which became most important in determining its values and goals. This stage saw the advent of a new inflection in consciousness, one distinctly more complex than the consciousness of the previous stage with its emphasis on simple perceptual experience. This was the appearance of self-consciousness, which brought with it an increased sense of distance between the inner life of the ego and outer life of the world. It was associated with striving to inflict one's will on others and the struggle to become the master of nature itself.

In the next stage there was a transition from the mind that attempts to master to the mind that strives for freedom. This came about as the thinking mind withdrew into its own process, free of the outer world. The idea is reminiscent of the ancient stoic philosophy with its emphasis on the ability of even the slave to achieve personal freedom and integrity within the sanctuary of one's own inner life. There was a tendency, however, for the mind to pass beyond this attitude and continue into skepticism, where it began to question even its own productions. According to Hegel, this was the dominant mind in late antiquity when the Roman Empire was declining. The rise of Christianity was an effort to overcome this uncomfortable state of affairs by seeking a transcendent God outside of human experience and attributing to Him all that is good. It was the beginning of the next stage of the evolution of consciousness.

Consciousness becomes invested in external, or exoteric, religions such as Christianity. This was ultimately unsatisfactory, however, because it radically cleaved the spirit into an inward aspect over and against a separate outward God, creating what Hegel termed an 'unhappy consciousness.' Finally, in the culminating stage of evolution, the emergence of 'absolute knowledge' allows the spirit to come to fully realize its own true nature.

Hegel sets the stage for a theme that will become increasingly familiar as we come to more recent theorists both in the East and in the West, the idea of an indwelling spirit, mind, or consciousness that presses for increasing expression. It is the theme of Being unveiling itself through human history. In Hegel's writing there is a strong sense of a preestablished plan for history, a plot in which the essentials are destined from the beginning. This idea leaves little place for the spontaneous creation of new and unexpected expressions of the spirit — e.g., new forms of mental, or spiritual life — since the single upward path is predestined from the beginning. In this regard Hegel's thinking is diametrically opposed to more evolutionary thought as seen in the grand evolutionary synthesis. It will later be necessary to examine the differences in more detail.

Another point of interest with Hegel is that the past, once finished, is over and done with. Previous modes of the spirit are said to be 'fulfilled' in later ones — 'nothing is lost' wrote Hegel — but in practical terms older expressions are submerged beneath newer emergent ones. More recent evolutionary views of consciousness, as well as systems theory in general, as seen in the grand evolutionary synthesis, tend to view earlier evolutionary stages not as lost, but as continuing to express themselves at lower levels of constantly complexifying systems.

We will return to these ideas later. For the moment, however, let us move on to two giants of early evolutionary thinking, Henri Bergson and Teilhard de Chardin. The first was a philosopher and the second an anthropologist. Both were French. Taken together they form such a continuous development of thought that it is difficult to see where one stops and the other begins. Both viewed evolution as a creative ascent toward higher and more complete expressions of consciousness or the spirit.

Creative evolution: Henri Bergson

Man only progresses by slowly elaborating from age to age the essence and the totality of a universe deposited within him.

Pierre Teilhard de Chardin, 1959

Abundance is the way of nature. Trees produce many more leaves than necessary for their survival. The brain of the human fetal infant produces, in certain regions, five to six times as many budding nerve cells as will survive until birth. Birds continue to sing when the mating season and nest building are long past. Humpback whales sing long intricate songs that can last for forty minutes or more without repeating, and they will change them from year to year. These songs seem outpourings of the sheer richness of life, going far beyond a simple communication of the whale's location. Evolution, likewise, seems prone to profusion and abundant creativity, and even to risks, so that the rule of thumb is to create first, to create richly, profusely, and without limit, and then let the results fall as they will.

The biggest difficulty with the Darwinian view of evolution as a creative process propelled solely by the emergence of random variations is to explain how it led to highly complex organisms such as human beings. This is a serious problem for the Darwinian model. Robert Richards, a prominent writer on evolution, puts it like this: 'An evolutionary process guided by material forces cannot guarantee progress.' To emphasize the magnitude of the problem, it has been said that the chance evolution of an organism as complex as a modern mammal is about like a wind sweeping through a junk yard and assembling by chance a Boeing 747!

Many evolutionary theorists of the late nineteenth and early twentieth centuries searched for means other than random variation that could lead toward ever higher levels of complexity. Lamarck and others, for example, believed that the benefits of the experiences of individual organisms could be passed on to descendants, and further that 'effort' could lead to inherited change. For instance, the cheetah might be seen as a product of many generations of predator cats, straining, as it were, to run down their prey.[5]

Many biologists opted for some inner guiding principle in what has been characterized as 'psychic evolution.'[6] Von Hartmann, for example, believed in the heritability of an 'unconscious purposive and formative activity' that resulted in inherited behavior. Hans Driesch proposed a purposive principle for which he adopted the Aristotelian term *entelechy*. This principle was said to influence organic processes by selectively moving energy between the potential and the kinetic states.

Most notable among this group, however, was the prominent French philosopher, Henri Bergson, whom we will spend some time with, as he was the first to elevate evolutionary thinking to the status of a major philosophy that includes both the outer dimension of biology and the inner dimension of consciousness.[7] Bergson argued eloquently for the idea that the cutting edge of evolution is propelled by a subtle non-material force which insinuates itself into organic matter. He referred to this force as a vital impetus, or *élan vital,* that operates to maximize evolutionary creativity and nudge organic matter ever forward toward a diversity that gives birth to higher and more complex forms. The essential nature of this vital impetus, according to Bergson, is not hard to find, for it is consciousness itself.

Bergson associated consciousness with an organism's power of choice, and thus with the breadth of freedom that is accessible to it. It operates in evolution as a pressure, gradually forcing its way to higher levels of expression. He wrote:

> Consciousness, even in the most rudimentary animal, covers
> by right an enormous field, but is compressed in fact in a
> kind of vise: each advance of the nervous centers, by giving
> the organism a choice between a larger number of actions,

calls forth the potentialities that are capable of surrounding
the real, thus opening the vise wider and allowing consciousness to pass more freely.

The direction and purpose of evolution, then, is to free up consciousness from the strictures of organic matter. This is achieved by the
development of large, flexible, nervous systems:

The more complicated the brain becomes, thus
giving the organism greater choice of possible actions,
the more does consciousness outrun its physical
concomitant.

Bergson believed evolution to be a truly universal process, so that life
evolves not only on the Earth but throughout the cosmos. At home,
however, consciousness clearly reaches its highest expression in the
human being. Indeed, Bergson's emphasis on the role of the human
as the highest expression of the evolutionary ascent led to the criticism
that he was a 'finalist,' that he believed evolution to be pulled forward
toward a predestined goal, and that his notion of evolution was not
free at all.[8] Certain comments made by him in the Second Introduction
to his foremost book, *Creative Evolution,* seem to point in this
direction. For example, he states there that the appearance of the
human is the *raison d'être* for life on Earth.

This zoological chauvinism may seem offensive to many today, but
we must realize that such statements were very much in keeping with
the heady intellectual atmosphere of pre-war Europe, one in which
leading thinkers were intoxicated with the success of the industrial
revolution and, along with it, the apparent supremacy of human reason
over nature. At the same time, however, they were also confronted
with the Darwinian reality of the human's intimate connection with
the world of animals and nature. The result, in Bergson's case, and
that of many others, was an evolutionary philosophy that placed
humankind at the pinnacle of nature.

All this aside, Bergson took pains to make it clear that what he
really meant by suggesting humankind as the reason for life on Earth
was that consciousness strives toward fulfilment in a form that can

give it maximum freedom of expression, and on the Earth this form
is that of the human.

Bergson's ideas about evolution were widely discussed, both in
Europe and in the United States, and his book, *Creative Evolution,*
was translated into more than twenty languages. Upon reading it just
after its publication in 1907 William James wrote:

> Oh, my Bergson, you are a magician, and your book is a
> marvel, a real wonder ... But, unlike the works of genius of
> the Transcendentalist movement (which are so obscurely
> and abominably and inaccessibly written), a pure classic in
> point of form ... such a flavor of persistent euphony, as of a
> rich river that never foamed or ran thin, but steadily and
> firmly proceeded with its banks full to the brim.

Bergson's lectures at the Collège de France were so popular that a
larger lecture hall had to be provided. Even it overflowed, however,
leading one wit to comment that the problem could best be solved by
moving them to the Paris Opéra house! When Bergson came to the
United States he was treated like a celebrity in New York, with well-
to-do society members vying for seats at his lecture.

Bergson made significant contributions to many areas of philosophy. Introducing him at Columbia University, the prominent
American philosopher John Dewey commented that 'No philosophic
problem will ever exhibit just the same face and aspect that it presented before Professor Bergson.' His most important contribution for
us, however, was his creation of a major evolutionary perspective
which placed the inner dimension of consciousness on an equal footing with external material organic processes.

Despite his fame during the first decade of this century, however,
Bergson's popularity after the First World War began to decline,
eclipsed by a new order of theorists. The grand and optimistic philosophical systems popular before the War gave way to a more sober
climate of specialization and philosophical positivism. The intellectual
life of the West changed dramatically. Fortunately, however, Bergson's way of thinking was not to lie fallow. The rich soil of
his thought was to nurture an evolutionary system that was to be

developed further than his own, and elaborated into a sweeping system of evolutionary thought by a brilliant paleontologist and Jesuit priest, Pierre Teilhard de Chardin.

Teilhard de Chardin

A little biographical information will help us understand Père Teilhard de Chardin's unique perspective on evolution. Teilhard was born in 1881 in Auvergne, France, where his father was a small landowner and also an archivist with an interest in natural history. At ten years of age Teilhard de Chardin entered a Jesuit College where he was to become fascinated with the fields of geology and mineralogy. He also felt the maturing of a deep spiritual calling, and at the age of eighteen entered the Jesuit order. By twenty-four he was assigned to teach physics and chemistry at a Jesuit College in Cairo, where he remained for three years before moving to England to study theology.

By this phase in his life he had begun to develop a real competence in geology and paleontology. This competence was supplemented by a reading of Bergson's *Creative Evolution,* which was to inspire him to a profound interest in evolution. In 1912 he was ordained a priest and in 1918, after serving as a stretcher-bearer during the First World War, he took the triple vows of poverty, chastity, and obedience.[9]

By 1919 the three major influences of Teilhard's life were in place. These were his career in geology and especially paleontology, his growing vision of an evolutionary cosmos, and his deep religious conviction. Within three more years he had received a doctorate in geology from the Sorbonne, and had become a Professor at the Catholic Institute of Paris, where his lectures were said to have attracted much attention among the students.

In 1923 Teilhard de Chardin spent a year in China on a Museum assignment. He returned to discover that his religious superiors had found unacceptable certain of his ideas about original sin and evolution, and had forbidden him to teach. Not long after that he returned to China. There he was destined to stay, with the exception of several trips around the world, for twenty years. Ironically, those years of isolation led to a great deepening and enrichment of his thinking about evolution. During this period, in fact, he wrote a variety of essays and books on different aspects of the topic, all of which lead up to his monumental work in 1938, *Le Phénomène Humain (The Phenomenon of Man)*. He was, however, not given permission to publish his writings. He returned from China in 1946 and during the last decades of his life became actively involved in the intellectual life of the West. *The Phenomenon of Man* was finally published in 1955.

Teilhard de Chardin worked out his evolutionary concepts several decades after Henri Bergson had published *Creative Evolution,* but the progression of ideas developed by these two men dovetail to such a remarkable degree that it is useful to think of the one as a continuation, refinement, and ultimately a vast expansion of the other.

Bergson, for instance, had suggested that consciousness influences the organic process of evolution by 'insinuating' itself into the chemistry of matter. This is good rhetoric, but does very little toward getting us down the road to a concrete understanding of what actually happens when this subtle inner force asserts its influence on the material events of a real organism. Teilhard's thinking on this question, however, was very clear, and is as interesting today as when he first conceived it.

The key to this problem, Teilhard de Chardin realized, is that very small amounts of work or energy can go a long way toward the creation of complex form. In Teilhard's own words, 'a highly perfected arrangement may only require an extremely small amount of work.' This notion, which may seem illogical on first nod, is in fact quite true. Many processes in nature start on a very small scale, one that may readily be influenced by the most minute quantities of energy. Consider, for example, the creation of a snowflake. The geometry of the first few water molecules that form the seed of the snowflake could be altered by very small influences. Once these first molecules are in place, however, the unique shape of the snowflake begins to form about them. One might even argue that the configuration of the initial molecular structure is, in fact, more a matter of probability than of energy. It would certainly seem to be the case that snowflakes differ not in energy levels, but in the myriad of complex shapes that they happen to take. A similar argument can be made in terms of embryonic development. The initial molecular events in the growth of, say, a lily, differ in form but not in energy from those of a rose. At this early stage in development it is not a matter of energy so much as of information. The genetic code for the rose contains unique information that is different from that of the lily. And, as demonstrated by precisely these molecular codes, a very small amount of work or energy can represent a very large amount of information.[10]

For Teilhard de Chardin, the small amount of work that makes the critical difference in the evolution of organic complexity is supplied by what he called *radial energy*. The term points to the idea that such energy emerges radially, as it were, from the inner center of the living organism. The effect of radial energy on evolution is to draw it 'towards ever greater complexity and centricity — in other words, forwards.'

Teilhard de Chardin believed that the cosmos presents us with two faces. One is the exterior, material, reality of conventional science, and the other is an interior reality, or consciousness. He thought this to be true of all levels of material existence, from the single atom through complex chemical structures and simple living organisms such as bacteria, on up to highly complex organisms, leading in a direct line to humankind. 'The exterior world,' he wrote, 'must inevitably be lined at every point with an interior one.' Thus, a progression is established in the exterior world running from the simple to the vastly complex, and simultaneously, in the interior world of consciousness, from the separate and elemental to that which is large and rich in quality.

> Whatever instance we may think of, we may be sure that ...
> a richer and better organized [physical] structure will
> correspond to the more developed consciousness.

Such notions, while contrary to the conventions of materialistic science, are not unknown to many of today's physicists and biologists, as well as certain philosophers. For instance the prominent philosopher Karl Popper observes that 'Dead matter seems to have more potentialities than merely to produce dead matter.' Likewise, Thomas Nagel, a philosopher who has spent many years considering the problem of how a physical system like the brain can give rise to conscious awareness, concludes that matter must contain some kind of 'proto-mental' properties. He further suggests that matter and mind, or at least the proto-mental properties referred to above, are essentially two sides of the same coin. This understanding would 'have the advantage of explaining how there could be necessary causal connections in either direction, between mental and physical phenomena.' In the same vein, quantum physicist David Bohm states that 'the mental and the material are two sides of one overall process that are (like form and content) separated only in thought and not in actuality.'

Very much in agreement with Teilhard's views, theoretical physicist Freeman Dyson recently wrote:

> I think our consciousness is not just a passive epiphenomenon carried along by the chemical events of our brains, but as an active agent forcing the molecular complexes to make choices between one quantum state and another. In other words, mind is already inherent in every electron.

Other examples could be given.

Teilhard de Chardin believed the evolution of complexity in the physical world to be accompanied by the evolution of quality in the world of conscious experience. This idea that consciousness is tied to complexity has, since Teilhard's day, become a familiar one, especially among members of the artificial intelligence community, who speculate that large computers, by virtue of sheer complexity, might give rise to conscious experience. Unlike Teilhard de Chardin, however, most of these individuals strongly favor reductionistic explanations of consciousness, and would not agree with the idea that consciousness exists at all levels of creation, from atoms to humans.

Teilhard de Chardin, like Bergson, not only believed that consciousness ascends to greater richness and depth as the physical organism achieves greater complexity, but that this was the very purpose of evolution. This theme runs throughout *The Phenomenon of Man,* taking many forms, but always returning to the idea that 'at the heart of life, explaining its progression, [is] the impetus of a rise of consciousness.'

And this impetus is manifested through the continuing enlargement and improvement of the nervous system.

This does not mean that Teilhard de Chardin did not believe that chance variation occurs in evolution. Indeed, to deny such a belief in the face of the evidence that the neo-Darwinians had accumulated by the end of the first few decades of this century would have been foolish.[11] He would have agreed with E.F. Schumacher, however, that the presence of random variation does not prove that there is no purpose anywhere in the process.[12] As the latter humorously put it, the fact that a man is seen picking up coins from the street does not mean that he makes his living by doing so. Teilhard de Chardin believed that despite random variation the direction of the grand sweep of evolution toward consciousness and intelligence was visible above the fray and confusion and the incredible variety of small-brained creatures which nature has brought forth.

This somewhat brazen disregard for the amazing diversity of life on earth as secondary to the primary agenda of evolution is perhaps the most difficult aspect of Teilhard's thinking for the modern scientifically minded reader to accept. Let it not distract us, however, from the force and luminosity of the vision he gives us of a cosmos in which life and consciousness are not secondary or incidental, but play an essential role in the drama of existence.

Like his contemporary, Sri Aurobindo, of whom we will have much more to say, Teilhard de Chardin viewed modern humankind to be a transient stage in the evolutionary ascent of life. In a vision of unprecedented grandeur he saw the future destiny of humankind tied to the destiny of the planet itself.

According to Teilhard de Chardin, just as the evolutionary web of organic life on Earth spans and transforms the entire planet, forming a *biosphere,* likewise the ever-expanding and interconnected mental life of humanity begins to encircle the earth forming a web or membrane of inner life which he termed the *noosphere,* or sphere of mind. This noosphere is the inner side of nature, the side of consciousness and mind. He argued that there is an increasing globalization of this internal dimension. As people come closer together in their activities, interactions, and communications, this process, so apparent today in our global culture, takes on an internal dynamism, a fusion on the inner dimension of the conscious life of humankind, and indeed all conscious life. This internal fusion of awareness on a planetary scale gives birth, in Teilhard's vision, to a new and higher level of being, a planetary consciousness, which he termed the *Omega Point.*

The achievement of the Omega Point represents a quantum leap in the planet's evolution. The Omega Point is to the individual human minds that form it what the individual mind is to the neurons of the brain. Like the individual mind, the Omega Point has its own emergent properties that go as far beyond the individual minds which support it as these minds go beyond the neurons of the brain. The Omega Point unifies and 'centralizes' the activities of its constituent minds in a fashion not unlike that in which the activity of the individual human mind draws together and centralizes the activities of the nerve cells of the brain. This process occurs, however, not through loss of individuality, but through a mutual enfolding of the most personal inwardness of each individual. Teilhard de Chardin identified this most personal inwardness with the experience of love.

> Love alone is capable of uniting living beings in such a way
> as to complete and fulfil them, for it alone takes them and
> joins them by what is deepest in themselves.

Teilhard de Chardin recognized love as a biological universal, 'easily recognized in its different modalities: sexual passion, parental instinct, social solidarity, etc.' Its highest expression, however, is selfless love, which Teilhard de Chardin understood through the Christian faith.

It is important to realize that the Omega Point is not something that might possibly come into existence in some ideal future. It is taking form during this very moment of evolutionary time, and its deep personal and mystical dimensions tend to draw us toward it as an organizing principle already felt as a presence in the world. In St Paul's words: 'God shall be in all.'

Today, Pierre Teilhard de Chardin's ideas are discussed primarily among philosophers and theologians. The face of biology is changing, however, and we may again see the appearance of subtle forces and even consciousness itself in biological circles.

5. The Ever-Present Origin

The diaphanous landscape of Jean Gebser

Behold! It is the eve of time, the hour when the wanderers turn toward their resting place. One god after another is coming home ... Therefore, be present ...

Friedrich Hölderlin

In this chapter we examine the first of two contemporary pioneers of the study of consciousness, Jean Gebser and Ken Wilber. Like Henri Bergson and Pierre Teilhard de Chardin of the previous chapter, these theorists also form a single fabric of thought, the one building upon the work of the other. Having said this much, I hasten to add that both also have unique views, especially of the highest forms of human consciousness.

Though rarely explicit in their writings Gebser and Wilber represent two different but related intellectual traditions. For Gebser it is the Neoplatonic tradition, particularly as shaped by the fifteenth century intellectual and mystic, Nicholas of Cusa, who believed all potential to be contained implicitly in God, the divine spirit, from which source it is projected, or explicated, out into the human world — a theme we will return to below.[1] Wilber, on the other hand, can trace his lineage to Hegel, who emphasized the realization of the spirit through history. Of Hegel's influence on his own work, Wilber once observed, 'his shadow falls on every page.' Wilber was also deeply influenced by Indian thought, especially Vedanta philosophy, as we will see.

Jean Gebser

Still largely unknown in English speaking countries, Jean Gebser (1905–73) was a cultural philosopher in the grand tradition of such intellectual giants as Giambattista Vico and Arnold Toynbee. His writings unfold a broad vision of the evolution of human consciousness comparable to that of Teilhard de Chardin, but with a much more contemporary flavor. Let us begin with some personal notes about Gebser's history.

Jean Gebser was born to an aristocratic family in Poland. He studied in Berlin, but at the age of twenty-four left Germany after encountering the Nazi Brownshirts, taking up residence in Spain. There, in the winter of 1933, the insight that was to become the core of his subsequent life's work came to him as a 'lightning-like inspiration.' This was the realization that a new and radically different form of consciousness was asserting itself in the world. Its influence could be seen in the art, literature, and science of his day. This form of consciousness, which he came to term *integral consciousness,* had the potential to transform the fabric of civilization from top to bottom.

In 1936, during the Spanish civil war, Gebser took flight from his home in Madrid just twelve hours before his residence was bombed. He was subsequently arrested and nearly executed by anarchists before reaching the border of France. Settling in Paris he became associated with a group of artists and intellectuals that included Pablo Picasso and André Malraux. He did not feel at home in France, however, and in August of 1939 crossed into Switzerland two hours before the border was closed. There he remained for the rest of his life.

Gebser's early writings had been in the realm of poetry and literature. After 1939, however, he increasingly devoted his energies to exploring the full implications of his vision of the new integral consciousness. Investigating its origins he was led to the discovery of several historically older structures of consciousness forming an evolutionary progression down to the consciousness of modern humankind. We will examine these below.

Ironically, Gebser was opposed to the characterization of his ideas as *evolutionary.* There were several reasons for this. One was that while Darwinian theory views evolution to be a process of continuous change, Gebser's structures represent more or less discrete or quantal jumps in the nature of consciousness. Another is that, for Gebser, the notion of evolution implied a progression toward increasingly higher and better forms, while he wished to emphasize that his historical sequence of structures did not form a movement from inferior to superior modes of consciousness. Gebser's most basic objection, how-ever, had to do with the nature of the concept of evolution itself. It is a concept rooted in a particular structure of consciousness, the mental-rational structure, which we will examine below, and according to his own theory this is but one of several possible forms of consciousness and thus of understanding the world, one to which he did not wish to be constrained.

My own feeling is that, while Gebser's objections may hold true for classical Darwinian ideas about evolution, they do not constitute a strong case against including his theory in the broad evolutionary context of the present discussion. First the notion that major evolu-tionary changes occur gradually, rather than in discrete leaps, is now in question. There is considerable evidence to the effect that species often remain virtually unchanged for substantial periods of geological time and then undergo relatively abrupt alterations. This type of quantal evolution, termed *punctuated equilibrium,* seems widespread and accounts for common fossil records that consist of sequences of related but distinctly different species, records in which the intermediate stages are often not found.[2] There are a number of factors that seem to contribute to this state of affairs, one of which is that evolutionary changes are thought to come about as the consequence of alterations in individual genes. Certain genes, termed regulatory genes, play a major role in governing the expression of whole sequences of other genes. Modifications in these genes, due, say, to single mutations, could alter the course of development of an organism in a major way, resulting in abrupt or *saltatory* (literally 'leaping') evolutionary change. Aside from genetic explanations, it has been pointed out that even slow transitions between relatively stable forms of life seem abrupt when viewed from the point of view of the extremely long periods of geological time.[3]

Gebser's second objection, that the concept of evolution implies a progression to increasingly higher or superior forms, is not one that most biologists would themselves agree with today. In fact, some of them have nearly bent over backwards to express the idea that no organism is in any fundamental way superior to any other. Robert Travis writes:

The chimpanzee and the human share about 99.5 per cent of their evolutionary history, yet most human thinkers regard themselves as stepping-stones to the Almighty. To an evolutionist this cannot be so. *There exists no objective basis on which to elevate one species above another.* Chimp and human, lizard and fungus, we have all evolved over some three billion years by a process known as natural selection.

This to my mind is a bit extreme, but the point is clear.

Gebser actually viewed each new structure of consciousness as both a gain and a loss. It is a gain in that it elevates the human to a new level of knowledge and competence, indeed a new and enlarged awareness of the world. At the same time it is a loss in that it carries him one step further from the root source of consciousness which Gebser termed the *origin,* a source that will be regained only at the final stage of development. I will have more to say about the origin shortly.

Gebser's third objection, that the concept of evolution itself is the product of a single type of consciousness, the mental-rational structure, is based in large part on the fact that linear notions of time derive uniquely from this type of consciousness and do not apply to others. In other words, to characterize his thought as evolutionary is to frame it and contain it in a single structure of consciousness, the mental-rational one. In my own opinion this may be the case, but it is indeed necessary to have some platform from which to start one's exploration, and for most of us, and Gebser too for that matter, this platform is the rational mind.

The structures of consciousness

The varieties of consciousness described by Gebser include five major structures. These are the *archaic, magic, mythical, mental,* and *integral* structures. They have emerged during human history as successively dominant patterns of experience, but in fact have overlapped considerably during periods in the past. All the structures are animated by the *origin* itself, the original spiritual impulse of life. Gebser begins his preface to *The Ever-Present Origin* with the observation:

> Origin is ever-present. It is not a beginning, since all beginning is linked with time. And the present is not just the 'now,' today, the moment or a unit of time. It is ever-originating, an achievement of full integration and continuous renewal. Anyone able to 'concretize,' i.e., to realize and effect the reality of origin and the present in their entirety, supersedes 'beginning' and 'end' and the mere here and now.

Jean Gebser conceptualized the structures of consciousness in terms of how each leads us to understand the world. Each structure is truly a knowledge or *noetic* process. Each has its own unique perspective or outlook. In particular, the perceptions of space and time change from structure to structure.

Gebser refers to the emergence of each new structure of consciousness as a *mutation* to indicate that it represents a relatively abrupt transition from the previous form. In Gebser's writing, however, it is not always clear whether we are dealing with a crisply defined historical sequence of transitions, or an ontological sequence. According to Gebser it is both. And though he often tended to emphasize the sequential order of the structures, a changing archeological record has moved strongly toward suggesting that the structures actually emerged during long periods of overlap.

Indeed, over the years that I have pondered and admired Gebser's work I have come increasingly to the opinion that the most fruitful way to understand the structures of consciousness is ontologically, or in other words as patterns of conscious experience which, like the states of consciousness mentioned in Chapter 2, are sufficiently separate to be viewed as fundamentally distinct — though more than one may exist at the same time. As we noted in that chapter, each structure of consciousness can be understood as an attractor, a process pattern of the brain and mind that produces a unique configuration of experience. Such patterns can become enfolded, or nested, like a movie within a movie, a wave riding on a wave, or a vortex moving within a vortex. The attractor of the dominant structure of consciousness, whether it be magical, mythical, or some later structure, has such a self-similar nature, the most recent and dominant pattern containing earlier structures as reflections of itself. But these are not perfect reflections, for each structure of consciousness is unique, and historically each successive structure is more complex than the one proceeding it. Thus the magic structure is more complex than the archaic, while the mythical structure is more complex yet.

At times Gebser himself seemed very nonchalant about just when, historically, the structures emerged, implying considerable periods of overlap in their appearance. Part of the apparent confusion here comes from his effort not to become bound up entirely in the modern rational structure of consciousness, and so he was caught in the paradox of trying to express himself in the linear mental edifice of written prose while struggling to reach beyond it. Perhaps poetry would be better for this, and as we know, Gebser was an accomplished poet. But poetry has its own limitations, for it is a creation of the mythic mind just as music is a creation of the magic mind, and prose of the logical mind. In this effort to operate the train off its tracks, to use Feuerstein's analogy, Gebser was occasionally prone to seemingly unreasonable statements. He once commented, for example, that:

> How far back we wish to place [the magic structure] into
> prehistory is not only a question of one's predilection, but,
> on account of the timeless character of the magical, is
> essentially an illusion ... It is pure speculation if we attempt
> to locate something timeless in a temporal framework that
> we have subsequently devised.

I will leave it to the reader to assess this comment. I will say in Gebser's behalf, however, that such statements are not as illogical as they may seem, as he, like Kant, David Bohm, and contemporary brain theorists such as Larry Vandervert and Ben Goertzel, considered reality to be an experienced construction, in his case a construction of the dominant structure of consciousness. Space and time are simply ways of experiencing reality; they did not exist before the evolution of the structures of consciousness that utilized them to understand the world. The archaic structure had no sense of space or of time, and so was zero-dimensional. The magical structure had no sense of time, but did contain the beginnings of spatial awareness. In this respect it was one-dimensional.

Gebser's five structures of consciousness in the order of their historical development include:

1. The *archaic structure of consciousness*. On the historical scale, this structure is essentially prehuman. It is also the least separated from the origin itself. It is the historical analog of the mythological state of purity at the beginning of history — life in the Garden of Eden before the Fall. It was a time when our hominid ancestors were still entirely at home in the natural world. The Jungian psychohistorian Eric Neumann referred to this period in terms of the mythological serpent oroboros that swallows its own tail, a symbol for self-enfolded consciousness (Figure 8).[4] Ken Wilber, who in *Up from Eden: a Transpersonal View of Human Evolution* achieves a substantial synthesis of the evolutionary views of Hegel, Gebser, Neumann and others, describes the symbolism of the serpent oroboros as signifying a form of awareness that is 'self-possessed, all-enclosing but narcissistic, "paradisiacal" but reptilian (or embedded in lower-life forms).'

Attempts to establish dates for this structure of consciousness are risky given the rate that changes occur in the field of human paleontology, and not entirely in keeping with Gebser's own view of it. He considered it as much an ontological condition, an original and continuing ground from which all consciousness arises, as a historical epoch. Still, it is interesting to speculate.

By modern archeological accounts we would need to go back amazingly far into prehistory to locate protohumans whose life styles exhibited such pristine unity with nature, that is, who did not exhibit a recognizably human culture or a tool-based technology. The gorilla-sized vegetarian ape, *Australopithecus,* that foraged the African savanna for food from five to one million years ago would certainly qualify. Its brain capacity of 450–700 cubic centimeters was roughly half that of the modern human, and it is unlikely that they developed anything like a human society. Whether they were actually an ancestor of the modern human is a matter of speculation, though it seems

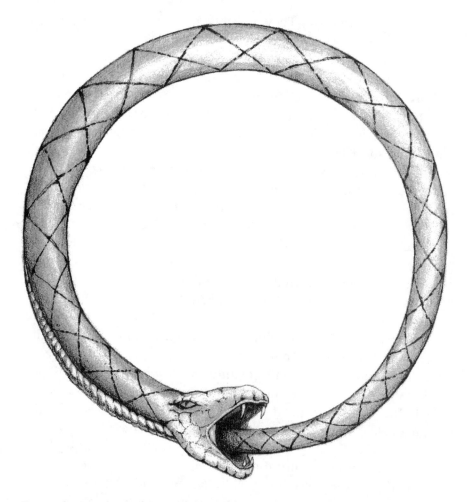

Figure 8. Artist's rendering of the serpent oroboros, symbolic of consciousness absorbed in itself in the archaic period.

likely. *Homo habilis,* who dates from roughly four to one and a half million years ago, should probably also be included in this category. Unlike *Australopithecus,* they were meat-eaters, and apparently the first to intentionally make and use tools (choppers or pebble tools). Small characters, about four to four and a half feet high, they had a brain capacity of 650–800 cubic centimeters. It was, however, a brain with a difference, because the left temporal lobe, an area associated with language ability in the modern human, was developed beyond that of *Australopithecus.*[5] They probably already had some precursors of language.

Homo erectus (the 'Peking man'), who spanned a period from one and a half million to seventy-five thousand years ago is also a candidate for the archaic structure of consciousness. On the other hand, they may represent a transitional case. At 800–1200 cubic centimeters, their brain at its maximum approached that of the modern human. They were adept tool users, including hand axes, which during their late period were very well crafted. Even with all of this, however, there still remains in the sparse geological record no indication that consciousness had moved beyond the confines of its immediate physical surroundings.

It is difficult to characterize the archaic structure of consciousness because it is the least differentiated of the five structures that Gebser described. He often likened it to a state of deep dreamless sleep. Here he cites the ancient Taoist philosopher, Chuang-tzu, who wrote: 'Dreamlessly the true men of earlier times slept.' This primitive awareness, however, was strongly suffused with the light of the origin.

According to Vedanta philosophy, in deep dreamless sleep consciousness is closer to the pure condition of *Brahman,* or Being as we would say in the West, than in any other state except the very highest, though the conscious mind does not know it. Likewise, of the dreamless sleep of the archaic human Gebser observes:

> It is akin, if not identical to the original state of the biblical paradise: a time where the soul is yet dormant, a time of complete non-differentiation of man and the universe.

One is reminded of Ovid's description of the Golden Age, in which humankind was said to live in perfect harmony with nature.

2. The *magical structure of consciousness.* While modern humans relate to their world in terms of logic, and ancient humans in terms of myth, dawn humans related to their world through magic. This was their posture for interacting with the cosmos. In this magic structure we encounter the first fully human mode of consciousness.

The key to understanding Gebser is to realize that each structure of consciousness contains a unique outlook on the world, in other words each embodies its own form of perception. This has to do with dimensionality, the number of dimensions accessible to consciousness, and the form that they take.[6] This will become clear as we go along. For the archaic human, perception was zero-dimensional, representing a posture of *identity* with the natural world, a sense of being completely embedded in it. For the magical human, perception was one-dimensional, allowing a sense of *unity,* but not of complete identity. In the latter case distance is not experienced as a primary aspect of the world. Objects separated in space can be made to substitute for each other. Gebser observes that the basis for virtually all magic, even today, is the substitution of one object for another. Another feature of this mode of experience is that part of a thing can substitute for the whole object. Poking pins in a doll that contains hair taken from someone far away in order to hex him at a distance is a crude but illustrative example. The doll substitutes for the actual person, and the hair from that individual adds an essential ingredient by substituting for the whole. Gebser would consider this type of magic to be a degenerate expression of the original magic structure of consciousness, but it makes the point.

Several instances of this type of *sympathetic magic* are found in the great cave sanctuaries of southern Europe, such as Lascaux and Les Trois Frères, which date from the paleolithic period thirty to ten thousand years ago. These include paintings of animals that have been struck repeatedly by stone projectiles, presumably spears.[7] In such instances the representations of the animals in the caves evidently substituted for the real thing. Hunters attacked and slayed them there, then later, almost incidentally, went out to attack them in the wild.

In another example, the paleolithic cave at Niaus in the French Pyrenees displays the painting of a bison with several arrows drawn on its side, as if to suggest the killing act of the hunter (Figure 9). Gebser recounted a similar situation that was observed in Africa by the French writer Leo Frobenius. In Gebser's words:

In the Congo jungle, dwarf-sized members of the hunting
tribe of Pygmies (three men and a woman) drew a picture
of an antelope in the sand before they started out at dawn to

hunt antelopes. With the first ray of sunlight that fell on the
sand, they intended to 'kill' the antelope. Their first arrow
hit the drawing unerringly in the neck. Then they went out
to hunt and returned with a slain antelope. Their death-
dealing arrow hit the animal in exactly the same spot where,
hours before, the other arrow hit the drawing.

We might note that recent discussions of the animals in paleolithic
cave paintings have tended to place hunting in a secondary role.[8]
Instances such as those suggestive of hunting magic, above, are relatively few. What is more, the animals for the most part seem relaxed
or pictured in spontaneous displays of movement, rather than running
from hunting bands or being driven over cliffs. Also, the most frequently depicted animals are not necessarily the ones that were most
commonly hunted. All of this lends greater mystery to these extra-
ordinary works of art, but does not deny the magical mentality that
created them.

Another aspect of magical consciousness is that perception is point-
centered, each part complete in and of itself. This is not alien to our
own experience, as we can easily look at a small part of, say, a
painting and allow it to grow in our awareness to consume the whole

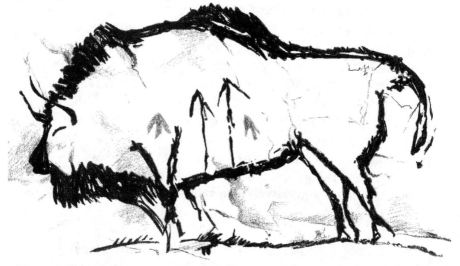

*Figure 9. Paleolithic cave painting of a bison at Niaus, in the French Pyrenees.
What appear to be several arrows can be seen on its side.*

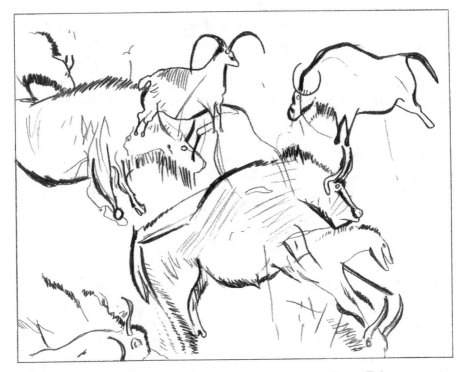

Figure 10. Paleolithic drawings such as these at Les Trois Frères cave in southern France, often overlap in a seemingly haphazard fashion.

of our experience. It is not, however, our usual mode of perception, which ordinarily places the part in the context of the whole. The absence of this larger context is a hallmark of magical consciousness and the world that is experienced by it.

The paleolithic drawings of animals, for example at Trois Frères cave near the Pyrenees in southern France, overlap to form a rich and in some locations almost haphazardly overlapping network of figures unlike anything most modern humans would draw (Figure 10). Such an arrangement is not surprising if the consciousness of the original artists was focused exclusively on each individual animal to the exclusion of others while it was being created.

Scattered throughout the paintings of animals in such caves are also many instances of 'sorcerers,' evidently the paleolithic counterparts of modern shamans. These figures display a curious collection of animal parts such as horns, tails, feathers, and so on, very much resembling the ceremonial attire of some modern shamans. Here again perception must be directed separately to each part to understand the way such costumes were apparently experienced by their original creators.

Gebser scholar Georg Feuerstein characterizes the magic structure of consciousness as having five principal features.[9] These include, first, an egolessness in which one's primary sense of identity is with the tribe or group. Second, perception is one-dimensional, or point-centered, as we saw above. Third, space and time have not yet unfolded as fully conscious realities. Gebser believed that phenomena such as telepathy and synchronicity (meaningful coincidences) may have been commonplace for people living in this mode of experience. Fourth, life is deeply and richly interwoven with the experience of nature. Fifth, the human's main vehicle for asserting himself is magic. This is important, because with the first awakening of the experience of separation from the world of nature comes the first need to dominate and control, expressed at this stage through magic.

Gebser believed that there may actually have been several stages between the archaic structure of consciousness and the fully developed magic structure. He observed, however, that the archeological record available to him did not allow any further clarification. *Homo erectus* may well have been a transitional case between the archaic structure and the magic structure. We do not, however, have a clear case for the latter until the advent of *Homo sapiens,* and in particular the Neanderthal man some half a million years ago.

The Neanderthal had a brain of 1400–1600 cubic centimeters, fully as large as that of a modern human. They made a variety of tools, and probably engaged in some form of speech, though judging from their throat development it was most likely poor by modern standards. In what appears to be the earliest evidence of religion of any kind, some apparently practiced a form of bear worship. Late in their reign, the Neanderthal also seem to have been the first to discover the great mystery of death. This was the first species to bury its dead, and did so ceremonially, as if to issue the deceased into an afterlife.[10] Bodies were sometimes placed in sleeping postures, lying on one side, legs curled up and head cushioned on one arm, as if to suggest a sleep from which one might awaken. In other instances the legs were tucked tightly upward and bound, perhaps emulating a return to the fetal posture. In one grave in Israel a man was buried among flowers, many of known medicinal value, suggesting that he may have been a healer. More than one instance has been found of what appear to be family units in which a man and woman were placed, heads together, with children at the woman's feet and other children nearby.

Joseph Campbell cites Giambattista Vico as writing that all nations, 'barbarous as well as civilized,' engage in three human customs: religion, solemn marriages, and burial of the dead. According to these, observes Campbell, the Neanderthal must surely be considered human.

It was the *Cro-Magnon* man, however, that brought magical consciousness into full bloom. This slimmer, more delicately proportioned species that came on the scene between forty and seventy thousand years ago was almost definitely our own ancestor.[11] While the cranial capacity was roughly equivalent to that of the Neanderthal, the throat cavity and tongue were significantly longer. The extension of these anatomical structures, vital to speech production, indicate without doubt that this was a human with language. It was they who created the cave paintings discussed above, and it is we, their descendants, that most of this book is about.

It is important to keep in mind that the older structures of consciousness, the archaic and the magical ones, are not simply archeological relics that have no relevance to modern life. They continue to exist beneath, or behind, the newer dominant structures and exert a lively influence even today. Indeed, we would not want it otherwise, for it is the light of the origin itself that shines through magic consciousness. It is this light that glows in the eyes of our beloved and leads us to that feeling of unity experienced in romantic love. A deep sense of community also comes from this consciousness, of belonging to a family or any other group of people. Music, with its ability to transport us out of the moment is also the product of the magic structure of consciousness.

Even in the modern world there are occasional eruptions of paranormal phenomena associated with the magic structure of consciousness — telepathy, precognition, synchronicity, and the like — and it is not surprising that these tend to exhibit themselves when rational consciousness is reduced to a minimum as, for example, during intense emotional states, in dreams, or in trance states.[12]

On the negative side, there is a tendency for the magic structure to overindulge in the security of the oneness experienced in close relationships, holding too tightly to other persons and sometimes refusing to allow them space to breathe. There is also a very dangerous tendency to follow the drum-beat of totalitarianism and collective ideological and religious movements, as was experienced so widely prior to the Second World War and all too much in today's world as well. The only remedy to these tendencies is to shift one's attention to the more recent structures of consciousness.

3. The *mythical structure of consciousness.* With the mythical structure came the beginnings of time experience, making it two-dimensional. This was not abstract Newtonian time, but what Gebser termed *temporicity,* the feeling of being *in* a certain time — living during the reign of a certain king, for example. Mythic tales take place in a time steeped in temporicity — for example 'long ago and far away,' or 'once upon a time.' There is often a sense of nostalgia connected with this feeling of time so that, for instance, the days of King Arthur are surrounded by and encapsulated in an enchanted time, one that has long since escaped the world of day-to-day affairs.

The origins of the mythic structure of consciousness seem, by the evidence of modern archeological findings, to be quite old, dating well back into the paleolithic age. While emotion is the force behind the magical structure of consciousness, it is imagination that propels the mythic, and we find evidence for such imagination even in the Neanderthal. Indeed, it is hard to imagine any truly human experience that does not involve imagination. The Neanderthal, for instance, buried their dead in sleeping or birth postures as if to return them to the womb of the earth, or perhaps to launch them into another world, in either case demonstrating an ability to empathize with the dead and to project them into the still unformed future. The reverence of the northern European Neanderthal for the great cave bear is further evidence of the presence of a mythic imagination.

As for Cro-Magnon man, even today one cannot look at the paintings in the cave sanctuaries mentioned above without being awed by the imagination of the artists who created them. The most enduring expression of the human imagination, however, and one that was to come down in a continuous stream all the way into the earliest periods of recorded history is the worship of the feminine principle in the form of the goddess. Starting well before 20000 BC the archeological record displays an increasing number of feminine figures that strongly suggest some form of symbolic worship of the feminine. One of the earliest and most graceful of these is the seventeen inch high *Woman with the Horn,* (Figure 11) carved into an overhanging limestone wall in Laussel France. She is holding a bison horn in her right hand and her left hand rests suggestively on a seemingly pregnant abdomen. At about this same time history saw the appearance throughout Europe of small statuettes of women no more than three to six inches high, typically faceless and footless, with exaggerated breasts and buttocks, often manifestly pregnant (Figure 12). They seem to symbolize the fertility of the feminine itself. Considering the meaning of these figurines, Joseph Campbell observed that:

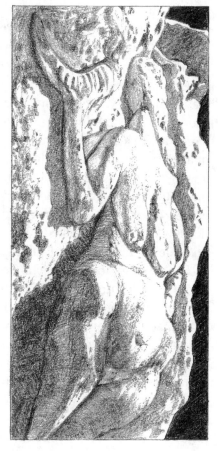

Figure 11. The graceful seventeen inch high Woman with the Horn, *carved in an overhanging limestone wall at Laussel France.*

> The evidence is now before us of a late Stone Age
> mythology in which the outstanding single figure is the
> Naked Goddess. And she can readily be recognized in a
> number of her best-known later roles: as Lady of the Wild
> Things, Protectress of the Hearth, Consort of the Moon-bull,
> who dies to be resurrected — with herself thereby a
> personification of the mystery of the moon, which has the
> power to shed its shadow (as the serpent sloughs its skin) to
> appear reborn.

The full sweep of the mythic imagination, and along with it the entire mythic structure of consciousness, did not break free of the older structures and come into its own, however, until the advent of the neolithic farming revolution. Sometime around 10000 to 8000 BC, perhaps even earlier, the first plants and animals were domesticated. During the next few millennia an entire *Old European* civilization based on agriculture developed in regions of Eastern Europe and the Near East, bringing with it artistry, commerce, copper metallurgy, and even what appears to be a rudimentary script.[13] Archeological excavations of that era have yielded a 'galaxy' of female figurines 'of bone, clay, stone, or ivory, standing or seated, usually naked, often pregnant, and sometimes holding or nursing a child,' along with ceramic wares painted with associated symbols. According to Campbell, these sacred images of the first agricultural civilization, and the bountiful earth goddess that they represent, point 'not to a new theory about how to make the beans grow, but to an actual experience in depth of that *mysterium tremendum* that would break upon us all even now were it not so wonderfully masked.' The richness of this experience was made possible by the faculty of the human imagination.

The deep mythic experience of the neolithic carried over into the ancient civilizations of the first few millennia before Christ, civilizations such as Egypt, Sumer, and Homeric Greece, where struggles of supremacy were waged between the goddess of the old religion and the new male insurgents such as Horus, Marduk, Zeus, and Yahweh.[14] The outcome of these struggles gave us the familiar mythologies of the ancient world in all their exquisite richness and color. Indeed:

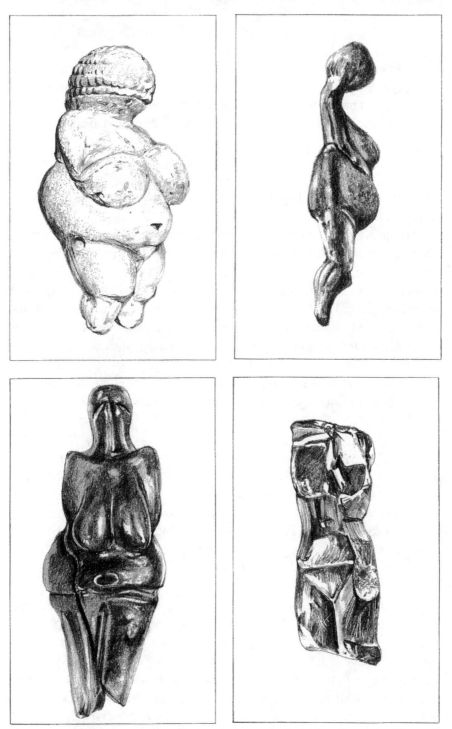

Figure 12. Examples of the many female figurines from late Stone Age Europe.

> The mythic consciousness moves and unfolds in sacred
> space and sacred time. It knows nothing of secular space-
> time. The mythical structure of consciousness is the source
> and medium of religion. It is religious consciousness *par
> excellence.*

It is the wellspring of religion even today, though in the modern world
it has been partially displaced by the rationally conceived god of the
mental structure of consciousness.

The profound richness of the human imagination derives from the
fact that it is no less than the outward projection as imagery of the
deep psyche, that is, of the human soul. In mythic consciousness
humankind discovers the inner wealth of its own depths. Imagination
expressing itself through myth, 'renders the soul visible so that it may
be visualized, represented, heard, and made audible.' Gebser often
emphasized this audible aspect of mythic consciousness. As music is
the purest expression of magical consciousness, so the outward expression of the soul in spoken poetry is the quintessential production
of mythic consciousness. In the words of Giambattista Vico, written
in 1744:

> Poetic wisdom, the first wisdom of the gentile world, must
> have begun with a metaphysics not rational and abstract like
> that of learned men now, but felt and imagined ... all robust
> sense and vigorous imagination. This faculty was their
> poetry, a faculty born with them ... Their poetry was at first
> divine, because ... they imagined the causes of things they
> felt and wondered at to be gods.

Historically, the pouring forth of the rich mythic imagination had quite
another aspect as well. It was the internal combustion engine in the
rapid acceleration of technology so characteristic of the first millennia
of the neolithic era. *Homo erectus* had lived for over one million years
making no more dramatic technological statement than some
moderately well crafted stone tools. Later the Neanderthal spent half
a million years developing what appears to be a modestly rich culture,
but one still lacking in aesthetic and technological expression when

judged against modern standards. With the Cro-Magnon these aspects of culture began to accelerate, as in the art work of the paleolithic caves. With the advent of full-blown mythic consciousness, however, artistic and technological development accelerated exponentially. Propelled by the outflow of inner creative imagery during the first millennia of the neolithic — as Feuerstein writes:

> Humanity embarked on a new decisive adventure in its
> millennia-long odyssey of awakening: the domestication of
> animals; the institution of sedentary communities (involving
> intense and comprehensive cooperative living); the
> expansion of villages into cities ... and with it the invention
> of professional specialization (including a professional
> sacerdotal class); the creation of an elaborate religious
> symbolism, focusing on the ideas of sacrifice and fertility;
> the invention of the temple; the formation of social classes;
> the institution of communal property; the introduction of the
> concept of work and trade; the institution of centralized
> political authority and the invention of the idea of law; the
> introduction of crafts (like pottery and weaving), and the
> invention of the potter's wheel, writing, poetry, and musical
> instruments; the invention of metal technology, boats, and
> the wheel, and a thousand other amenities without which
> our present-day civilization would be unthinkable.

Feuerstein points out that this enormous creative energy needs to be appreciated, because in his own works Gebser tends to stress the introverted aspect of the mythic consciousness, by which the human discovered the meaning of his soul.

4. The *mental structure of consciousness.* This structure emerged as the dominant way of assimilating reality during the final centuries before the birth of Christ and remains dominant today. It first reached a full expression in classical antiquity when Parmenides, in 480 BC, could say *to gar auto noein estin to kai einai,* 'For thinking and being is one and the same.' Plato, in the *Phaedo,* attributes a similar attitude to Socrates, who seems to equate the soul and the afterlife with pure

thought. The identification of being with thinking would be expressed again in the Renaissance times by René Descartes as: 'I think, therefore I am.'

Feuerstein estimates that the roots of the mental structure actually go back as far as ten millennia before Christ, in other words, to the beginnings of neolithic agriculture. If this is the case the emerging mental structure, like the mythic structure before it, overlapped greatly with its predecessor. Feuerstein supports his estimate with several instances of early writings that seem clearly to communicate an emerging sense of reflective awareness. Most prominent among these is the epic of Gilgamesh, composed around 2000 BC, in which the hero Gilgamesh in his failing quest for immortality seems to experience something very close to an existential crisis.

The mental structure underwent further elaboration during the late Roman empire when the ego first became fully established as a self-reflective center of the inner life. At this point in history individual personalities were systematically explored for the first time in art and literature. Busts of Roman citizens became studies in character, in contrast to the earlier Greek ideal of universal perfection. The biographer, Suetonius, attempted to capture the uniqueness of his subjects, such as Augustus Caesar. Indeed, it has been said of Augustus himself that with him individualism reached an early peak among rulers, for he managed to create an entire government fashioned on his own personality style.[15] At the same time the writings of Plotinus, the late Roman spokesman of Neoplatonism, represented one of the highest ascents of self-reflective awareness in the ancient world.[16] Saint Paul, as well, was taking religious thought and inspiration in a new direction with his implosive and introspective emphasis on Christ within ('Not I but Christ in me').[17] Later, Saint Augustine's *Confessions* would become a watershed in self-reflection.

Evidently the gains of late antiquity were all but lost, however, in the dark ages that followed the fall of Rome. During that time there was a notable weakening of the self-reflective inner life from which the ego finds support. Historian Morris Berman comments on a 'loss of interiority, or self-consciousness,' during this period. In his remarkable book, *Coming to Our Senses: Body and Spirit in the Hidden History of the West,* he has traced the historical development of self-awareness in terms of the history of mirrors and their role in reflecting externalized representations of the self. He observes that 'Periods of strong self-awareness are curiously accompanied by sharp increases in the use, distribution, or manufacture of mirrors.' Seeing our own image in a mirror gives us a sense of how others see us, and thus confronts us with ourselves as social objects. Such confrontations seem to engender an increased sense of self-awareness. Berman notes that, 'Mirrors became so popular in Rome that they were even owned by servants; and Seneca (first century AD) reported his disgust at one Hostius Quadra, who had himself constantly surrounded by mirrors.' But during the dark ages little or nothing was heard of mirrors.[18]

The advent of the Renaissance heralded a major transformation in the structure of consciousness, one that went far beyond the gains of the Roman world. The emergence of spatial perspective for the first time gave consciousness the ability to fully accommodate a three-dimensional or *perspectival* worldview. This new awareness of perspective is seen clearly in the paintings of the Renaissance, but also appears in its literature, philosophy, and mathematics. The geometric laws of perspective were finally worked out to near perfection by Leonardo da Vinci in the mid-sixteenth century. Within a few decades René Descartes would create the spatial mathematics of analytic geometry. Autobiographical documents such as personal diaries also began to imply an internal subjective referent equatable to a personal self or ego. Objectivity began to take on a new meaning as the ego identified its location as a point separated and distanced from the rest of the world.

The achievement of such objectivity was essential to modern analytic thought in general, and science in particular. It has, in a multitude of ways, created the world we know today with its powerful technologies and its political, ecological, and personal crises. Berman observes that after centuries in which nothing was heard about mirrors, they reappeared during the early Renaissance, and have more or less continually increased in popularity up to the modern period.

It is important to understand that Gebser did not consider perspectival consciousness to be an improvement on the original mental structure, as exhibited, for example, in ancient Greek thought. In fact, he believed each structure of consciousness to have both an *efficient*

and a *deficient* form. For example the efficient form of magic consciousness involved spell-casting, as illustrated above in the use of
sympathetic magic for hunting. This use of magic allows the human
to direct nature, but at the same time remain in accord with it. The
deficient form of magic consciousness involves witchcraft, by which
Gebser meant the immoderate use of magical power to manipulate
nature. For the mythic structure of consciousness, the efficient form
involved myth as imagery projected outward from the soul. The
deficient form involved myth as spoken narrative — mythology as it
is ordinarily understood today, for example, in the stories of the gods
of ancient Europe or Greece.

For the mental structure of consciousness the efficient form is epitomized by *menos,* balanced directional thought as seen, for instance,
in the dialogues of Plato. Its deficient form — and Gebser was
adamant about this — is reason, rational consciousness, or *ratio.* It is
characterized by divisive, immoderate, hair-splitting reasoning. Gebser
comments:

> *Ratio* must not be interpreted ... as 'understanding' or
> 'common sense'; *ratio* implies calculation and, in particular,
> division, an aspect expressed by the concept of 'rational
> numbers' which is used to designate fractions and decimals,
> i.e., divided whole numbers or parts of a whole. *This
> dividing aspect inherent in ratio and Rationalism — an
> aspect which has come to be the only valid one — is
> consistently overlooked, although it is of decisive
> importance to an assessment of our epoch.*

Perspectival consciousness places the sense of self in objective space
somewhere in the head, as contrasted with the experience of the
ancient Greeks and Native Americans who would point to the heart.
The heart, noted Gebser, is the source of the experienced soul, as the
head is the source of *ratio.*

The discovery and articulation of perspective was equivalent
to becoming fully conscious of the deep geometry of space, thus
adding a third dimension to human awareness. The fixed location of
the ego in objective perceptual space led, however, to rigidity and a

self-centered inability to go beyond one's own narrow confines. In Gebser's words:

> Compelled to emphasize his ego ever more strongly because of [its] isolating fixity, man faces the world in hostile confrontation. The world in turn reinforces this confrontation by taking on an ever-increasing spatial volume or extent (as in the discovery of America), which the growing strength of the ego attempts to conquer.

This sense of isolation is reflected in many forms.

> Isolation is visible everywhere, isolation of individuals, of entire nations and continents, isolation in the physical realm in the form of tuberculosis, in the political in the form of ideological monopolistic dictatorship, in everyday life in the form of immoderate, 'busy' activity devoid of any sense-direction or relationship to the world as a whole; isolation of thinking in the form of the deceptive dazzle of premature judgments or hypertrophied abstraction devoid of any con-nection with the world. And it is the same with mass pheno-mena: overproduction, inflation, the proliferation of political parties, rampant technology, atomization in all forms.

This is the condition to which *ratio* has brought our world. Is it any wonder that Gebser saw hope for the future only in a large-scale shift to a new and more holistic structure of experience, the integral con-sciousness?

5. The *integral or aperspectival structure of consciousness.* This is the structure that Gebser saw emerging in his own lifetime.

Each structure of consciousness contains its own experience of time. In the magic structure time is vaguely experienced simply as the pres-ent. In the mythic structure, time, as we have seen, is experienced as temporicity. In the mental structure, however, time becomes an ab-stract quantity. This is particularly so in perspectival consciousness, which treats it, in Newtonian fashion, as a scalar linear quantity ana-

logous to a spatial dimension. In integral or aperspectival consciousness time, however, is experienced as a concrete aspect of the world.

Gebserian scholar Algis Mickunas explains the apparent paradox of
this experience of time as follows. Suppose you awaken one morning
and look out the window to find that it has been snowing during the
night. You see the blanket of newly fallen snow on the ground, the
trees, and your window sill. Though the snow had not yet fallen when
you went to bed the night before, and though you were not awake
when it came, the event of the night snow is enfolded in the very
experience of its presence in the morning. There is a poetic aspect to
this form of the experience: this is the night-fallen snow, the gentle
blanket of cool whiteness that fell quietly during sleep.[19] If you want
a Newtonian account of the snow, you can turn on the weather station.
'Two inches of snow fell on the western counties this morning
between three and five a.m. as another cold front moved through our
area from the north.' Here you have the essential coordinates for
complete perspectival space-time. But what a bore!

The tangible grasp of time by the integral consciousness is
comparable to the tangible grasp of space experienced first by the
perspectival structure of consciousness and retained by the aperspectival structure. Gebser observed the awakening of this sense of
time in writers such as Rilke, T.S. Eliot, and Hölderlin.

Living with time as a tangible reality means living in the manifest
world of the present. As is known to virtually every mystical tradition
in the world, living fully in the present is equivalent to a revolution
in one's entire life experience. It is a tribute to Gebser's genius that
he achieved this insight, not through the study of wisdom traditions or
Eastern philosophies, but by sheer force of insight. Georg Feuerstein
once referred to Gebser as a Jnana yogi, that is, one who seeks to
know the true nature of reality by sheer penetrating insight.

Gebser found evidence of the aperspectival view appearing in both
science and the arts. In *The Ever-Present Origin* his enquiries spanned
a wide range of fields including physics, mathematics, biology, and
sociology, as well as philosophy, jurisprudence, and music, painting
and literature! His treatment of these, moreover, is not casual, but
detailed and lucid, having spent years searching these fields for
evidence of the emergent structure of consciousness.

Though the awakening of integral consciousness is 'accompanied by an increasing reification or materialization of the world,' its overall effect is not only an increased sense of concrete time and space, but paradoxically, a transparent, or *diaphanous,* experience of reality, one in which perspective, no longer anchored to the perspectival ego, becomes fluid. This is witnessed in the paintings of Pablo Picasso and Paul Klee, where multiple viewpoints appear simultaneously as integral wholes. It is also evidenced in the quantum physics where, in contrast to mechanistic Newtonian thinking, time and space become fluid.

It is perhaps apparent that there is a spiritual depth to integral consciousness. Indeed, its transparent or 'diaphanous' quality is suffused with the light of the spirit, the animating radiance of the *origin,* and to a greater degree than any dominant structure since the archaic consciousness, but here with a solid clarity previously absent.

Although Gebser preferred to avoid comparisons with Eastern philosophies — most likely because the atmosphere in which he worked was less liberal in this regard than it is today — he noted a fundamental similarity between integral consciousness and Zen *satori.* In this respect it is worth noting that though he did not often emphasize it, as with the other structures of consciousness there is a distinction between an efficient and a deficient form of integral consciousness. He termed the deficient mode *diaphainon,* referring to the shining-through of the spiritual light of the origin. The efficient mode he simply referred to by the Buddhist term, the *Void.* A sense of the quality of this experience is given in his comment that in it:

> The pre-temporal becomes time-free, vacuity becomes
> plentitude, and in transparency the spiritual comes to
> perception: origin is present. In truth we ware [experience]
> the whole, and the whole wares us.

Gebser used the term 'waring' *(Wahren)* to refer to category-free perception, beyond the ordinary constraints set by time and place. He felt that such perception is possible when the perspectival ego is transcended.

Georg Feuerstein believes that the full-blown experience of integral consciousness is best understood, not as a structure of consciousness at all, but as an open and fluid condition of being, one through which all of the rich variety of human experiences, including the previous structures of consciousness, might flicker without disturbing or destroying it. If this is the case it is equivalent to the highest forms of realization in both Hindu and Buddhist traditions.

As to the future, Gebser held little hope for a world controlled by men's and women's egos. Only with the emergence of integral consciousness on a large enough scale to change society did he see the possibility of a positive outcome. He wrote:

> The future will definitely establish itself, our role being at the very most that of participants. But one thing must be said: the coming decades will decide whether the fundamental transformation will occur during the next two generations, or not for the next two millennia.

Gebser was clear, however, that large-scale mutations in individual consciousness are accompanied by widespread suffering and chaos. He believed today's world to be in such a transitional state, struggling to give birth to the new consciousness. He wrote in 1949:

> If mankind can endure the new tensions that are becoming acute as a result of the irruption of new heavens and the earth's migration through new regions of the universe — tensions which are becoming acute on the earth and thus in man as well — then the impending collapse will only mean the end of the exclusive validity of the hitherto dominant mental structure. But if man and the earth are unable to endure these tensions, they will be torn apart by them.

It is apparent that we live in an age of a transition, one leading either to self-destruction or perhaps into a new age of human freedom and growth. William Irwin Thompson, as we have already seen, conceptually models this historical moment on Vico's notion of a cyclic return of the Age of the Gods. Gebser, however, would most likely identify the Age of the Gods with the mythic structure of consciousness, and thus consider it a regressive and impractical solution to the problems of today's world, problems which require a step forward to a new integral consciousness.

What does the new landscape of the emergent integral world look like? In Georg Feuerstein's words:

> No (mythical) world-*view* can frame it, just as no (mental-rational) world-*conception* can grasp it. But it is nonetheless accessible and understandable to us — through direct (integral) participation in it. Such *participation* renders self and world diaphanous so that their spiritual foundation becomes obvious.

Projection and the advance of evolution

Gebser's view of evolution, like Hegel's, and also like that of Sri Aurobindo, holds the ultimate potentials of human consciousness to be enfolded in the origin (the Spirit for Hegel and the Divine for Sri Aurobindo) from the beginning, needing only time and history to exfoliate them as manifest realities. Perhaps this statement is too strong, since Gebser himself criticized Hegel for viewing the process of history — we would say the evolutionary process — as rigidly predetermined. It is clear from what we have seen so far that Gebser considered the dawning of each new step in the evolutionary movement, the birth of each new mutation of consciousness, to be laden with difficulties and in many ways indefinite. All this in the balance it is still the case that for Gebser the sequence of the structures as well as their essential forms appears to be inflexible.

Gebser differs from Sri Aurobindo, however, in that the latter, as we will see, viewed the highest level of the individual being, the Atman, to be complete from the beginning, so that the human problem is one of transforming the lower aspects of human nature — the body, the mind, the emotions — and bringing them up to their highest potential. Reading Gebser, on the other hand, one has the definite impression that, more consistent with Hegel, the highest potentials exist in the origin only as potential, not yet actually complete until expressed in human nature.

The mechanism by which potentials latent in the origin become manifest is of more than casual interest, as it also supplies the vehicle for evolution itself. This mechanism is *projection*. Gebser's use of this term is not unlike its use in psychology, namely as an outward displacement of something originally located within the psyche itself. In psychology, however, and especially in Freudian theory, there is usually an implication of something undesirable such as memories, feelings, or urges that are unacceptable to the ego and have been repressed only to appear later as a projection.

For Gebser, however, projection is the mechanism by which latent potentials of the origin first appear in human experience.[20] It is easier, it would seem, to recognize new facets of reality if they first appear as external and objective facts. Only later in evolution is their source recognized to be within ourselves. Magic, for instance, was first projected outward as a characteristic of the world of nature, only later to be associated with persons and their abilities.

The experience of space likewise developed in stages. The early Greek sculptors and architects, for instance, were very much aware of space, but not yet of geometric perspective, which was consciously perfected only much later by Renaissance artists. Consciousness of time developed by degrees as well, beginning with a vague sense of the present in magical consciousness, and continuing through the abstract metric and quantitative time of *ratio*. In integral consciousness the projections of space and time are *retracted,* withdrawn and re-integrated back into the psyche, yielding a world that is paradoxically at once more solid and more fluid. This fluid quality is seen in the conscious manipulation of spatial and temporal perspectives of Picasso, Klee, and Cézanne. It is experienced in the music of Stravinsky and Stockhausen, in the poetry of Eliot and Rilke, and in the science fiction of Roger Zelazney and Gene Wolf.

Gebser wrote that 'no awakening of consciousness can take place without projection,' and further, that the retraction of the projection 'is itself an act of the awakening consciousness.' Since such a retraction 'can be realized only out of a new consciousness structure' the retraction itself heralds the advent of a mutation, the coming of a new structure of consciousness. For example, the fluid experience of space characteristic of aperspectival consciousness is possible only by retracting and integrating the geometric perspective typical of the mental rational structure. But the very act of reintegration is a revolution, propelling consciousness toward the aperspectival attractor.

One wonders what we can do individually to bootstrap ourselves into the integral structure of consciousness. Unfortunately Gebser has no explicit agenda for growth. He gives only general advice, indicating, for instance, that it is necessary to overcome the inflated ego of modern rational consciousness by reintegrating the projection of individuality and separation.[21] This is a big order! Moreover, Gebser does not recommend the techniques of Eastern traditions. Even though he experienced a temporary but genuine satori state himself, one which he identified as authentic integral consciousness, he believed the European mind to differ too dramatically from the Eastern mind to benefit from such practices.[22] Whether this is actually true or not is a matter of vital interest to many contemporary Westerners. We will return to it later in the book.

Nicholas of Cusa, and Plotinus

In Gebser we reconnect with a line of thought that goes all the way back to Plotinus. Although he rarely mentioned it, Gebser seems to have been influenced by a remarkable philosopher and man of letters of the fifteenth century, Nicholas of Cusa (1401–64).[23] Nicholas, in his turn, had been deeply influenced by the writings of Plotinus and, in fact, played a major part in revitalizing Neoplatonism in the face of Aristotelian ideas that had dominated western Europe since the thirteenth century.[24]

Nicholas advocated certain ideas that were strikingly advanced for his day. For instance, he believed that the universe has no circumference, is boundless and undetermined. These were revolutionary concepts in the Church-dominated cosmology of his time. Moreover, he did not subscribe to the notion that the Earth is at the center of the universe, but believed that it moves in space with a motion that is relative to the observer. In these ways he anticipated modern cosmology and broke with the Ptolemaic and Aristotelian views according to which the earth is at the center of a circumscribed spherical cosmos.

Influenced by Plotinus' concepts of *nous* and the One, Nicholas believed in a higher source of wisdom than the rational intellect, stressing the importance of knowing the limits of the ordinary mind.[25] He referred to conventional knowledge as learned ignorance *(docta ignorantia)*. Also in line with Neoplatonism, he proposed the doctrine that all potential exists within God, who alone is infinite. Because God is the absolute maximum, he contains all things 'enfolded' *(complicatio)*, and is also their source or 'unfolding' *(explicatio)*.

The latter notions anticipate the ideas of quantum physicist David Bohm, who argues that the material world is supported by a vastly deeper and larger process which he terms the *implicate order*.[26] This hidden order can be thought of as a holographic process of cosmic dimensions, similar to a deep ocean on which the universe, the *explicate order*, rides like waves. Strictly speaking, little that is truly new or creative comes from the explicate order itself, as it is only a surface phenomenon. The implicate order is the wellspring of creativity, expressing itself not only in the physical world, but through human intelligence and even life itself. These are precisely the processes that Nicholas of Cusa, using different language, attributed to God; namely that novel aspects of reality come into existence by unfolding outward from their divine source. Let that divine source be Gebser's origin, and let projection be the mechanism for the unfolding, and we have Gebser's concept precisely.

We may note that with Jean Gebser we have come full circle in terms of Western concepts of the nature of consciousness. The first profound Western system concerned with consciousness was that of Plotinus, and in Gebser we return again to Neoplatonic ideas, now transformed into modern concepts.

Integral consciousness in today's world

The most important and nagging question concerning Gebser's work, the one which he himself was most concerned about, is whether humankind is really moving in a tangible way toward integral consciousness. Is integral consciousness a realistic hope for the future? At this moment of personal, economic, and global ecological crises, we cannot afford to delude ourselves with idealistic illusions.

As we saw above, Gebser was quick to point out that a transition to a new human order would be achieved only at the expense of great strain and suffering. To what extent does the strain and suffering so obvious in today's world evidence this transition? My own impression is that much of the intellectual and ideological ferment so apparent today can be understood, at least in part, as a struggle of the conservative perspectival world against the emergent and threatening play of the aperspectival experience. This newly fluid consciousness can be seen in the whole intellectual panorama of the postmodern world.[27] I believe it to be most apparent, however, in the softening of the borders of perspectival reality on all fronts.[28]

Beginning with philosophical deconstructionism — a sort of unraveling of the written texts upon which knowledge is based[29] — and continuing through contemporary moral, political, and religious relativism, there is an increasingly widespread disposition to see issues through the protean vistas of integral awareness.[30] People often become disoriented and paralyzed by the welter of perspectives, but on the positive side the new consciousness offers a delightful play of creativity. One thinks of the new physics with its conspicuous disregard for ordinary causality and Newtonian space-time; with its particles which have color and flavor, its quarks, its quantum foam, and its multiple universes. One thinks of writers such as Jorge Luis Borges, Milorad Pavic, Doris Lessing, and Olaf Stapledon, who play with realities as if manipulating shafts of light, to say nothing of the many science fiction writers from Isaac Asimov to Roger Zelazney who explicitly fabricate alternative realities by way of science and fantasy. One could go to the music of Philip Glass, George Crumb, and the juxtaposition by Enigma of ancient Gregorian chants with modern erotic rhythms, or the elevating creations of 'new age' composers such as Kitaro. The story is the same everywhere. There is a fluid and luminous, often lyrical, but sometimes dark play of the postmodern consciousness that makes and dissolves realities with the same vigor and delight with which previous generations created representational landscapes on canvases. We will see the play of this consciousness again in Chapter 11 where I will attempt to shed light on states of realization or enlightenment.

All the above in mind, however, my own impression is that aperspectival consciousness typically appears through specific talents; in one person through artistic acumen, in another through music, and so on, rarely becoming revolution of the entire consciousness. Thus, an artist, writer, scientist, or even an executive or gardener, might experience integral awareness in his own domain of expression. But this experience is just a foot in the door. It does not mean that he or she has become a Zen master, or in other ways has revolutionized his life. This is disappointing. One hopes that the great artist or writer will carry over the wisdom of his work into the world of daily life, but it is often not the case. Sometimes, however, the door opens and a wider light enters the personality. Wisdom is gained. This certainly was the case for Gebser, whose intellectual quest led him to an enriched consciousness.

Nevertheless, I suspect that the newly emerging integral consciousness may become an important player in the world culture of the twenty-first century.[31] Like all chaotic attractors its effects are difficult to foresee in detail. We can anticipate, however, that short of a major regressive trend, opinions and perspectives in all realms of culture will continue to become more fluid and playful, while conservative perspectival factions resist these trends as if their very existence were threatened to its roots, as indeed it is.

6. Through 'Every Possible' Grade

Eden and beyond

*The subconsciousness of matter and body gives way to the
self-consciousness of mind and ego, which in turn gives way
to the superconsciousness of soul and spirit — such is the
'big picture' of evolution and history, and such is the
context of man's history as well.*

Ken Wilber

In Ken Wilber we come to a modern scholar of consciousness of
major importance. During a period of just nine years Wilber wrote a
series of exploratory books beginning with *The Spectrum of Consciousness,* published in 1977, that shaped a systematic tradition of
transpersonal psychology in the United States.[1] In his first book he
reviewed a wide range of spiritual traditions from throughout the
world, developing a common model of shared knowledge. Later, in
The Atman Project, he systematically cross-referenced the results of
this synthesis with a variety of mainstream theories of psychological
development including Piaget's psychology, Maslow's needs hierarchy, Kohlberg's stages of moral development, psychoanalytic theory,
and others. Here our main interest will be with Wilber's exploration
of the evolution of consciousness, which he developed in his book *Up
From Eden: a Transpersonal View of Human Evolution.* In this book
Wilber gives us a substantial synthesis of several major perspectives
on human evolution, all viewed from the framework of traditional
wisdom schools, or in Wilber's terms, the perennial philosophy. Since
this philosophy plays a central role in Wilber's thinking, and indeed
is important throughout much of this book as well, I will take a
moment to describe it in terms that may be helpful.

The perennial philosophy

In his classic collection of edited readings, *The Perennial Philosophy,* Aldous Huxley described the philosophy as:

> *Philosophia perennis* — the phrase was coined by Leibniz; but the thing — the metaphysic that recognizes a divine Reality substantial to the world of things and lives and minds; the psychology that finds in the soul something similar to, or even identical with, divine Reality; the ethic that places man's final end in the knowledge of the immanent and transcendent Ground of all being — the thing is immemorial and universal.

The term *philosophia perennis,* and related ones such as *prisca theologia,* and *philosophia occulta,* actually came into use in the Renaissance to refer to a tradition, partly historical and partly mythical, of esoteric wisdom that was said to have flowed through many lineages from ancient sources.[2] Wilber, however, uses the term to refer to a more metaphysical doctrine by which the cosmos is understood to be comprised of levels or tiers. It is an old story. In his classic 1936 work, *The Great Chain of Being,* Arthur Lovejoy observed:

> The conception of the universe as ... ranging in hierarchical order from the meagerest kind of existents ... through 'every possible' grade up to the *ens perfectissimum* ... has, in one form or another, been the dominant official philosophy of the larger part of civilized mankind through most of its history.

Both Ken Wilber and the eminent scholar of religion and contemplative spiritual traditions Huston Smith point out that virtually all such traditions assume such a series of layers of being ascending from the material world of multiplicity up to a single absolute reality.[3] In fact, the idea that the cosmos is stratified, and further that this stratification is reflected in our own inner being, was written down over twenty-five centuries ago in what is still perhaps the most elegant expression of this idea, the Vedantic philosophy of India. This philosophy in its various forms continues to permeate the entire spectrum of spirituality on the Indian subcontinent and is mirrored in Buddhist traditions scattered throughout the Far East.

In Vedanta the absolute undivided reality of the universe, *Brahman,* is experienced in the individual man or woman as the *Self* or *Atman,* the eternal and unchanging source at the apex of the multiple layered structure which is the human being. This Self is surrounded and eclipsed by a series of sheaths, or *koshas,* as shown in Table 1. Each represents a lower vibrational level, so to speak, or a denser form of substance than those above it.[4] There are five such sheaths beginning at the most subtle level with the causal body, also termed the *anandamaya kosha* or the sheath of bliss. It is said that to experience this level is to enter a state of rapture. According to Wilber, it is possible to mistake this experience for the highest reality itself, the radically unconditional experience of the Self. This can happen if the student is not forced to make this discrimination by a teacher and tradition that clearly recognizes it for what it is. Indeed, in some traditions the experience of the causal realm is taken as the very goal itself.[5]

Next is the subtle body, termed the *vijnanamaya kosha* or the intellect. The term 'intellect' as used here, however, does not carry the usual meaning it takes in the English language, but refers to a source of high intuition or *gnosis* associated with elevated or true knowledge.

Anandamaya kosha	(sheath of bliss)	causal body
Vijnanamaya kosha	(intellect)	subtle body
Manomaya kosha	(mental sheath)	mental body
Pranamaya kosha	(energy sheath)	pranic body
Annamaya kosha	(food sheath)	physical body

Table 1. The sheaths (koshas) of Vedanta that surround the Self.

This is the source of 'yogic intuition,' which is valued far more highly than the rational productions of the ordinary mind. Such intuition, it would seem, is accessible not only to sages, but occasionally to great creative geniuses. Mozart, for example, was able to write entire orchestral compositions just as they came to him. Indeed, such intuition can be cultivated to a greater or lesser degree by anyone who wishes to do so, and seems to be a general aspect of transpersonal development.

The next level below the subtle body or intellect is the mental sheath, termed the *manomaya kosha* or mind. This sheath represents the level of ordinary mind. Here is found the domain, for instance, of the developmental theories of knowledge such as that of psychologist Jean Piaget, as well as the many cognitive studies of memory, decision-making, and so on.

Below the mental sheath is the prana or energy body, the *pranayama kosha*. Comprised of pranic energy, this level is the object of yogic practices that work with subtle energies, practices such as *pranayama,* which represent an entire technology for molding them. It is the conscious control of energies at this level that accounts for some of the remarkable feats of physiological self-control exhibited by yogis, such as the ability to stop the heart. It is also the control of these energies that allows certain yogis to heal others. In the case of Sri Aurobindo, for example, it was said that when he was healing, one could actually feel the Force, or shakti, flowing from him.

At the most dense or gross level of this hierarchy of being is the physical body itself, also termed the *annamaya kosha,* or food sheath, because it derives literally from food.

Few traditions are as specific about these planes of being as is Vedanta, but many agree that the cosmos exhibits an inner vertical order comprised of a greater or lesser number of levels.[6] Huston Smith, for example, suggests four such levels, though I doubt that he intends them to be taken as rigid categories. The first is the terrestrial or physical realm. The second, intermediate level, is the already familiar realm of mind. The third is the celestial level, which would seem to correspond more or less to the subtle realms of Vedanta. And finally there is the infinite, which clearly to refers to the unconditional Self or the One.

Mahayana Buddhist tradition, which has its origins in first century AD India and later spread throughout Asia and Japan, speaks of the 'three bodies' of the Buddha. The highest is the *dharmakaya* or the 'body of the great order.' This 'body' is identical with transcendental reality and seems to correspond to the level of the Self of Vedanta. The second is the *sambhogakaya* or 'body of delight' which seems analogous to the causal level, the sheath of bliss of Vedanta. The third body is the *nirmanakaya* or 'body of transformation,' which corresponds to the physical body itself. Comparing this three-part system to Vedanta discloses several of the levels or sheaths to be missing. This is not a simple omission. The Mahayana tradition in many of its forms is not a path of yogis, and so is less interested in the intermediate levels associated with subtle energies and mental phenomena than in ultimate levels of being.

In the West, the concept of a cosmos stratified according to 'The Great Chain of Being' was influential in Renaissance Europe and again during the seventeenth and eighteenth centuries. According to this system, which is summarized in Lovejoy's quote above, the entire cosmos is ordered into tiers that descend from God and the celestial beings at the top, down to the human and the animal worlds, on through plants, and at the bottom to the world of inanimate matter. Thus, the orders of being formed a pattern in which humankind had a rightful place. This concept is also found in the philosophy of Neoplatonism, with its historical roots in the writings of the third century mystic, Plotinus. The latter, however, was more interested in inner levels of being than in categories of outward appearances. The esoteric philosophy that unfolded in his writings was to become a source of inspiration for many artists, intellectuals, and mystics down through the ages.

Plotinus himself seems to have been the inheritor of a stream of Western esoteric wisdom that flowed down from the ancient Greek Pythagorean and Orphic mystery schools.[7] These teachings were imparted to him in the city of Alexandria by an enigmatic teacher named Ammonius, who like Socrates did not write, but simply discoursed with his students.[8] It was a contemplative wisdom which, to be fully appreciated, had to be imparted by direct experience with a realized master, one such as Ammonius himself.[9]

In Neoplatonism we again find the grand tiered cosmic scheme reminiscent of Vedanta. According to Plotinus, the eternal wellspring of all existence is termed the *One*. It represents a vital and boundless power that 'overflows' in its richness, making possible the multiple levels of being, all but the lowest of which are themselves vital and active.[10] The first of these levels beneath the One is the intellect or spirit, termed *nous*. This is not the intellect as we ordinarily know it, but a level of eternal being in which consciousness is completely at one with its object. This level in turn makes possible a multiplicity of living forms called *souls*. The soul is related at one end to the absolute, and at the other to the sensory world. The human being in its essential nature is a soul, and as such can, in its highest octave, directly experience the absolute One from which it is derived and with which it is still fundamentally identical. Plotinus himself was said to occasionally enter a state of rapture beyond any sense of duality or self-awareness, a state that seems very much like the yogic samadhi. In its lower octave, however, the soul can become involved with the passions and desires of matter, losing itself in them as is humankind's plight.

These three levels — the One, the *nous,* and the soul — are not actually separate, but are mutually enfolded within each other as different aspects of a single reality. According to the Neoplatonic scholar E. Bréhier:

> The One includes everything without any distinction.
> Intelligence [*nous*] contains all beings; but if they are
> distinct therein, they are nonetheless unified, and each of
> them contains all others potentially. In Soul, things tend to
> be distinguished from each other, until at the borderline they
> are dissipated and scattered into the sensible world.

In Plotinus' worldview, the entire cosmos is an organic whole, but one that is hierarchical. Moving from the One down to the material universe is a series of steps through diminishing degrees of reality accompanied by increasing multiplicity. The human soul participates in virtually all of these levels.

Comparing Plotinus' levels of being with those of Vedanta it seems clear that the One corresponds to Vedanta's Self, or perhaps the Self and the causal level as experienced through a state of rapture. Beyond this, Plotinus' level of intellect or *nous* corresponds remarkably well with the sheath of intellect, as both represent a higher form of intuitive knowledge or *gnosis.* It seems that in Plotinus' system, as in Mahayana Buddhism, we have discovered levels of reality that correlate well with those mapped by Vedanta.

Back to Wilber

Ken Wilber begins with the traditional Vedantic tiers of being, or sheaths, and brilliantly blends them together with Gebser's analysis of the history of consciousness to produce a working model for evolution. In honor of Gebser's influence he hyphenates Gebser's term for each stage of the evolution of consciousness to his own term, up through the mental structure. For example, Wilber identifies the first epoch as the *archaic-oroboric* stage. This is followed by a *magic-typhonic,* then a *mythic-membership* stage, and a *mental-egoic* stage.

Other major influences on Wilber's thought include the existential archeology of E. Becker and Norman O. Brown, the mythological studies of Joseph Campbell and others, and the Jungian archetypal analysis of the history of the psyche by Erich Neumann.[11] Wilber utilizes a careful reading of these to enrich his historical interpretation of Gebser's structures of consciousness. Beyond this, he takes advantage of his own rich understanding of the perennial philosophy to project a map of the evolution of consciousness up to the highest forms of human experience.

Wilber's model differs from Gebser's in that it provides a specific impelling force, a particular motivation that pushes the evolutionary process from level to level, striving always for the highest ascent. This is in agreement with Sri Aurobindo's contention that the highest indwelling spirit, ultimately *Brahman,* is what draws evolution forward. Wilber, however, approaches this notion from a psychological point of view. He terms the impelling force the *Atman project,* and develops it in detail in his 1980 book of the same name. The central idea is that the human constantly struggles to escape a sense of isolation, striving toward a state of original unity with the absolute. The *Atman project* is a yearning for a return to wholeness. It derives from the notion that the essence of life itself, the absolute, has become involved in matter and yearns to recover its true nature. Wilber writes:

> Evolution, then, is the remembrance of involution — a rediscovery of the higher modes which were enwrapped in the lower ones during the soul's flight from God.

For Wilber the path of evolution involves, first, an outward arc away from the *prepersonal* consciousness of the archaic state toward the personal consciousness of the egoic mental structure. The arc then bends inward, leading toward the transpersonal levels. The mechanisms by which consciousness transforms itself from epoch to epoch along this arc are complex and will not be dealt with here in detail. His model of growth, however, is richly informed by psychodynamic concepts. In overview, it involves the essential idea that consciousness progresses through a series of identifications, first with the grosser aspects of being, and then in stages moving toward the subtler aspects. This idea is well known to many wisdom traditions such as Neoplatonism and India's Vedanta philosophy, but has rarely been articulated as clearly as by Wilber, and never in a context that includes concepts from Western psychology.

I will summarize Wilber's model in a few lines, then return to explore its stages in greater detail below. According to his view the oroboric stage of consciousness identifies with the natural world in the immediate present. Later, consciousness comes to identify with the physical body and its energies, then with the social community, followed by the ego, and ultimately with the aspects of being that correspond to the most subtle inner sheaths of Vedanta. Before examining this progression in detail below, let us note that evolution as Wilber sees it is mirrored in the development of the human from infancy to adulthood. The situation is that 'ontogeny recapitulates phylogeny.' Wilber's book, *The Atman Project,* tracks the individual developmental sequence in detail, while *Up from Eden* tracks the evolutionary process.

The stages

1. The *archaic-oroboric* epoch. Wilber uses the term *oroboric,* which he appends to Gebser's term, *archaic,* to indicate the image of the serpent that swallows its own tail. During this early, essentially pre-human period of evolution, consciousness was self-consuming or self-absorbed. As we have seen, Gebser likens this mode of consciousness to deep dreamless sleep. Wilber refers to it also as 'cosmocentric,' meaning that it is invested in nature as a whole. He cautions, however, that this condition must not be confused with modern mystical or transpersonal experiences. It is rather a prepersonal infantile-like unity in which awareness of oneself as a separate mind and body system has not yet emerged. It is associated with the mythical paradise of Eden when the anguish of separation and with individual existence and death was not yet known.

During each epoch the Atman project expresses itself differently. In this most primitive period it was expressed simply through the search for food and moment-to-moment survival.

2. The *magical-typhonic* epoch. This epoch is named after the Titan called Typhon, or Typhoeus, the youngest offspring of the Earth Goddess Gaea, and said to have the upper body of a man but the lower body of a serpent. Half man, half animal, this figure represents the mid-point in transformation from the animal or oroboric consciousness into full human consciousness. Wilber suggests that it corresponds historically to the Neanderthal and Cro-Magnon men, extending down historically roughly to the origins of agriculture.

In the typhonic epoch, consciousness identifies primarily with the physical body and its energies. Wilber likens this to Freud's infantile *body-ego,* the first sense of a separate self experienced by the child. During this epoch there is an increased awareness of time, heralding an awakening awareness of the inevitability of personal death.

While much shorter in duration than the oroboric period, this epoch encompasses the major transitions from the earlier animal and protohuman worlds into the rich human consciousness of the mythic epoch to follow. In it the Atman project expresses itself in a variety of forms, but prominently hunting and the practice of magic, both of which meld together in paleolithic societies. Hunting and the laying up of food for the future provides a degree of insurance against death. Magic is a way of gathering power or *mana,* and thus increasing one's sense of security as well as distancing oneself from death.

Wilber observes that a residue from this epoch can surface in modern times as neurotic behavior. As Freud himself pointed out, the psychological defense mechanisms such as projection and repression are nothing short of magical strategies to rid oneself of unwanted impulses.

3. The *mythic-membership* epoch. Wilber's description of this epoch closely follows Gebser's depiction of the mythic structure of consciousness. Wilber, however, explores in detail certain historical aspects of it, including the development of a high degree of proficiency with language and the evolution of a truly transcendent religious mythos.

Wilber concurs with psychologist Julian Jaynes, who believes that the original function of language was to provide a powerful mechanism for personal self-regulation:

> It is only language, I think, that can keep [a man] at his
> time-consuming all-afternoon work [e.g., farming]. A
> middle-Pleistocene [magic-typhonic] man would forget what
> he was doing. But lingual man would have language to
> remind him.

Wilber notes: 'It is, I think, this added linguistic mentality ... that resulted in agriculture.' Thus, according to Jaynes, language provided the mechanism necessary to keep a person on-task during the many long hours of hard work that are so much a part of farming, and indeed a part of virtually all of the professions on which civilizations are built. These require that individuals commit their full time to being soldiers, builders, scribes, artists, and so on.

Language also provided the cognitive machinery necessary for long-range planning, so much a part of the ancient agricultural civilizations in which planting and harvesting had to be accurately coordinated with the changes of the seasons. Perhaps even more important, however, is that language provided the mechanism for the smooth coordination of the diverse social roles that came with the large and complex societies such as Old Europe, and later ancient Mesopotamia, Egypt, the Indus Valley. This was possible because language gave the individual a new sense of identity, one grounded in a profession and role in society, a role based on lingual labelling. Wilber notes that in this process of discovering a language-based identity, an important watershed was crossed for self-identity. The sense of self shifted from the body-ego of the earlier typhonic human to a language-based self defined by one's role in society.

At the same time, newly acquired cognitive abilities led to an intensification of the awareness of human mortality. It became increasingly difficult to ignore or deny one's own eventual death. Wilber speculates that the horror created by such an awareness resulted in a psychological rejection of the finite self, leading to a self-hatred, repressed and projected on to others in the form of the urge to war and destruction. Indeed, organized warfare was practically invented around the third millennium before Christ in Sumerian city states such as Ur, Uruk, Kush, and Lagash. During this period regular and bloody campaigns were waged between the kings of these cities, sometimes involving the wholesale slaughter of entire populations. Thus was the Atman project perverted by the mythic-membership human, attempting to murder those who, like himself, were all too mortal and vulnerable.

Other means to the Atman project also became prominent during the membership epoch. The hording of commodities, and later of money, by the well-to-do became a new means to personal, almost magical power. Becker observed that:

> Gold became the new immortality symbol. In the temple
> buildings, palaces, and monuments of the new cities we see
> a new kind of power being generated. No longer the power
> of the totemic communion, but the power of the testimonial
> of piles of stone and gold.

For the privileged few, wealth became a kind of condensed mana, a hedge against mortality. It is still so today.

Late in the membership period, preparation for the afterlife came to be an obsession. Egypt, especially, devoted a great part of its national resources to life beyond death. In this, the Atman project asserted itself as the denial of death. Here, however, as in the other forms of the Atman project we have so far seen, the effort could only fail, or at best be only partially successful. The best laid preparations for an afterlife do not return anyone to the original oneness that is the source of life any more than does laying up wealth in warehouses or banks, or slaughtering others to eradicate their disgusting vulnerability.

Wilber takes particular care to track the development of the dominant myths through this epoch. He notes the virtually universal worship of the Earth Goddess that was gradually transformed in certain times and places into the worship of a truly transcendent image which he calls the Great Goddess. Later, male deities would be seen in similar light, but the first penetration of religion into the subtle realm, the realm of the *vijnanamaya* sheath of Vedanta, was guided by the image of a goddess.

4. The *mental-egoic* epoch. Wilber's description of this epoch closely matches Gebser's historical rendition of the development of the mental structure of consciousness, but with certain important differences. He does not, as did Gebser, stress the importance of the visual perspectival worldview for this mode of experience. His own approach to the evolution of consciousness, rather, emphasizes the changing objects with which consciousness identifies itself. Thus, he characterizes the self of the egoic epoch as a mental construction, one closely tied to memory. In this mode there arises an almost palpable sense of a self formed of memories, one that existed since one's first childhood memories and which, by dint of the imagination, can be projected out into an indefinite future.

The mental-egoic epoch characterizes the world today, although Wilber and Gebser are both aware that it is simply the dominant mode. Certain groups, pockets as it were in the theater of contemporary world culture, still exhibit a high degree of magical and mythic thinking. We might note, however, that Gebser went to pains to point out that these should not be equated to the inhabitants of the historical epochs that first discovered these structures. Though he viewed native peoples who still engage in magical thinking and rituals as representing evolutionary backwaters, such backwaters evidently occur in the presence of at least some degree of development of the more advanced structures.

This is a view that might well meet with opposition today, with the current emphasis on cultural relativity, and with a growing awareness of the need to understand diverse cultures in their own terms rather, for example, than in terms only of our own objective and analytic *(ratio)* worldview. Perhaps a more neutral statement of the same principle can be drawn from evolutionary biology, where it has long been known that certain species which seem to have changed little over vast periods of evolutionary time — for example ants or turtles — are not in fact the same creatures as were their ancestors. They simply seem to have achieved, early on, an optimal external form, while in terms of internal processes such a metabolism, digestion, and muscle and neural efficiency, they have continued to evolve. The ant on your front porch is not the ant in the block of amber on your desk. Likewise, the modern Australian Aborigine, despite his participation in the magical world of the *dream time,* is not the fellow who painted the animals on the walls of Lascaux, and indeed may turn out to be a very complex character.

Both Gebser and Wilber view the ego as a major cause of the modern human's self-alienation. Gebser stresses that ego-based *ratio* is dramatically removed from the light of the Origin, while Wilber in similar fashion concludes that the tendency of the ego toward self-aggrandizement and emotional detachment causes it to be the most desperately isolated and lonely of all structures of consciousness.

In the mythic structure the sense of self was located in the heart. This was the felt location of the soul, which is the very root of mythic consciousness. This felt quality of the heart is still present, for the older structures do not disappear. The historical displacement of the subjective sense of self away from the heart, however, and to the location of thought and memory in the head was tantamount to creating a psychic disconnection from the wellspring of human meaning. An interesting commentary on this arose in a conversation that once took place between Carl Jung and Chilean writer and diplomat Miguel Serrano, later recorded and published by Serrano himself. Jung observed:

> I once remember having a conversation with the chief of the
> Pueblo Indians, whose name was Ochwiay Biano, which
> means Mountain Lake. He gave me his impressions of the
> white man, and he said that they were always upset, always
> looking for something, and that as a consequence, their
> faces were lined with wrinkles, which he took to be a sign
> of eternal restlessness. Ochwiay Biano also thought that the
> whites were crazy since they maintained that they thought
> with their heads, whereas it was well-known that only crazy
> people did that. This assertion by the chief of the Pueblos
> so surprised me that I asked him how *he* thought. He
> answered that he naturally thought with his heart.

And then Jung added: 'And that is how the ancient Greeks also thought.'

In the tradition of Erich Neumann and others, Wilber emphasizes the connection between the historical emergence of the ego in the first few millennia BC and the rise of the great mythologies of solar and sky-dwelling gods. This occurred near the end of the mythic-membership epoch when the mental-egoic structure of consciousness was just beginning to surface on a wide scale. These patriarchal figures displaced the images of the Great Goddess with their ancient connections to the Earth Goddess, the earth itself, the night, the moon, and the feminine. Examples of such patriarchal deities included the Egyptian sun god, Ra, and Horus the hawk, who vied with Isis for the central place in Egyptian religion. Others included Zeus, 'shower of light,' associated with the eagle, Mount Olympus, and all atmospheric phenomenon, but especially lightning and thunder, and Yahweh, who disclosed himself to Moses on Mount Sinai.

The transition to dominantly patriarchal mythologies seems to have accompanied a comparable transition in human culture to the rule of patriarchal warrior heroes, the appearance of a dramatically hierarchical social order, as well as the promoting of war and conquest as noble and heroic activities.[12]

The ascendence of the male principle did not come without a struggle, as seen for example in the story of the great Mesopotamian god Marduk, 'Sun of the Heavens,' who did battle with and literally dismembered Tiamat, goddess of the sea. In like vein, the ancient Mesopotamian epic of Gilgamesh tells how the hero Gilgamesh spurned the advances of the goddess Ishtar (Inanna), goddess of love and war and representative of the old Earth Goddess. In anger, she arranged to send down the Bull of Heaven to avenge her humiliation, but Gilgamesh and his powerful friend Enkidu made short work of it, ripping out its right thigh and flinging it back at her. Not only this, but they took its horns and hung them up in Gilgamesh's 'room of rulership.' Now the horns of the bull were widely understood to symbolize the Earth Goddess herself, because the bull was her consort. For Gilgamesh to hang them in his own throne room was an act of sacrilege against the old religion of the Earth Goddess and the feminine. Of this act, mythologist William Irwin Thompson comments:

> The old conservative religion of the women is being
> mocked in a celebration of male ambition. The battle
> between the sexes could not be clearer ... Contained in the
> conflict between Ishtar and Gilgamesh is the conflict
> between the institutions of temple and militaristic monarchy,
> the conflict between the civilized remnants of the old
> neolithic religion and the new masculine order of
> civilization.

The important point in all of this, according to Wilber, is that the female principle, embodied in the old paleolithic Earth Goddess, was not only overcome by male patriarchy, but absolutely crushed by it, so that the status of the feminine, both in heaven and on earth, became entirely suppliant to male domination.

Now the feminine principle as an aspect of the human soul and as an aspect of the experience of nature can in reality no more be destroyed than can any other fundamental dimension of consciousness. It can, however, be repressed, and Wilber makes a good case that this is exactly what happened. Not only did worship of the great feminine deities virtually disappear, but the entire feminine principle was forced underground and out of consciousness. In other words, it was repressed. The price that we, a civilization that derives in large part from those ancient cultures of the Middle East, have paid for this crime is enormous. On a personal level we have become less than whole human beings. We elevated the masculine values of dominance and control far above the softer, more caring, feminine values of nurturance and cooperation. Descriptions of the costs of the damage done by this state of affairs, damage in terms of self-alienation, ineffective and broken personal relationships, and power-mongering on all levels, would fill a library of books in philosophy, psychology, and psychiatry. On a planetary scale, the loss of the deep sense of connection with the earth in favor of the strong analytic and manipulative values of *ratio* have given us an ecological situation which, if allowed to proceed on its present path, will soon lead to our extinction as a species.

Wilber notes that this great suppression of the feminine was at least partially avoided in Eastern cultures. In modern Japan, for instance, a respect for the earth and a sense of belonging to it remain even to the present. This goes along with a trust in what is natural and spontaneous in human nature as well. These themes come together in the beautiful Zen gardens found in Japan, which seem both carefully groomed and at the same time a celebration of spontaneity. They can be contrasted with formal European gardens which attempt to exclude the wild, spontaneous, aspect of nature. During the Age of Enlightenment the effort to exclude wild nature reached such heights that bushes were trimmed to resemble human-made objects such as carriages!

Returning briefly to the mental-egoic epoch, let us note that the flexibility of the ego allows it to approach the Atman project in a variety of ways, drawing even on styles rightly appropriate to older evolutionary stages. It can indulge in gluttony, as if harkening back to the oroboric concern for survival through obtaining food. Or it can engage in excessive emotional and sexual gratifications, echoing the magical-typhonic emphasis on the body and its energies. Most basic to the concerns of the ego, however, are self-esteem and self-aggrandizement.

It is the central project of the ego to promote itself. Indeed, with the ego's astounding ability to project images of itself into the future, even beyond death, it is common for the egoic individual to attempt to create self-legacies in the form of empires, estates, family names, works of art, and so on, that will by association imbue a kind of immortality. It was the rise of the ego in the late mythic-membership period that led to such egotistical extravaganzas as the construction of huge stone monuments by kings and pharaohs to remind all eternity of their greatness.

5. The *existential-centaur* stage. This stage can be viewed as a transition between the mental-egoic structure and the psychic structure, described below.

As we go beyond the mental-egoic epoch Wilber departs from Gebser and outlines several evolutionary stages based on his composite study of modern psychology and the major forms of the perennial philosophy. These stages are indicated in Table 2. I will refer to them as stages rather than epochs because it remains to be seen whether they will ever become dominant structures of consciousness for human-

Vedanta (sheaths/koshas)	Wilber (epochs/stages)	Wilber (identity)	Gebser (structures)
(Self, Atman)	(Self, Atman)		Origin/integral*
Anandamaya	Causal	Formless self-realization	
Vijnanamaya	Subtle	Overmind	
	Psychic	Astral-psychic	
Manomaya	Egoic	Mental ego	Mental
	Membership	Verbal Self membership	Mythic
Pranamaya	Typhonic	Body ego	Magic
Annamaya	Oroboric	Nature	Archaic

* This is technically not a structure but the Original awareness which the structures invest.

Table 2. Comparison of the constructs from Vedanta, Ken Wilber, and Jean Gebser.

kind as a whole. Wilber's emphasis at this point shifts to the evolution of the individual and away from historical periods.

The existential-centaur stage is mentioned only in passing in Wilber's *Up From Eden,* where he focuses mainly on the historical and archeological record of humankind. For more detail about this stage one can go to *The Atman Project,* or to Wilber's only informally written book, *No Boundary: Eastern and Western Approaches to Personal Growth.* This stage heralds a softening of the identification of self with the ego and a re-owning of the body and its energies. A larger perspective is taken of the place of the self in the landscape of existence. In psychology the existential-centaur stage is represented by the humanistic-existential thought of Abraham Maslow, Carl Rogers, Eric Fromm and others, as well as in Gestalt and various bioenergetic therapies. It is philosophically represented by existentialism.

Each stage of consciousness carries its own liabilities and risks, and its own potential pathologies. Wilber has made a study of the latter, which he explores in *Transformations of Consciousness: Traditional and Contemplative Perspectives on Development.* In the case of the existential orientation, the dawning realization that the seemingly important agendas of the ego really amount to very little when all is said and done can lead to existential despair. The individual may appear very small and meaningless and all too mortal, resulting in anxiety and a deep sense of self-alienation. There is no easy solution to this dilemma, but as Abraham Maslow once observed, to fully accept one's real situation with no holding back usually leads in the long run to the release of bound-up psychological energies and increased optimism. Interestingly, certain schools of traditional wisdom, such as Zen Buddhism, intentionally force the student relentlessly against the impenetrability of the existential situation, precisely in order to break the stronghold of the ego. This is the meaning of the Zen parable of the flea that bites the iron bull. The insect of the intellect simply cannot penetrate Reality.

6. The *psychic* stage. From this point onward as evolution progresses the subjective self identifies with increasingly more subtle inner structures until all of them are put aside in favor of unconditional

reality. Throughout these stages the Atman project is felt as a desire to approach the absolute.

Wilber observed that in each major evolutionary epoch a small number of individuals achieve a quantal leap to a much later stage. These represent the evolutionary pathfinders, achieving a degree of personal advancement often literally millennia ahead of their time. Thus, the first persons to achieve the psychic stage lived during the domination of the mythic-membership structure of consciousness, probably in the paleolithic age. These were the shamans. Their ability to move into and manipulate the energies of the psychic (subtle energy) realm made them healers and sources of power and wisdom for their stone-age cohorts. These are roles that true shamans play in primary cultures even today. Wilber does not pretend to imply that all sorcerers or witch doctors were, or are, masters of the psychic level of consciousness. To the contrary, he suggests that probably relatively few were. These few, however, set the standard for the rest, and for the tradition of shamanism itself, which, interestingly enough, is practiced today in a very similar way in primary cultures throughout the world.

According to Wilber, the self of the psychic stage identifies with the astral-psychic level, the lowest of the major subtle energy levels that reside behind manifest reality. This level puts one in touch with subtle energies of the body such as prana, that can be manipulated in psychic healing. This level is also said to be associated with various psychic paranormal powers. It is the first of two levels that Wilber identifies with the *vijnanamaya* or subtle sheath of Vedanta. He refers to this level as the lower subtle, as contrasted with the higher subtle which for convenience he simply calls the subtle.

7. The *subtle* stage. At this stage consciousness releases its identification with the body and the ordinary mental self, so that the resulting condition might be termed the 'over-mind' or 'over-self.' This is much like referring to the ego as the 'over-body,' since its source of self-identification is beyond the physical body. Wilber emphasizes that this level of consciousness is the source of much authentic religious inspiration. Dante, for example, described his experience of it as follows:

Fixing my gaze upon the Eternal Light
I saw within its depth,
Bound up with love together in one volume,
The scattered leaves of all the universe ...
Within the luminous profound substance
Of that Exalted Light saw I three circles
Of three colors yet of one dimension
And by the second seemed the first reflected
As rainbow is by rainbow, and the third
Seemed fire that equally from both is breathed.

As seen in this passage, the subtle level of consciousness is associated with an experience of divinity or God as unity. Here consciousness can come into mystical identity with the Divine. The absolute can take the image of the Divine Mother, as it often does in Hinduism, or of the Divine Father, as it does in Christianity. Wilber suggests that this level of consciousness was first experienced by rare individuals of the mythic-membership epoch, 'saints,' who transformed the identity of the Earth Mother into that of the Great Goddess, as was the case with Isis. The Divine Mother represents the nurturing and sustaining aspect of the Divine. The Father image, on the other hand, represents God the creator and ruler, as expressed in many images from the Judaic and Christian traditions.

8. The *causal* stage. Ascending to the causal level there is a shift from an experience of God as the source of all forms, to a transcendence of form itself, combined with an experience of 'Boundless Radiance.' In the words of Lex Hixon:

There is now perfect release into the radiance of
formless Consciousness. There is no ishtadeva
[divinity], no meditator, and no meditation, nor is
there any awareness of an absence of these. There is
only radiance.

Wilber speculates that this level of consciousness was first achieved by advanced individuals of the early mental-egoic epoch, whom he terms 'sages.' These include such spiritual pathfinders as Jesus Christ, the Buddha, Shankara of India, and Lao Tzu.

9. The *ultimate* stage. This final level is the pure Self or Atman, no longer shrouded by even the subtlest of the sheaths. It is the condition in which consciousness awakens entirely to its ...

> original Condition and Suchness (Tathata), which is, at the same time, the condition and suchness of all that is, gross, subtle, or causal. That which witnesses, and that which is witnessed, are only one and the same. The entire World Process then arises, moment to moment, as one's own Being, outside of which, and prior to which, nothing exists ... At that point, the extraordinary and the ordinary, the supernatural and mundane, are precisely one and the same.

This stage is depicted in the final drawing of the famous Zen series of oxherd pictures. These portray the oxherd (seeker) setting out to find the lost ox which represents his Original Nature. After a considerable time he finds it and rides it home, the various stages of his progress depicted in the series of drawings. In the last one he is often shown as an old man with an unassuming smile and a begging bowl. The accompanying poem reads something like: 'He has forgotten the gods, he has even forgotten his enlightenment. Quite simply he goes to the market-place begging, but wherever he goes the cherry trees blossom.'

Involution and evolution

Reading *Up From Eden* one gets the sense that the sequence of evolutionary stages is more or less predictable in the sense that, 'The higher modes ... were enfolded, as potential, in the lower modes to begin with [involution], and they simply crystalize out and differentiate from the lower modes as evolution proceeds.' This view, or something like it, we have seen in Hegel, and we will see it again in

Chapter 7 with Sri Aurobindo. Let us look more closely at what it means.

In Indian thinking, of which Sri Aurobindo will be our principal example, the evolutionary pathway is fairly clear. All the grades of being represented by the material and subtle bodies of Vedanta exist continuously behind the material body, and for the most part behind ordinary consciousness as well. The agenda for evolution is to bring these back into conscious expression. What this means in practical terms is that during the sequence of lives that is the destiny of all living beings, consciousness brings each of these grades of being sequentially into its sphere of operation. This process can be accelerated by certain practices such as yoga. In this philosophy the course of evolution is entirely determined, at least in the spiritual sense.

Returning to Ken Wilber, we find agreement with this view of evolution as a successive realization of the subtle planes of being. Wilber, however, has observed that involution, and thus evolution, can be understood in more than one sense. First, it can mean the descent of the spirit into matter, creating the manifest universe. Evolution, then, becomes the movement of the spirit back toward its origin. This is the exact idea that we have been discussing in terms of the subtle planes of being. A second idea of involution, however, occurs in each lived instant 'as we separate ourselves from the Ground or the Source.'[13] This meaning is essentially phenomenological, pointing to the continuous presence of the Origin in each instant of experience, a presence that paradoxically is also limited within each instant, giving us the illusion of limited existence. It suggests that the release from this limiting process can best come about by a reordering of the structure of experience itself.

The first meaning, above, implies the necessity of a historical evolutionary process that leads consciousness back through ascending levels of being. This is what we have found in Wilber's model and will see again with Sri Aurobindo. The second requires an evolutionary process of quite a different sort, one that operates within the immediacy of the lived moment. In Chapter 11 we will find that these two agendas represent two major types of spiritual tradition. I will call the first the *ontic path,* because it is vested in levels of Being, and the second I will call the *noetic path,* because it is founded on insight or knowledge.

We now leave Ken Wilber, but before doing so I note that his work forms an important bridge between scientific ideas of evolution on the one hand and the traditional knowledge of wisdom traditions on the other. I will have reason to disagree with certain of his conclusions, but let us keep in mind that this work is of inestimable value and as such we will return to it frequently.

7. They Climb Indra like a Ladder

The tiers of being

They climb Indra like a ladder. As one mounts peak after peak, there becomes clear the much that has still to be done. Sri Aurobindo, *Taittiriya Upanishad*

In November of 1859 the British naturalist Charles Robert Darwin published a book titled *On the Origin of Species by Means of Natural Selection.* The entire printing of 1,500 copies sold out within a day. From that moment humankind's conception of itself was irrevocably altered. Aside from its jarring implications for conventional religion, the theory of evolution placed the human in the midst of a stream of biological development that began with the historical origins of life on Earth and continues through the present day and on into the future. In the world scientific community the definition of human nature itself was altered from top to bottom. Not only did the physical body come to be understood as the product of a long history of adaptation and change, but the human's psychological constitution came to be seen as the product of this same evolutionary process. In the United States, for example, the dominant view of psychologists came to be represented by the 'Functionalist School' of the University of Chicago, which regarded the mind and its faculties, such as perception, memory, and rational thought, in terms of biological adaptation and survival.

Darwin's concepts were not entirely new. As indicated in the Foreword to this book, evolutionary trends were already present in early Indian philosophical thought. The term *evolution* was actually coined by the French biologist Jean-Baptiste Lamarck, who in 1809 had published a well-reasoned theory of biological evolution based on the notion that organisms could genetically benefit from the experiences of their ancestors. For a time Lamarck's ideas retained considerable popularity before ultimately being rejected by the scientific community during the early years of the twentieth century.

Darwin's chief contribution was the notion of natural selection. According to this, each new generation of a species exhibits considerable variation. For instance, each generation of giraffes displays a variety of neck lengths. If there is an advantage to having long necks, say, for eating foliage from the topmost branches of trees, then those with the longest necks would be most likely to thrive and reproduce, passing on the tendency for long necks to future generations. Darwin had no concept of genetics as understood today, but he assumed that the mechanism behind variation was thoroughly physical. Thus, in a straightforward fashion he was able to account for the amazing diversity of life and for its adaptation to different environments. This, coupled with a talent for detailed and persuasive writing, was sufficient to convince most scientifically minded persons of the validity of his theory.

The classical Darwinian emphasis on the survival of the fittest, however, was not to be the only legacy born of Darwin's theory of evolution. The widespread recognition of a long and continuous historical development behind all forms of life led many people to entertain similar ideas beyond the realm of biology. One individual who thought deeply about evolution and its meaning for the destiny of humankind was the Indian yogi and sage, Sri Aurobindo Ghose. We will examine Sri Aurobindo's ideas in some detail, as they represent a monumental effort to understand the traditional wisdom of the perennial philosophy from an evolutionary perspective.

The evolutionary pathfinder: Sri Aurobindo Ghose

The extent to which Sri Aurobindo (1872–1950) may have been directly influenced by Darwin's writings is difficult to say, as he was less than generous with biographical information. He once commented to a biographer: 'neither you nor anyone else knows anything at all of my life; it has not been on the surface for men to see.' Despite such disparaging remarks, certain facts are well known and worth mentioning.[1] He spent his entire youth from the age of seven to twenty in England, where he received a thoroughly British education at Cambridge before returning to India in 1892. This was a time when evolutionary ideas were widely and vigorously discussed in England and elsewhere. It is inconceivable that he was not aware of the growing influence of the theory of evolution. Moreover, although in his writings he was sometimes critical of Western science, he treated Darwin surprisingly well when he had occasion to speak of him at all. It is clearly more than coincidence that Sri Aurobindo was the first and greatest philosopher sage of India to bring evolutionary ideas to the core of his thought.

During his student years in England Sri Aurobindo read widely, not only English literature, but French, Latin, and Greek as well. Later he also became a master of Sanskrit. As a student he developed a vital interest in the liberation of India from British rule. He committed himself to the Indian student movement at Cambridge, and after returning to India became involved in numerous activities dedicated to this cause. His most important contribution to the Indian independence movement was a very active journalistic career dedicated to the revolution. On May 4, 1908, however, he was arrested by the British police and placed in jail. An attempt upon the life of a British official had involved a bomb that had been traced to the activities of Sri Aurobindo's younger brother, Barin.

Sri Aurobindo's interest in spiritual matters had, in fact, begun much earlier. Immediately upon his arrival in India in 1892, at Apollo Bunder in Bombay, he was overtaken by a spontaneous and profound experience of silence that lasted for several months. At that time he was twenty years old. His arrest occurred in his thirty-sixth year, and during the years between he became increasingly interested in discovering a yogic practice suitable to his busy life of journalism and political activism. After his arrest he was to spend a year in prison, much of it in solitary confinement, before he was acquitted. During that year he devoted most of his time to the study of the *Bhagavad-Gita* and to meditation. His sense of purpose changed dramatically. Yoga had previously been a means for acquiring energy and divine guidance for his work in the world. Now he became absorbed completely in the inner purpose of finding a spiritual pathway for all of humankind, an evolutionary passage.

Sri Aurobindo did not give up his political activities immediately. In April of 1910, however, when he got word that he would again be arrested — this time on a charge of subversion — he felt an inner prompting to leave British India entirely. In ten minutes he was on his way to Pondicherry in French southern India where he would be safe from arrest. There he settled down and devoted the rest of his life to evolutionary yoga.

Sri Aurobindo's use of the term *evolution* is, in fact, different than its use in biological circles, but much more along the lines of Hegel and Wilber's usage. The word 'evolve' (from the Latin *evolvere)* means literally to roll out, or to unroll, and carries the implication of something that has previously been rolled up and hidden from view. The thing that has been rolled up, according to Sri Aurobindo, is the Self, the divine spark.

> Before there could be any evolution, there must be an involution of the Divine. Otherwise there would be not an evolution but a successive creation of things new, not contained in their antecedents, not their inevitable consequences or processes in a sequence, but arbitrarily willed or miraculously conceived by an inexplicable Chance, a stumbling fortunate Force, or an external Creator.

Here, Sri Aurobindo seems to be speaking directly to Darwinian notions of evolution as well as to Western religion. His reference to 'a successive creation of things new' is surely an allusion to the scientific view of evolution, while the reference to an 'external Creator' seems an apt description of the traditional Hebraic and Christian concept of a God beyond nature, one who created the cosmos like an artist creates a painting or a sculpture. The central idea in the above quotation, however, is that of 'involution'; that from the very beginning the highest order of the cosmos, the divine spark, is rolled up and hidden in the stuff of matter itself and is latent in all life.

According to Sri Aurobindo it is the task and goal of evolution to unroll this dormant potential in matter and organic life. Quite simply, 'Evolution is nothing but the progressive unfolding of Spirit out of the density of material consciousness and the gradual self-revelation of God out of this apparent animal being.' This process, unlike Darwinian evolution, is not driven by laws of chance, but is dynamically propelled by the indwelling spirit striving for self-expression, and ultimately yearning to rediscover itself in its own creation. According to Sri Aurobindo: 'All evolution is the progressive self-revelation of the One to himself.' This is very suggestive of Hegel's notion of the forward striving of the indwelling spirit — so much so, in fact, that one cannot help but wonder the extent to which Sri Aurobindo may have been influenced by Hegel's thoughts, already written down for nearly a century when the young Aurobindo moved to England for his education. If there was such an influence, however, it is not mentioned in his major writings. The index to Sri Aurobindo's eleven-hundred page work on evolution, *The Life Divine,* lists no entry under Hegel, though Darwin is mentioned more than once with favorable comments despite his decidedly materialistic approach to evolution.

Sri Aurobindo departs from Hegel, however, in at least one important respect. While for Hegel the spirit becomes infinite only through its struggle to overcome the finite, for Sri Aurobindo the spirit is already complete from the beginning. The aim of evolution is not so much to create a state of perfection, *but to recover it.* Moreover, that portion of the Divine which became involved in matter encompasses only a part of the whole. There is a higher part — *Brahman* in Indian terms, like the One for Plotinus — that was not ensnared in the first place. It is the intervention of this latter part, its pull on the material universe, that calls evolution forward. Without it the material universe would remain inert. It is also this latter aspect of the Divine that the yogin calls upon in his practice, its shakti and its grace, which draws forward the development of the yogin in a personal evolution that recapitulates the future evolution of the entire human species.

These ideas are very familiar in Ken Wilber's work as well. Like Sri Aurobindo, Wilber also sees evolution as the unfolding of a previously enfolded inner spirit. And also like Sri Aurobindo, he sees individual spiritual growth as reflecting the future spiritual evolution of the human species, which he sees as still far from complete.

Sri Aurobindo, likewise, believed that humankind as we know it is not the final product of evolution, but rather only an intermediate step to a higher form. 'We are in respect to our possible higher evolution much in the position of the original Ape of the Darwinian theory.' Moreover, continues Sri Aurobindo, if that ape were somehow to learn of its future destiny as human, its limited capacities could imagine but the faintest and most limited idea of the fullness of human experience. So it is with us, who without resort to divine intuition, can only project our present experience, writ large, into an unknown future.

For Sri Aurobindo evolution assumes two separate forms. One is the outward visible process that corresponds to Darwinian evolution. The other is an invisible inner development that asserts itself over a sequence of rebirths. Coupled to this latter process is a larger movement that represents the cutting edge of the evolutionary pathway, a cutting edge that is defined by the progress of a very few persons. Indeed, one or two persons can open the way to the next stage of development for the entire species. This was precisely Sri Aurobindo's own self-assigned task during the latter years of his life; to lay a groundwork for the forward movement of humanity to the next stage of its evolutionary ascent. This labor was shared by his companion Mirra Alfassa, known best as the *Mother.*

The idea that a few individuals, or even a single person, can break evolutionary ground for the entire human species seems, at first glance, to be unwarranted. Evolutionary progress in the realm of physical morphology is encoded in the genes and is passed on only to an organism's immediate descendants. How then could it be possible for Sri Aurobindo and the Mother, sitting in their ashram in south India, to open an evolutionary gateway for the rest of humankind? To my knowledge Sri Aurobindo never directly answered this question. The answer, however, may in part have to do with the idea, above, that the direction of the evolutionary ascent is already contained in matter itself. From this point of view, Sri Aurobindo and the Mother were simply vehicles, and as such were, in a sense, test cases for the entire species.

Sri Aurobindo and the Mother, however, spoke of their work in stronger terms than one would expect if they considered themselves as merely models that others would follow. They spoke as if they were literally struggling to bring new levels of being into the reach of human experience. Such ideas were not in empathy with the mechanistic worldview that dominated science during the early years of this century, when Sri Aurobindo was writing his major works on evolution. Today, however, they seem a bit less strange. Quantum physics, for example, has shown that separate events can be interconnected in ways that go far beyond the limitations of Newtonian dynamics.

Recently, for example, two Western scientific theorists, Rupert Sheldrake, a molecular chemist and historian of science, and the already familiar Ervin Laszlo, a systems philosopher and the architect of the grand evolutionary synthesis, have advanced carefully considered hypotheses which support the idea that a few persons, or even a single individual, could conceivably alter the entire future of the human potential.[2] These hypotheses are of such enormous potential importance to the whole topic of evolution, especially where it touches issues of consciousness, that I will spend a little time describing them here, and return to them again in Chapter 8.

Rupert Sheldrake's *hypothesis of formative causation* was originally intended to explain certain unaccountable facts concerning biological shapes, or forms, and their embryonic development. The essential idea is that when a new form first comes into existence — for example a new snowflake, flower, or animal — a patterning field is created which Sheldrake calls a *morphic field.* This field tends to promote future recurrences of that form. Moreover, each time, say, the snowflake recurs, the field is strengthened. Thus nature forms habits, and there is a tendency for morphology to become stable with repetition. These morphic fields are not contained within the usual Newtonian restrictions of time and space. Once created, they can exert influence at distant points in space as well as later in time. All this is not to deny the importance of the genetics, but Sheldrake views the physical genes as not the primary factor in defining morphology, but as a kind of antenna that tunes into the morphic fields.

Such fields do not only influence morphology. There is a particular type of field, which Sheldrake terms a *motor field,* that organizes activity in the nervous system. It represents a subtle patterning force that causes brain states, once experienced, to be more likely to recur in the future. Such fields are equivalent to gentle attractors that nudge the overall activity of the nervous system in one direction or another. Sheldrake observes that these fields may be the basis for memory.[3] The implication, however, is broader than this, suggesting that it is possible for a particular motor field, embodying a particular memory, to be accessed to some extent by others, even at a distance in space or at a later time. In his three books, *A New Science of Life, The Presence of the Past,* and *The Rebirth of Nature,* Sheldrake makes a forceful case for such effects based on research with both animals and humans.

Ervin Laszlo's *psi-field* hypothesis has much in common with Sheldrake's hypothesis of formative causation. While Sheldrake's primary interest, however, has been in establishing the reality of morphic fields, and exploring their effects, Laszlo developed an entire theory of the physics behind such fields. The term, *psi-field,* for instance, refers partly to Schrödinger's probability wave function. More on this aspect of the theory in Chapter 8.

Whether we choose the term morphic or psi-fields, the implications go well beyond what has been considered so far. For example, if such fields exist then each of us carries a certain moral responsibility with regard to just what conditions we entertain in our own inner lives. In other words, what we become may influence others. This also means that great individual achievements are not lost irrevocably, but in some degree remain accessible to humanity as a whole. Laszlo observes of such a possibility, 'It lends substance to the notion that an exceptional person makes a remarkable contribution to humanity, and indeed to all creation.'

In words that could have been written about Sri Aurobindo himself, Laszlo continues:

> Personal growth and development are more than the self-centered striving of an individual toward subjective goals; human goals can have 'objective' dimension, and their achievement can signify a value transcending all selfish and egotistic purposes ... The [psi-field] hypothesis suggests that a fully developed person makes a more significant contribution to the field that conserves the traces of all that is felt and thought than an immature or underdeveloped individual.

The latter conclusion is based on the curious but reasonable idea that a fully developed person manifests a greater range and clarity of inner experience than one who is less developed. Along these same lines but on a grand scale, Sri Aurobindo's notion that individual achievement

can foreshadow the advancement of humankind seems consistent with
this thinking, in fact anticipating it by three-quarters of a century.

Standing back for a moment from Sri Aurobindo's vision, we see
in overview that it is a monumental effort to reconcile the idea of evolution with traditional Indian thought, especially Vedantic philosophy
with its subtle vehicles or 'bodies.' As we saw in the previous chapter,
these also played an important role in Ken Wilber's thinking. In Sri
Aurobindo's words:

> In my explanation of the universe I have put forward this
> cardinal fact of a spiritual evolution as the meaning of our
> existence here. It is a series of ascents from the physical
> being and consciousness to the vital, the being dominated
> by the life-self, thence to the mental being realized in the
> fully developed man and thence into the perfect conscious-
> ness which is beyond the mental.

Here, the vital corresponds to the pranic or energy sheath, the mental
to the mental sheath, and perfect consciousness alludes to higher
sheaths and the Atman itself.

The Integral and Supramental Yogas

For Sri Aurobindo the vehicle for individual development was the practice of yoga. First comes the *Integral Yoga,* also referred to as *Purna*
Yoga, which strives not to release the spirit from matter toward some
higher transcendence, but to integrate and spiritualize the entire mind-
body system on all levels. Then, for those rare individuals who have
made substantial progress in the above work, comes the *Supramental
Yoga,* which strives to bring down into human experience the transcendent energies and supreme knowledge *(gnosis)* that are rooted above
in that aspect of the Divine which was never shrouded in matter.

The basic method of Integral Yoga is simple to describe but most
difficult to follow. It can, and indeed should, be practiced continuously, not only during special periods such as sitting or walking meditations, but also while one goes about one's ordinary daily routines.

Sri Aurobindo, in fact, is best known among the sages of modern India for carrying yoga into an active life in the world. In his method,

> It is necessary to lay stress on three things: (1) an entire quietness and calm of the mind and the whole being, (2) a continuance of the movement of purification ... (3) the maintenance in all conditions and through all experiences of the adoration and bhakti for the Mother [the feminine expression of the Divine].

This practice amounts to a living meditation that can be carried out only by developing an alert and steady habit of calm self-observation. In time it unfolds into consciousness a widening inner landscape, expanding to disclose a number of layers of being.

The hierarchy of minds

As the yogic work progresses, an entire hierarchy of inner levels unfolds. These correspond roughly to the sheaths of the perennial philosophy. In Sri Aurobindo's writing they are referred to as *minds,* each depicting a more or less distinct level of consciousness experience and, more importantly, a distinct way of reaching for truth. In approaching these matters it is useful to realize that for Sri Aurobindo mind is no more than an information manager that receives knowledge and gives it form. Therefore, a superior mind is not one that is a better thought machine, but rather it is a better receiver, one that adds minimal distortion to the signal. This is quite a different notion than that taken by Western psychology, always in search of a more efficient cognitive engine.

The progression of minds described by Sri Aurobindo is listed in Table 3. These represent an entirely different psychology than we are used to seeing in the West, one discovered during years of profound meditative introspection rather than through external, 'objective,' observation, as is the accepted way of Western psychology. For these reasons, and because Sri Aurobindo is recognized as one of the foremost visionaries of twentieth-century India, and also because they are

Sri Aurobindo's levels	Vedanta
7. supramental (supermind)	Self/Atman
6. overmind	causal
5. intuitive mind	subtle/intuitive
4. illumined mind	(transitional)
3. higher mind	mental
2. life-mind (vital mind)	pranic
1. sense-mind (physical mind)	physical

Table 3. Sri Aurobindo's hierarchy of minds and the Vedantic levels.

fascinating, I will take the time to describe them in a little detail. I will describe them in Sri Aurobindo's original terms.

1. The *sense-mind* or *physical mind.* For Sri Aurobindo this most basic level of mind is rooted entirely in the material operations of the brain. It is the day-to-day intellect of the average person as he or she goes about meeting the demands of physical reality. Sri Aurobindo calls it the 'instrument of understanding and ordered action on physical things.'

This mind can become quite highly developed in its own way, as in Piaget's adult or *formal operations* level of intellectual development. Its primary limitation, however, is that it has no access to illumination from higher levels of being. Such illumination comes ultimately from the overmind and above. At best it builds logical structures in a careful step-by-step fashion. In doing so, it takes its models from the physical world of objects. This is especially apparent in the logic structures, or schemata, developed during Piaget's *concrete operations* period, the final stage of transition into *formal operations* or adult intelligence. The cultivation of concepts dealing, for instance, with the understanding of the conservation of volume and number is nothing short of an interiorization into thought itself of relationships that characterize the physical world of objects.

2. The *vital mind* or *life-mind*. The first of the more subtle levels of mind is identified with the energy of the pranic sheath. Not surprisingly, it is associated with vitality and emotion. While the physical mind is bound entirely to the material brain, the vital-mind derives from *prana,* the subtle source of all energy in many esoteric traditions. At its lowest level this is the emotional mind, melodramatic, unruly, and constantly goading us toward a hundred sources of satisfaction. In its highest form, however, it is a source of compassion and love.

3. The *higher mind.* This level represents the first of several of what Sri Aurobindo refers to as truly mental planes of being. It is associated with the mental sheath of Vedanta. It is also, however, a transitional mind in the sense that it is the lowest to respond to the illumination of knowledge from the higher levels of being. Indeed, this is its defining feature. Unlike the physical mind, which gropes in ignorance, it receives knowledge directly, though in bits and pieces. This level of mind is experienced by many creative individuals. An example of its operation is evidenced in the description by the great French mathematician Henri Poincaré of how ideas occurred to him while seeking the solution to a problem in mathematics. He states:

> Never in the field of his [the mathematician's] consciousness do ideas appear that are not really useful, except some that he rejects but which have to some extent the characteristics of useful combinations. All goes on as if the inventor were an examiner of the second degree who would only have to question the candidates who had passed a previous examination.

He goes on to give a more detailed example:

> One evening, contrary to my custom, I drank black coffee and could not sleep. Ideas rose in crowds; I felt them collide until pairs interlocked, so to speak, making a stable combination. By the next morning I had established the existence of a class of Fuchsian functions, those which come from the hypergeometric series; I had only to write out the results, which took but a few hours.

The higher mind seems capable of a greater degree of detachment from the thought process itself than is the physical mind. This allows it a broad overview of the mental process, seeing, for example, multiple causes of a single event. Such abilities appear to represent a step beyond formal operations. They are consistent with what Herb Koplowitz terms general systems thinking, in which multiple causes are the rule.[4] In this mode of thought one understands circular causation as it is seen, for instance, in situations involving feedback loops. Koplowitz rightly considers this thinking ability to be a step in intellectual development beyond the linear and mechanistic limitations of the formal operations mind.

4. The *illumined mind.* This mind is transitional between the higher mind and the intuitive mind. It is 'simply higher mind raised to a great luminosity and more open to modified forms of intuition and inspiration.'

5. The *intuitive mind.* This seems most clearly associated with the subtle sheath, sometimes termed the sheath of intellect. It represents a distinct further step toward the reception of truth or *gnosis* from the higher planes. It grasps truth directly, but in much larger chunks than does the higher mind. It does not depend on a step-by-step progression of ideas, but proceeds by strides or leaps, 'like a man who springs from one sure spot to another point of sure footing.'

This mind is characteristic of certain extraordinarily creative individuals. In it, ideas and insights emerge full-blown, ready to be put to use. Thomas Edison evidently had such a mind. His wife once commented: 'he believes that his inventions come through him from the infinite forces of the universe — and never so well as when he is relaxed.' Another such person was George Washington Carver, who discovered a remarkable number of uses for peanuts and their chemical derivatives, as well as evidencing a remarkable degree of creativity in other aspects of his life. He was, for example, a self-taught painter and pianist. At an exhibition of paintings done with brushes and pigments that he had made himself, he was asked what methods he used when confronted with a problem. He replied: 'I never grope for methods. The method is revealed the moment I am inspired to create something new.'

Since the intuitive mind derives its illumination from above, those who experience it typically have some sense of the higher levels of being. Edison, though considered to be an atheist, believed the well-spring of his intuition to be the 'infinite forces of the universe.' Carver was a deeply religious man and, as we will see below, was actually well in touch with the overmind.

6. The *overmind*. This very subtle level seems most clearly associated with the causal sheath of Vedanta. It is the transition point between the human and divine reality. All levels of mind down through the higher mind are progressively limited expressions of it, receiving knowledge from this level. It acts as a lens for the illuminating knowledge of the Divine above, transmitting to the lower minds.

The overmind is a purely transpersonal level of experience. In it, aspects of higher truth may be experienced in mythic visions. For example, 'The beings native to the Overmind are gods.' And, 'While in the overmind ... they appear as independent beings.' Carver lived much of his life at this level, as evidently have many saints. For Carver, the manifestation of the overmind occurred effortlessly along with the intuitive mind:

> I live in the woods. I gather specimens and listen to what
> God has to say to me. After my morning's talk with God I
> go into my laboratory and begin to carry out his wishes for
> the day.

And: 'When I touch that flower, I am not merely touching that flower. I am touching infinity.' In Integral Yoga, the goal is to develop this level of mind simultaneously with all others. Carver seems to have achieved just this.

Koplowitz describes a mode of cognition he terms *unitary thought* that seems to correspond to this level of mind. It is one in which space and time are experienced as artificial constructs. At this level problems as they are ordinarily experienced are seen to be illusions and self created. Koplowitz considers this to be a step beyond general systems thinking. He observes:

> When the thought in spiritual traditions is considered
> characteristic of unitary thought, those traditions become
> less mysterious, more understandable, and less in conflict
> with scientific thought. Mysticism, a discipline of unitary
> thought, becomes not a rejection of science ... but rather a
> transcendence of it.

The overmind would seem to be capable of what William Irwin Thompson calls *hieroglyphic thought* which, in the spirit of Vico, is said to be mythic and archetypal. It is expressed, for example, in the music of Bach, in the architecture of the cathedral of Chartres, and in the equations of Pythagoras ('The All is number'):

> The archetypes of melody, figure, equation, and mythic
> image are like seed crystals from the causal plane; as they
> are dropped into time, they take time to exfoliate all their
> compressed possibilities.

Despite the grandeur of the overmind, it also has a limitation. Even it is founded to some degree on the physical, and exhibits a characteristic flaw: the tendency to divide the universe into parts, however large. The overmind,

> Keeps from us the full indivisible supramental Light ...
> divides, distributes, breaks it up into separated aspects,
> powers, multiplicities of all kinds, each of which it is
> possible by a further diminution of consciousness, such as
> we reach in Mind, to regard as the sole or the chief Truth
> and all the rest as subordinate or contradictory to it.

This sense of fragmentation is escaped only in the supramental.

7. The *supramental (supermind)*. Here we achieve a dramatic shift in the ground of the being. While all the lower minds rest to some extent on the support of the physical, the supramental, like the fabulous inverted tree of alchemical mythology, has its roots not in the earth but above in the Divine. It is supported by luminous energies that

have never invested themselves in matter. The supramental is synonymous with the highest form of truth or *gnosis,* untainted by lower forms of knowledge. At the supramental level the gods return 'into the One and stand there united in a single harmonious action as multiple personalities of the One.'

Of this level, Sri Aurobindo comments:

> If supermind were to start here from the beginning as the
> direct creative Power, a world of the kind we see now
> would be impossible; it would have been full of the divine
> Light from the beginning, there would be no evolution in
> the inconscience of Matter, consequently no gradual striving
> evolution of consciousness in Matter.

The supramental seems to correspond to the highest level of being in Vedanta, the Self or Atman. This, however, may be an oversimplification, since the Self is said never to invest itself in matter. Perhaps the supramental is best understood as the highest form of consciousness attainable to a corporeal being.

The path of development

A unique feature of Integral Yoga is that while, by Sri Aurobindo's own account, evolution builds from the lower or denser levels of being toward the higher and more subtle ones, the course of personal transformation in his yoga is in almost the reverse order. This is because the subtle transformative energy that is drawn upon is divine shakti, associated with the levels of being above the material mind. Sri Aurobindo referred to it as the *Force.* As the yogic practice continues, it descends, both figuratively and literally, animating first the higher cakras[5] associated with the subtle mental levels, then descends through the middle of the body activating the cakras associated with the vital life force. It continues down to the levels most strongly associated with the physical body. It is common, in this process, for students to first experience a quickening of the mental abilities, and only later the awakening of compassion associated with the heart cakra. Most difficult of all is to transform the lowest cakras associated with power, sexuality, and survival.

This progression is the reverse of what is seen in those types of yoga that strive to awaken the dormant kundalini energy at the root of the spinal cord and to guide it upward, quickening the cakras from the base up. There is a disadvantage to the ladder, however, because the ascending energy activates the primitive sexual and competitive impulses before the tempering effects of compassion and *gnosis* are awakened and firmly established from the higher cakras. It is a problem that Integral Yoga avoids.

The idea in Sri Aurobindo's work is the now familiar notion that individual development anticipates the evolutionary future of the entire human species. At first this may seem contradicted by the fact that progress in this yoga proceeds from the higher, more refined energy centers, to the lower, seemingly more primitive ones, rather than in the opposite direction. It is, however, the role of the divine shakti, or the kundalini as is the case in more traditional forms of yoga, to purify and 'quicken' the cakras, not to create them out of the blue. They already exist in each of us. If this were not so, only saints and yogis would experience compassion, insight, unitive mystical states, and other expressions of the higher cakras.

Sri Aurobindo and the Mother considered the practice of the Supramental Yoga to be their most important contribution to evolving humankind. They saw themselves as evolutionary pathfinders, opening this way for others to follow, making available, by their own effort, the supernal transformative energies of the highest realms of the Divine available to human beings.

Here we leave Sri Aurobindo for the time being. We will return to his evolutionary thought often, however, as we continue to explore the connection between evolution and consciousness.

PART THREE

Emergence

8. Right in Front of our Eyes

The perennial philosophy

*On a visit to Leningrad some years ago I consulted a map
to find out where I was, but I could not make it out. From
where I stood, I could see several enormous churches, yet
there was no trace of them on my map ... It then occurred
to me that this was not the first time I had been given a
map which failed to show many things I could see right in
front of my eyes.*

E.F. Schumacher

Most works on the nature of consciousness are written from one of
two attitudes. The first treats consciousness from the conventional
point of view of science or philosophy and is interested in its ordinary
manifestations such as waking thought and perhaps the nature of
dreams. Many recent works of this type are to be found on the shelves
of local bookstores. Alternatively, there is a tradition of works on the
nature of consciousness that flows in a steady stream from antiquity
and concerns itself with non-ordinary states of experience. These
range from mystical and meditative states of consciousness to shamanic and healing trances and on to myriad unusual states such as out
of the body experiences, trance channeling, simultaneous multiple
states of consciousness, remote viewing, and other forms of extra-
sensory experience. The latter include the great writings of the mystical and esoteric wisdom traditions from throughout the world.

The first class of writers, above, typically ignore the second, if they
do not deny their validity outright. There is good reason for this, because if there is any validity whatsoever to what the latter have to say
then these scientific and philosophical leaders in the field of consciousness research need to think about throwing out some of their
most valued work and starting over on a considerably larger canvas.
On the other hand the latter writers, especially the mystical and

esoteric ones, are often aware of current scientific and philosophical views, but tend to operate in a different frame of reference, one steeped in traditional wisdom, and often grounded in direct experience.

The first class of writers above may or may not find the topics of the second class to be of interest to them personally, but as a group they find it convenient to leave these topics off their official maps of reality. This is not because they are small-minded, but because disciplined enquiry tends to value consistency over richness. A scientific theory is not a statement of final truth, as for example a religious testimony might claim to be, but is intended to gather within its purview the most extensive set of consistent and observable facts that it can stretch itself to reach. What lies beyond that reach is left off the map. Unfortunately, many scientists eventually come to confuse this map, which they had a hand in drawing, for reality itself. These are the ones who are most likely to deny the reality of what they do not understand.

I am reminded of an event some years back at the University of Georgia, involving a friend who was also a mathematical topologist. The topologist parked his car one morning in a muddy lot near his office, only to return later to find a citation for parking on the grass stuck under the windshield wiper. The topologist took this citation to the chief of police to protest, but the chief immediately showed him to a map of the campus and pointed out the bright green area where his car was parked. 'Yes,' said the topologist, 'I see what you mean, ... But you know,' he said as he leaned over the map to get a closer look, 'I don't see my car there!'

Like the churches in the Schumacher quotation above, one would like this car to be on the map, and one would also like the map to show the territory accurately. In our case the territory is not, however, geographical but the vast space of human experience in all of its manifold forms.[1] In plain English, we would like to sketch a picture of the nature of consciousness on a canvas large enough to incorporate its fabulous possibilities while honoring the best thinking of science and contemporary philosophy. This will have us walking the razor's edge between science and mystery, but it is a path well worth treading. In our era, for the first time since that of the ancients, there is enough of a convergence between science and traditional wisdom to open an honorable dialogue.

The many-tiered cosmos

One of the items which we would like to retain on our maps is the many-tiered structure of the cosmos represented in the various forms of the perennial philosophy. As previously noted, there are many variations on the basic motif. The problem we are confronted with, however, is that of honoring a multilayered structure without abandoning the context of evolutionary reality. In terms of the perennial philosophy this means that we do not reject the inner structure of the human being in favor of a thoroughgoing material evolution.

One solution to this problem is to conclude that only human beings have an inner architecture, while other species have no such structure at all. This quickly gets us into hot water. If this were the case, we would be forced to conclude that this inner structure came into existence only during the evolutionary history of our own species. Then we must ask questions such as, did it come about during the reign of the great vegetarian ape, *Australopithecus,* who vanished a million years ago and was probably one of our earliest ancestors? But this species had a brain capacity of only half that of the modern human, and virtually no technology. Perhaps we should move on and look to the first significant tool makers, *Homo habilis,* who date from roughly four to one-and-a-half million years ago. Still, its brain capacity was only slightly larger than that of *Australopithecus,* and its lifestyle was probably closer to that of a modern great ape than of modern human beings. What about the first true members of our own species, *Homo sapiens neanderthalensis,* the Neanderthal? Here we find a highly developed tool technology coupled with what appears without question to be a human culture, though one lacking the abundant imagination and ingenuity that would characterize the modern humans to follow. Or must we wait for the final stage of the biological evolutionary ascent, *Homo sapiens sapiens,* before crediting an inner structure? Such questions are impossible to answer and seem frankly foolish. Moreover, such an approach fails to honor our own experience with other species, many of which, though they cannot talk, communicate a most palpable impression of a very real inner life of their own.

A more radical form of the above notion, and one that seems to me even less acceptable, is the idea that only the human, of all species, is conscious at all. I object to this in spite of three centuries of cold-blooded materialistic science that has often supported such a view. It was René Descartes who in the mid-seventeenth century 'proved' by logic that only the human is a repository of a divine soul, thus reducing all other life forms to the status of organic machines. He was said to have stood looking at animals in rapt amazement, reminding himself that they were merely machines, biological mechanisms for which pleasure, pain, and suffering held no meaning. He might well have been amazed, for no one can honestly look into the eyes of a chimpanzee or a dolphin, or even a dog or a cat, and believe that there is nothing before him but a machine, that he is not, in Martin Buber's terms, engaged in an I-thou relationship. Only by the most intrusive imposition of the intellect (Gebser's *ratio*), an imposition which Descartes worked hard to achieve, could one believe such a thing. For ordinary persons it takes years of intensive training to achieve such a degree of callousness.

On the night of November 10, 1619, the very night before Descartes achieved his final formulation, he dreamed that he was walking in a strong wind that forced him vigorously over to his left, as if to crush the left side of his body. Others in the dream were strangely unaffected.[2] Later the same night he dreamed that some of the words were missing from his dictionary. Given the almost universal association of the left side of the body with intuition, creativity, mystery, and the feminine, it is as if these dreams foreshadowed the destruction of such qualities and the words to describe them. Only the right side of the body, associated with logic, analysis, and the masculine, survived to dominate. The inability of this side to empathetically interact and respond to the wild world of nature, a world beyond the boundaries of *ratio,* is part and parcel with an inability to see the light of consciousness in the eyes of animals. Indeed, it was even to become possible to view other human beings without seeing this light, as was the case with slave holders in pre-Civil War America. For many of them the black person, like Descartes' animals, was only an organic machine.

Returning, however, to the question at hand, it would seem that the only completely sensible recourse open to us at this point is to assume, as did Teilhard de Chardin, that the inner structure of being advances in richness and complexity as the outer organic support evolves to new levels of complexity, leading from the microbe (or perhaps even preorganic physical organizations such as molecules, atoms, or even elemental particles) up through organisms with nervous systems and on to larger-brained creatures such as humans and perhaps certain dolphins and whales. It seems hard to deny this trajectory, either on the basis of common sense and intuition, or on the basis of empathetic observations of animals.

If an outer evolutionary advance in complexity is paced by an inner advance in richness of structure and experience, then our next question must concern the nature of that inner advance. Here we come to an enigma. If we assume an evolution on the inner levels of being, are we not discussing them in patently materialistic terms? Certainly the ordinary mechanisms of biological selection, based as they are upon reproductive efficiency, may be inappropriate for such a discussion. More sophisticated concepts such as that of genetic drift, according to which slow evolutionary changes occur, not so much by the 'survival of the fittest,' but by gradual accommodation of the species to the environment, likewise seem inadequate.[3] In any event, is not the inner structure of the human tied to the outer structure so that it makes little sense to discuss its evolution as if it were broken off and separate?

On the other hand, is the inner structure so locked in place by the anatomy of the nervous system that the inner life has no latitude of its own for evolution (or even personal growth)? If we accept such a conclusion then we have gained little from the wisdom traditions, as we are back to something very close to mechanistic materialism. In particular, we seem to arrive at some form of epiphenomenalism in which the inner being amounts to no more than a by-product of the material brain and has no power or significance of its own. Not only is this repugnant, but contrary to the experience of accomplished practitioners of virtually all wisdom traditions. Such persons tell us that there is considerable freedom for growth and development on the inner levels of consciousness. Moreover, there is a universal observation among mystical traditions from Vedanta through Neoplatonism that the subtle inner realms are in fact *more* real than are the gross outer ones.

Here we seem at a dead end. If we allow that the inner subtle architecture of the human is the product of an evolutionary history, then either it is tied to the outer material evolution or it is not. If it is, we must deny the reports of the mystics and practitioners of wisdom traditions who tell us that true inner transformation is indeed possible. These are the same individuals who described such an inner architecture in the first place. If their reports are unreliable then this whole discussion is on a wrong footing. The notion, on the other hand, of an inner evolution independent of the outer material one, especially at the species level, makes little sense either. Such an evolution, for example, could drift off in directions entirely of its own. Between these two options we seem to be at an impasse.

One possible solution to this problem is to suppose the existence of a 'soft' connection between the various levels of being, one that allows a degree of movement in the form of personal growth and perhaps even species evolution. One would suppose, though, there are limits, however broad, to such flexibility, so that at a minimum the outer form sets constraints on inner possibilities.

This suggestion seems even more sensible if we construe the traditional levels of being in process terms. In particular, let us consider them in the framework of complex systems. My own inclination, as indicated in the first few chapters, is to view consciousness itself as a system near the edge of chaos, and states of consciousness as chaotic attractors by which the various aspects of the mind-body system, and especially the brain, are drawn into patterns of activity, or basins. From this point of view the inner sheaths of Vedanta (Table 1), for example, can be thought of as states of consciousness. This makes sense in the case of the pranic sheath *(pranamaya kosha),* the intellect *(vijnanamaya kosha),* and the sheath of bliss *(anandamaya kosha),* which have been described by contemplatives such as Sri Aurobindo. Indeed, the entire notion of a tiered inner structure of being, practically universal in wisdom traditions throughout the world, is in virtually every case said to arise from experiential accounts of contemplatives. The mental sheath *(manomaya kosha),* on the other hand, refers to the ordinary mind in which most of us live most of the time. This mind is the primary object of Ben Goertzel's cognitive equation, described in Chapter 3.[4]

My point here is not to question the metaphysical foundations of the perennial philosophy, but to point out that, *at a minimum,* it maps a hierarchy of states of consciousness. Whether these correspond to independent levels of reality in their own right is a separate issue that we will return to shortly.

Let us recall, however, that a system moving in an attractor basin, unless it is a point attractor, is not a static configuration like a gravitational or magnetic field, but a fluid process that moves within certain broad boundaries. Viewing states of consciousness in this way we see that each represents an entire landscape of experience, a world of reality. The mental world, for example, is one of hard, separate, objects suitable for objective science and the construction of machines: a world of reason and order. It supports a rich range of experiences such as excitement, pleasure, and pain. In time, however, it can grow boring and eventually even become hollow and empty, as it did for the European existentialists. By comparison, the intuitive world is much softer. It is one in which essences interpenetrate each other, and rather than solidified facts and units of information, entire intuitive horizons appear. Emotions become finer, more exquisite, and more deeply fulfilling. An important idea that will be explored later is that personal growth involves an increasing ability to move easily between such states.

The amount of variability in each state of consciousness depends on the size and slope of its attractor basin. Remembering that an attractor is a pattern of change, it is now possible to imagine a series of broadly constrained configurations of brain activity, each an attractor in its own right, that corresponds to the levels of consciousness described by the perennial philosophy. The existence of such attractors might, in fact, be measured to a satisfying degree by monitoring the EEG, the electrical patterns emitted from the cerebral cortex, while an individual is experiencing various states of consciousness. These patterns are known to differ for waking consciousness and for each of the four stages of non-dream sleep, as well as for the dream state.[5] A considerable body of research indicates that various meditative states produce similarly distinct EEG patterns.[6] Furthermore, a wide reading of contemplative literature strongly suggests that such meditative states correspond to the subtle levels of being, for example, the sheaths of Vedanta.[7] In yoga philosophy, for instance, meditative states are said to proceed from the gross to the subtle, and on to the most subtle states. It was apparently from such states that the Vedantic sheaths were described in the first place.

It is perhaps not surprising that the sequence of EEG patterns which emerges as a person drifts from wakefulness toward the deepest stages of non-dream sleep resembles, in approximate form, the sequence seen in progressively deeper states of yogic meditation. Indeed, the deepest state of sleep is said to closely resemble the state of *turiya,* the experience of absolute reality or supreme consciousness. The *Mandukya Upanishad* states that in deep sleep 'there is neither desire nor dream. In deep sleep, all experiences merge into the unity of undifferentiated consciousness. The sleeper is filled with bliss and experiences bliss ...' The drawback, of course, is that in deep sleep, unlike deep meditation, there is no reflective awareness, and upon waking there is no remembrance. Still, a few observers beyond the Vedic tradition have suspected the richness of deep sleep. In 1800 the romantic poet Novalis wrote:

> Daylight has got limits and hours, but the hegemony of
> Night penetrates through space and through time. Sleep does
> not end, sleep lasts. God-like sleep ... you are the
> messenger who opens mysteries that unfold forever, but
> avoids words.

Returning to our theme, it appears that the mind-brain system contains within its broad limits a range of possible states, or attractors, some of which are highly desirable and can be achieved through systematic practices such as meditation. In other words, personal growth is a natural implication of the perspective that views consciousness as a system near the edge of chaos.

The limits of growth are not known, but it is an implication of this view that such limits must exist as long as the gross structure of the physical vehicle itself is not altered. In this connection, it is perhaps not surprising that more than a few wisdom traditions work toward a significant transformation of exactly this vehicle. For example, it is common in yoga to stress the importance of physical health as almost a precondition for the achievement of high levels of transpersonal growth. Diet, exercise, and hatha yoga are viewed as important preparations of the body that will allow it to sustain the intense energies and demanding transformations that come with advanced yogic work.[8]

Sri Aurobindo and the Mother's highest form of practice, the Supramental Yoga, actually strives for a divine transformation of physical body right down to its individual cells. Working from a view of the body that emphasizes subtle energy channels, kundalini yoga strives toward a transformation of the subtle energies associated with the body.[9] Certain Buddhist traditions in historical Tibet, as well as traditional Chinese Taoist disciplines likewise worked toward transformations of the body's subtle energies.[10] It is hard to understand the importance of such disciplines if they do not ultimately yield new possibilities for human experience, in other words, new chaotic attractors.[11]

Before leaving our present topic, let us consider the evolutionary implications of a mind-brain system that, within broad limitations, is capable of supporting a range of attractors representing diverse states of consciousness. Such a system would seem capable of evolutionary change based on accumulated alterations of the genetic structure of the human species. Such changes, however, occur slowly, over vast periods of time. This traditional type of evolution does not seem to accommodate the dramatic changes in human consciousness suggested by evolutionary models such as those of Jean Gebser, Ken Wilber, or Sri Aurobindo, which involve known and, evolutionarily speaking, very recent human history. Moreover, all three of these theorists have expressed considerable interest not only in past evolutionary changes, but more importantly, in the potential for further changes in the not-so-distant future.

What is needed if evolution is to be accelerated is a mechanism to anchor the gains made by each generation, so that future generations can use them as footholds. As far as we know at the present, changes in the species genetic pool occur far too slowly for this. Still, if we wish to honor the record of history itself, a record that in the writings of Gebser, Wilber, and others, bears witness to a historical progression of structures of consciousness, then such a mechanism must be found. To appeal alone to ordinary learning as an explanation seems less than credible. This would need to postulate that each generation begins anew from scratch and gains whatever advances it can, based solely on its own merits and what it learns from the past. From this point of view a Cro-Magnon infant miraculously transported forty thousand years forward into the present would grow up as a thoroughly modern person. It seems to me that the fundamental differences in the structures of consciousness which separate us from our ancestors of forty thousand years ago are too profound to be explained in this fashion.

If we were facing these questions only a few years ago we would at this point be at a dead end as far as science is concerned. Fortunately, recent advances in a number of fields of inquiry have significantly expanded the horizon of possibilities.

Formative fields

Of particular importance here is the work of biochemist Rupert Sheldrake and philosopher and systems theorist Ervin Laszlo, mentioned in Chapter 7.[12] Sheldrake's notion of morphic fields, as well as Laszlo's comparable psi-field hypothesis, if proven correct, would provide strong support for the possibility of a relatively rapid advance in the evolution of the chaotic attractors that undergird states and structures of consciousness.

Sheldrake has, over a period of years, collected a considerable body of empirical evidence that supports such ideas. He began by asking some very difficult questions about the embryonic formation (morphogenesis) of plants and animals. Morphogenesis literally means 'the coming-into-being of characteristic and specific form.' In his first book, A New Science of Life, he presented a carefully reasoned argument that conventional scientific explanations of morphogenesis in terms of genetics and biochemistry are inadequate and fail to account for certain of the known facts of morphological development, even in principle.

Sheldrake's idea, as we have seen, is that the physical formation of a living organism is guided in part by a non-material field or force which he refers to as a morphic field, similar to Laszlo's psi-field. The early twentieth-century vitalists such as Bergson had also argued for the presence of a guiding non-material aspect in organic life. Beyond the largely philosophical arguments in favor of it, however, they were unable to muster the hard evidence necessary to convince the no nonsense scientists of the early mid-twentieth century of its viability. The situation has changed significantly since then. Though the hypothesis of formative causation, like Laszlo's psi-field hypothesis, will certainly benefit from further scientific research, it is far beyond the stage of pure speculation. We will review some of the evidence shortly.

Of primary interest here is Sheldrake and Laszlo's suggestion that morphic or psi-fields can influence not only embryonic development, but also patterns of electrical events in the brain. In other words, they can influence behavior and states of experience. The nervous system is a natural place to look for such subtle influences, because at the highest level of brain function critical neocortical processes seem so delicately poised that the smallest influences might alter them profoundly.[13] Moreover, increasing evidence that higher order brain functions can be understood as the chaotic or near chaotic attractor patterns makes the influence of subtle patterning forces seem even more possible. This is because chaotic systems are extremely sensitive to even minute influences. Even the slightest 'push,' timed properly, can send such a system gliding off in a new direction.[14]

The influence of such subtle fields, which Sheldrake terms *motor fields,* may be important in producing genetically programmed behaviors such as the tendency for a particular species of spider to spin a unique web, or for a bird to sing its own unique species song. They may also provide a new model for explaining learning and memory, a model in which memories are equivalent to motor fields built up from the past experiences of an individual organism. This idea is compatible with increasing evidence that particular memories may be equivalent in terms of brain activity to the activation of specific chaotic attractors, as we saw in Chapter 2.

Morphic fields have the seemingly paradoxical quality of not being limited by location. The implication of this is that, though a person's individual memories must match the unique pattern of his or her nervous system, one individual's experience could conceivably influence those of others. In other words, when something is learned once, it is more easily learned again later by others. In this way a pattern of thought or behavior, once established, becomes more easily repeated by others. Precisely here lies the possibility that forms of consciousness, supported by specific patterns of brain activity may advance in an evolutionary fashion. In other words, attractors that configure brain

activity into patterns that represent, say, Gebser's structures of consciousness, or Sri Aurobindo's ascent of minds (essentially equivalent
to the Vedantic sheaths) could undergo significant alterations within
spans of time much shorter than is usual in biological evolution.

As to the scientific legitimacy of such fields, the jury is still out,
but more than enough evidence has been presented to make the idea
credible. For instance, in the early years of this century, one of the
founders of American psychology, William McDougall of Harvard
University, discovered quite by chance that untrained rats were quick
to learn a task (escaping from a water maze) previously acquired by
many earlier generations of rats of the same strain. These findings
were strikingly confirmed several years later in both Scotland and
Australia, when researchers discovered that untrained rats picked up
the task almost immediately. The great Russian physiologist Ivan
Pavlov, best known in the West for his studies of conditioned reflexes
in dogs, observed a similar effect when he trained several generations
of white mice to run to a feeding station at the sound of a bell. While
the first generation required an average of about three hundred trials
to learn the task, the second generation required only about one
hundred trials. The third and fourth generations learned in thirty and
ten trials respectively!

In a recent test of Sheldrake's theory a picture containing the
hidden face of a Cossack to be presented on British television. As
viewers watched, its features, including a handlebar mustache, slowly
emerged from a puzzle background. Groups in America, Europe, and
Africa were later shown the picture, and their ability to recognize the
hidden figure was dramatically faster than when it had been viewed
by the British audience.[15]

In his book, *The Presence of the Past,* Sheldrake presents a variety
of lines of evidence in favor of the influence of motor fields,
specifically on human behavior. For instance, Gary Schwartz at Yale
University, presented students with a large number of Hebrew words
from the Old Testament. Some were presented as they are normally
printed, while others had their letters randomly rearranged. Though the
students did not know Hebrew, they guessed at the meaning of the
words, indicating their confidence in each guess. Schwartz found that
the real words were rated with considerably greater confidence than

those that had been scrambled. More than that, the confidence ratings were found to be about twice as high for the words that occurred frequently in the Old Testament compared to those that occur only rarely. Presumably, the real words had been learned by countless numbers of individuals throughout history, thus forming strong morphic fields. Beyond this, the most frequently occurring words had been seen and read the greatest number of times. The alternative explanation that the real words were simply *better words,* that is, that they were words that are more easily read and learned, was all but eliminated by the ratings of linguistic psychologists, who found the scrambled words to be as structurally as sound as the real ones. Experiments of a similar nature have also been carried out using Persian words and even Morse code.

Despite the preliminary success of these ideas, we are still left wondering just what could be the real substance of morphic fields. What are they made of? It seems unlikely that a satisfactory answer to this question will be found in the mechanistic framework of classical physics, with the strict spatial and temporal boundaries it places on causal influences. Quantum theory, however, is another matter. It offers an entirely different and more open set of possibilities for events related to each other at a distance in time and space. While Sheldrake has not been greatly concerned with this question, it is interesting to note that in a conversation between himself and quantum physicist David Bohm the latter suggested that morphic fields might be understood as something like the *quantum potential.*[16]

The concept of the quantum potential has its roots in an idea suggested back in 1927 by the French quantum physicist Louis de Broglie, who proposed that individual particles such as electrons are guided or directed by 'guide waves.' In the 1950s Bohm originated a similar idea in the form of the quantum potential, and worked with de Broglie to develop it. Bohm points out that the quantum potential has many of the properties of morphic fields. It exerts an effect that is non-local, meaning it is not restricted to the usual spatial constraints of classical physics. Moreover, it 'guides' the particle much like a radio signal guides an airplane or a ship, by supplying information rather than force.

Laszlo's conception of the psi-field articulates this notion in detail.

The idea is that wave functions equivalent to quantum potentials are built up into enormously complex higher-order, or nested, processes, retained in non-local psi-fields analogous to Sheldrake's morphic fields. Such processes could exert influences not only on single subatomic particles, or small sets of such particles, but also on large-scale real-world events such as those of the human nervous system. With such large-scale capabilities, Laszlo's hypothesis offers an approach, founded in quantum theory, to a field effect that could very well lie at the foundation of psychological evolution. Historical changes in dominant structures of consciousness could gradually gain substantial momentum through the mediating effect of psi-fields. Let us return, now, to our unfinished business concerning the Vedantic levels of being.

The levels of being

As I suggested above, perhaps these levels can best be understood as states of consciousness supported by particular chaotic attractors of brain activity. It would be unfair, however, to leave this topic without at least touching on the question of whether they represent actual strata of being as well, as real in their own right as the gross material level.

If in fact they are as real as the physical universe, or more so, then why do we not detect them with scientific instruments? One answer to this question offered by the pioneering researcher in the field of biological self-regulation, Elmer Green, is that we simply do not have instruments with parts that extend into these subtle realms.[17] They are all made of gross matter. Evidently there is only one instrument sensitive enough to detect and report these subtle realms, and that instrument is the human being. It alone has parts that extend into these regions. How reliable is this instrument? And is it able to distinguish states of consciousness from actual states of being? We can only conjecture.

Let us note, however, that when dealing with 'higher' states of consciousness there is a near universal consensus that these experiences contact larger and more substantial levels of reality than does ordinary consciousness.[18] The entire experience of the sacred is steeped in a sense of profound *realness* beside which ordinary reality pales by comparison.[19] This much we have from subjective descriptions of mystical and meditative states. Furthermore, we have from many wisdom traditions, but especially the yogic ones, descriptions of energies whose origins are said to lie deep in the subtle realms. It is said among yogins, for instance, that the subtle energy, prana, is the wellspring of all manifest energy in the universe. In this same vein, we have also touched on Sri Aurobindo's idea that the highest of the divine energies 'descends' from the supramental level, rather than rising from the gross physical.[20]

Aside from the above, there is at this time an increasing interest world-wide in the role subtle energies may play in health and healing. Subtle energies, of course, are at the heart of many ancient healing traditions, especially in the Far East. What is unique these days is the impressive spread of interest in such systems, and ways that they can be scientifically investigated. For example the recently formed International Society for the Study of Subtle Energies and Energy Medicine, founded by Elmer Green and others, grew from a few founding members to a global constituency of twelve hundred individuals, most of them physicians, professional healers, and scientists, before its first newsletter made it to press.[21]

I will leave it to the reader to decide whether all of this amounts to a proof of the existence of the subtle realms as domains of existence in their own right. Perhaps for practical purposes it does not really matter whether the subtle realms exist beyond the dimensions of human experience. One question for which an answer to this puzzle would be useful, however, concerns the possibility of life beyond the death of the body. If, indeed, the human being has a 'vertical structure,' to use Sri Aurobindo's phrase, then the subtle levels of that being might continue more or less unscathed after the bottom level, the gross physical body, drops off. Such a view is common in Eastern philosophies as well as in occult traditions world wide. Yogic philosophy speaks of the *jiva* as that part of the human being which continues from lifetime to lifetime, carrying with it certain unconscious memories and karmic 'seeds,' the latter having something in common with what modern depth psychology would call a *complex,* a psychological entanglement that clamors to be worked out.

The continuous existence of an inner structure apparently assures the conservation of individuality. That is, from incarnation to incarna-

tion we retain some inner part of ourselves. This notion is at the heart
of thinking about reincarnation which emphasizes the growth of the
soul, or inner person, over many lifetimes. This belief, in one form or
another, is so ancient and so widespread that it almost qualifies for
inclusion as part of the perennial philosophy itself. In many traditional
Eastern cultures it goes virtually unquestioned. Interestingly, it is not
entirely unusual in countries such as India and Sri Lanka for children
to report memories of previous incarnations, often lived somewhere
nearby such as in a neighboring village, and for their parents to take
them to that place, where they visit with previous relatives and ac-
quaintances.[22] Similar reports can be found in the West, though they are
rare, perhaps because Western parents do not take such talk seriously.
Perhaps, also, the Western psyche, especially the ego, is less fluid and
permeable than is its Eastern counterpart, even in childhood.[23] If this
is the case it would seem less likely that vague or weak memories of
a previous existence could leak through into consciousness.

Many cultures besides traditional Eastern ones have had some form
of belief in the advancement of an inner being across more than a
single lifetime. These range from the Aztec culture of ancient Mexico
to the Celts of ancient northern Europe.[24] After battling the Celts in
the first century before Christ, Julius Caesar wrote of them:

> They wish to inculcate this as one of their leading tenets,
> that souls do not become extinct, but pass after death from
> one body to another and they think that men by this tenet
> are in a great degree excited to valor, the fear of death
> being disregarded.

Julius Caesar should not have been surprised at the beliefs of the Celts
with whom he warred, for Cicero, the Roman orator of his own time,
wrote in *Hortensio:*

> The ancients, whether they were seers, or interpreters of the
> divine mind in the tradition of the sacred initiations, seem to
> have known the truth, when they affirmed that we were
> born into the body to pay the penalty for sins committed in
> a former life.

Rebirth was discussed seriously among certain of the ancient Greek mystery religions. The semi-legendary founder of the Pythagorean mysteries, Pythagoras himself, was said to recall a large number of previous existences.

Let us return, however, to our discussion of the inner levels of the perennial philosophy. If the subtle sheaths of Vedanta exist as independent realities in their own right, then they hold forth a further possibility for understanding states of consciousness. This is that certain of them might act as receptacles for consciousness in much the same fashion as does the physical brain. To take this idea further, suppose that the physical nervous system is not the primary support of the nonordinary states of consciousness of the varieties experienced in deep meditation. One version of this idea is that the physical brain is the lowest rung in a series of harmonious structures which coincide with the nervous system at more subtle levels of being. This is to say that the human body-mind system exists at many levels. Such an idea is in full agreement with Sri Aurobindo's contention that the human is a being with a vertical structure. It seems also to be in agreement with certain comments of the American yogic adept and trickster Da Avabhasa (previously Da Free John), who considers much of the agenda of yoga to be the development of experiences at these subtle levels.[25] In fact, we have here put into words what seems to be essentially the working philosophy of virtually all types of yoga, namely that consciousness can aspire to ascending levels of subtlety — from the mental, to the intuitive, to the blissful, and on to ultimate unconditional Reality.

Let us note at this point, however, that if consciousness can be configured within the subtle realms — if attractors can be mapped into them — we would still expect to see characteristic patterns of activity in the physical brain even during higher states of experience. This gives us an alternative interpretation of the EEG patterns associated with states of deep meditation.[26] The large, slow-wave, electrical patterns seen in these states could represent an idling brain, while consciousness is actually patterned in the subtle realms. All of this, of course, is highly speculative, but interesting.

Holism

For the moment we can push our explorations only so far and then must submit to mystery. In the case of the nature and evolution of consciousness one word for this mystery is holism. The increase in inner richness with the development of outer organic complexity is precisely the fruit of this wholeness. Evolution does not follow different rules for different orders of being, because there is only one process of evolution. We map it from the gross level, as with a topological map, and thus our theories are about the evolution of material forms. This is what we see. But the process may be deeper.

My own view is that it seems most reasonable to suspect that all levels of phenomena form a continuum of matter and energy in which the material and the subtle realms are but two opposite extremes of a spectrum, and that they obey some kinds of general principles, though we have only an inkling of what these might be.[27] Inner evolution, from this holistic perspective, is seen as the natural counterpart of outer evolution, and consciousness in its deepest essence remains untouched, experiencing the richness of what is created in mind and body. (Recall again the basic notion of consciousness as an unfettered living presence from the first chapter.)

Consciousness is akin to, if not identical with, Gebser's *origin*. In Sanskrit it is called *purusha*,[28] pure spirit, which the ancient Vedic poet described as follows:

> Purusha is the shining,
> yet formless cosmic spirit,
> the Self of the Universe.
> He is within everything,
> and without everything,
> unborn,
> untainted by either breath or mind.
> He is beyond even the tendency to take form.

Mundaka Upanishad

9. A Benchmark for Evolution

Complexity, evolution, and the farther reaches of human nature

Complexity provides a benchmark for evaluating the direction of evolution ... To contribute to greater harmony, a person's consciousness has to become complex.
                                Mihaly Csikszentmihalyi

Evolution is usually thought of as a progression of events in time, but in another sense it is the rise of complexity. At least this would seem to be the case if we take seriously Ilya Prigogine's contention that ordinary historical time is defined by the self-organizing activities of dissipative systems such as living organisms.[1] Indeed, it would seem to be the very nature of any complex self-organizing system, such as the mind or the brain, to evolve toward ever greater complexity. In the words of British evolutionary biologist Brian Goodwin, 'it has nowhere else to go.'

Does ontogeny recapitulate phylogeny?

This chapter is about two questions. First, does ordinary psychological development emulate the historical evolution of the human species? Second, do evolutionary theories provide a useful model for understanding the highest reaches of the human potential?

There is a certain romance to evolutionary thinking. The original power, simplicity and scope of Darwin's theory was a source of fascination to nineteenth-century philosophers, psychologists, anthropologists, and economists alike.[2] We have already covered some of this ground with Henri Bergson and Pierre Teilhard de Chardin. Well-known late nineteenth-century and early twentieth-century psychologists such as England's George Romanes, and Mark Baldwin and

G. Stanley Hall in the United States, turned to evolutionary explanations of human behavior as well as the psychological development of
children, seeing the latter as a recapitulation of the evolution of the
species. This idea had its biological counterpart as well, in which it
was observed that in certain phases of development the unborn fetus
exhibits the gills of a fish, and a two-chambered heart that transforms
into a human four-chambered heart only at birth. Thus comes the
famous phrase, 'ontogeny recapitulates phylogeny,' suggesting that
individual development follows along the track of species evolution.

Such notions fell out of favor during the early decades of the twentieth century. One explanation for this decline is that they were overly
simplistic, and all too characteristic of neophyte sciences that had not
yet developed mature theories of their own. The fact of the matter,
though, is that the rise of positivism, as well as an increasing specialization among academic disciplines after the Second World War made
virtually all such grand theories *passé*. In philosophy, Bergson's comprehensive evolutionary perspective gave way to constrained dis-
courses on logic and language. Broad evolutionary explanations of
human nature likewise fell out of favor to be replaced by reductionistic behaviorism. It was a new century.

In answer to our first question above, however, there is more than
a little truth to the idea that psychological development follows a path
parallel to the long haul of evolution. But the similarity is one of
principles, not of particulars. Growth from infancy through childhood
marks a course from an early undifferentiated condition through increasing stages of articulation in a general line leading to adult complexity and competence. In Chapter 3 we saw this line of development
worked out most clearly in Piaget's theory of the growth of intelligence in the child. In general terms, the idea that psychological
development follows a parallel course to evolution is consistent with
the observed appearance of complexity over the long spans of biological time. On the other hand, a much more useful understanding of
psychological development is obtained by viewing it in terms of the
grand evolutionary synthesis, in which we find that complex self-
organizing systems such as the human mind tend to grow toward
increasingly complex structures, as we saw in Chapter 3.

These issues can be confusing if for no other reason than that the fact that the term *evolution* does not have a single meaning, but is used in a variety of ways. Any discussion of growth and evolution involves both a theory of growth and a theory of evolution. With this in mind, before pushing on to the question of the development of higher human potentials it will be as well to stop briefly and consider what exactly is meant by evolution.

Evolution soup

The term *evolution* is commonly taken in at least three more or less distinct ways. The first, which I will call *biological evolution,* refers to a gradual change and diversification of entire plant and animal species.[3] The principles by which this type of evolution operates have been the subject of intense discussion among biologists since the time of Darwin. Contemporary biologists have tended to emphasize genetic selection, so that the study of evolution is basically the study of how population genetics change over time.

The second is an informal idea of *historical evolution,* which usually carries an implicit suggestion of some kind of growth, maturation, or improvement with time. We speak casually of the evolution of a civilization, or the evolution of an idea. In terms of consciousness and the mind, it suggests a progressive development of the inner person towards greater freedom, self-expression, and in particular toward a natural and harmonious way of being in the cosmos. This is closer than the first meaning to what we think of as psychological or spiritual growth. It is this notion of evolution that is expressed by virtually all the wisdom traditions.

The third is the *grand evolutionary synthesis,* described in Chapter 2. It does not derive from biology, but is an idea that came out of systems thinking and the sciences of complexity. (Nowadays it would be fair to include it among the sciences of complexity.) It attempts to account for the self-organizing properties of complex systems. Its range is enormous, spanning from the formation of matter in the early universe to the creation of the first molecules of life, and on upward to include increasingly complex hierarchical systems all the way through natural ecologies and human societies, including multinational political and economic structures. It tends to stress the role of energy in the formation of order in systems that exist far from thermal equilibrium, but a more fundamental theme is the creation of complexity.[4]

Several efforts have been made to bring together under a single conceptual roof the Darwinian ideas at the root of biological evolution with the self-creating systems notions at the heart of the grand synthesis. Brian Goodwin has recently made monumental steps in this direction as explained in his book, *How the Leopard Got its Spots.* His ideas are important to our own exploration, so I will say a little more about them.

Essentially, Goodwin goes to considerable pains to show that processes in nature are pulled by their own internal dynamics toward specific forms. This is evidenced, for example, by the fact that, of over two hundred and fifty thousand species of higher plants, only three basic distributions of leaves around the stems are actually seen, and all but twenty percent of these are of a single form, the spiral. Likewise, the bone structures of hands, paws, and fins have certain similar features in all vertebrate animals. Goodwin makes a strong case that these likenesses are due not simply to common genetic histories, but represent basic patterns, or attractors in the growth processes of plants and animals. In other words, only certain viable forms are available. The role of genetics is no more than to steer development into the right region of an extended morphological space, as it were, and natural self-organizing mechanisms take over. Goodwin's case is detailed, and based on computer simulations as well as natural observation, but the bottom line is fairly simple: 'there is an inherent rationality to life that makes it intelligible at a much deeper level than functional utility and historical accident.' Here, functional utility and historical accident refer to the two well-worn hinges of Darwinian evolution.

Goodwin's ideas are important because they demonstrate that nature does not take on indefinite numbers of forms, but assumes only certain stable patterns, or attractors. The metabolic processes that underlie the placement of leaves on the stem of a plant, or the formation of a paw on an animal, are complex, but nowhere near as complex as the exquisitely intricate events produced by the two hundred billion nerve cells of the human brain. Perhaps it is not surprising, then, that unlike the patterns of leaves on plant stems, the human mind, supported by this elaborate brain, is capable of an enormous number of thoughts, perceptions, feelings, and states of consciousness. Still, what Goodwin's work has to teach is that this variety, while rich, is not unlimited. Only certain patterns are viable, and among these some are more stable than others.

Here we are reminded again of Charles Tart's contention that states of consciousness are discrete. In Chapter 3 we noted that each state of consciousness is accompanied by an attractor in the complex processes of the brain, as well as a corresponding attractor in the process structure of consciousness. What we have from Goodwin is a further explanation for why such states of consciousness do not take on indefinite variety, but fall into a wide but discrete distribution of individual states. From this we might imagine a kind of periodic table of consciousness, representing a large but finite array of potential states. Chemically altering the excitable milieu of the brain with drugs, or employing technologies of consciousness such as meditation, or even listening to music, or dancing, can evidently alter this table, enlarging some regions and making them more accessible while diminishing others. With these ideas in mind, let us return to the question of whether the growth of higher human potentials — 'spiritual' growth — mirrors evolution.

Spiritual growth and evolution

It will come as no surprise that the history of ideas concerning evolution and consciousness presents a shifting ground, rife with confusions between the three types of evolution above — biological evolution, historical evolution, and the grand evolutionary synthesis. As we have seen, both Henri Bergson and Teilhard de Chardin considered the inner evolution of consciousness to be a counterpart if not a direct function of the evolution of complexity in the nervous system. Their descriptions of the progressive development of consciousness, however, owe more to their philosophical dispositions than to their dedication to evolutionary biology. Nor were they particularly interested in individual psychological or spiritual growth.[5] Their emphasis on the importance of complexity, however, anticipated to a remarkable degree the principles of the modern sciences of complexity, including the grand evolutionary synthesis. This was especially true for Teilhard de Chardin. They were scientific mystics making the best of both the scientific and spiritual worlds of their day.

Sri Aurobindo's evolutionary spirituality is of the second type, that is, historical. At bottom it is founded almost entirely on traditional Indian ideas of the progress of the spirit through many incarnations toward identification with subtle levels of being. How then did Sri Aurobindo come to frame so many of his thoughts in the language of evolution? It is my guess that he recognized something in the traditional Indian ideas that looked very much like evolution as progress.[6] During his years in England he may well have read Hegel, with his concept of the historical unfolding of the Spirit. He certainly was familiar with Darwin's writings. Indeed, educated people throughout the world were talking of Darwin and evolution. So it is not surprising that he would see something familiar in the notion of evolution as ascendence. Moreover, it was natural to think of individual development, particularly of the advanced yogic variety, as a guiding light for the future development of humankind. Beyond all this, it seems likely that Sri Aurobindo and the Mother intuited some process like Sheldrake's morphic resonance or Laszlo's psi-field, according to which, as we have seen, the gains of even one individual might well contribute to the potential wealth of the entire species.

Ken Wilber, like Sri Aurobindo, sees the evolution of consciousness as following a predestined path toward a progressive identification with subtle levels of being. He also sees this evolutionary progression in line with modern psychological theory, as involving increasingly complex structures, not unlike the structures of intelligence in Piaget's theory, or the increasing sophistication of moral judgments in Kohlberg's theory. Recently he has published a massive re-synthesis of his ideas in relation to the historical evolution of complexity.[7] The result has much in common with Henri Bergson and Teilhard de Chardin, but does not represent any basic changes in his thinking.[8]

Since Wilber's views have been very important in opening the door to the legitimate study of transpersonal growth by psychologists and philosophers alike, especially in the United States, let us spend a little more time with them. Wilber's essential notion, as we recall from Chapter 6, is that human development, beginning at or near birth, progresses through a series of stages similar to Gebser's historical structures of consciousness. Wilber refers to these as the archaic-oroboric, magic-typhonic, mythic-membership, and mental-egoic stages. If growth continues upward from the mental-egoic stage it progresses by a series of identifications with the inner planes of being, adopted essentially from Vedanta and the perennial philosophy as seen in Table 2 (Chapter 6). This Table shows Wilber's entire sequence of development, from the four Gebser-like stages mentioned above, through three stages — four if the Self, or Atman, is treated as a stage — derived from the innermost planes of Vedanta (also see Table 1, Chapter 6). These are viewed as forming a unified evolutionary and developmental sequence.

Now here is where I get off the boat. Gebser's structures of consciousness are one thing. Vedantic planes of being are another. To line them up on the same continuum is a *type error,* a 'category error' as it is sometimes called. Philosopher Alan Watts once described a type error as going into a restaurant and proceeding to eat the menu! Food is food; menus are menus. Even if we treat the Vedantic planes simply as *states* of consciousness, as suggested in the last chapter, this still does not make them fully blown *structures* of consciousness. This is an important point. (The complete distinction between *states* and *structures* of consciousness was developed in Chapter 3. We will return to it again shortly, and review its basic implications.)

Another difficulty I have with Wilber's model, and a serious one, is that he has individuals 'jump' stages of development. For instance, certain paleolithic shamans are said to have entered trance states that carried them directly into the lower subtle realms where subtle energies can be manipulated, for instance, to heal others. Wilber speaks very highly of these individuals:

> And we can only stand in deepest awe and admiration for those isolated souls, perched on the mountaintops far away from their fellows, who were quiet enough in their own hearts to hear the call of the Beyond.

According to Wilber, a few individuals of the late mythic period are said to have reached the higher subtle realms, where experience is characterized by a devotional sense first felt in the worship of the goddess. And during the early ascent of the mental structure a few gifted individuals are said to have achieved dramatic leaps into the causal realm, and even beyond to the original source of Being. These were religious geniuses such as Jesus Christ, Gautama Buddha of India, and Lao Tzu of China.

As intriguing as all this is, there is a fly in the ointment. Two of the most fundamental tenets of any stage theory of psychological development are, first, that every person pass through every stage and, second, that no stage can be omitted.[9] This is because each stage is literally built upon the gains of earlier ones. To skip a stage is like trying to build the upper stories of a house without first constructing the ground floor. A developmental theory based on stages simply cannot claim that certain individuals, no matter how gifted, can skip or leap to higher levels of development.[10]

Along these same lines it is worth noting that some wisdom traditions regularly seem to entirely omit certain stages, suggesting that they are not stages at all. The American master, Da Avabhasa,[11] once outlined three major paths to inner development. First is the *path of yoga* which focuses on the energies of the body, such as prana, and may continue to move toward the more subtle planes of Vedanta. Second is the *path of saints,* concerned primarily with the most subtle realms of being. And third is the *path of sages,* which strives for direct unconditional illumination. This latter path, when successful, seems to bound over the lower stages, as in the lightning-swift illumination characteristic of the Rinzai school of Zen Buddhism. Zen is a path of the third type and has little to say about the intermediate levels. It would seem that an alternative model for growth is in order here.

A process view of spiritual growth

Wilber is certainly right about one thing, people throughout history have experienced remarkable states of mind. Need we be reminded, however, that many states of consciousness can seem profoundly different from our normal business-as-usual reality while at the same time remaining curiously near? Indeed, the attractor of ordinary consciousness is more tenuous than we may realize, while possibilities for experiences beyond it are in equal measure larger. An inhalation of nitrous oxide (laughing gas), a moment of peace in the forest, a few chords of Beethoven's Choral symphony, the scent of tea in the garden at sunrise ... These and a thousand other events can trigger the collapse of mundane reality and send us gliding into states of experience we never before imagined. In the clumsy language of science, the minutest alteration in one of the control variables of consciousness can send it through one or more bifurcations, carrying us into profoundly different realities like Alice falling down the rabbit hole. In the words of William James:

> Our normal waking consciousness ... is but one special type of consciousness, whilst all about it, parted from it by the filmiest of screens, there lie potential forms of consciousness entirely different. We may go through life without suspecting their existence; but apply the requisite stimulus, and at a touch they are all there in all their completeness.

One contemporary theorist who has emphasized the large and fluid range of consciousness is the neuro-psychiatrist Gordon Globus, who on the basis of a penetrating examination of both neurological and psychological data argues that the brain is like a holonomic generator, able to produce a virtually unlimited variety of experiences.[12] He states that 'the brain in its unsurpassed complexity generates its own holoplenum of *possibilia* — a virtual holoworld of possible worlds.' In other words, 'human beings have the capacity to constitute *de novo* perfectly authentic worlds in the absence of input, worlds which have never previously been experienced.' Such worlds are experienced, for example, in dreams, shamanic trances, and so on.

Even in the late nineteen-eighties Globus wrote without the benefit of recent scientific work which suggests that the brain is a system on the edge of chaos. Neuropsychologist Larry Vandervert, whom we met in Chapter 3, is well aware, however, of the importance of chaos to the function of the brain. He believes that the physical brain carries a remarkable intrinsic capacity for a much larger natural intelligence than we ordinarily see.[13] According to his thinking, this is in part because the brain carries in its evolutionary inheritance internal process patterns, or algorithms, that match the subtle organization of the world itself. It is thus not entirely surprising that creations of the human mind such as mathematics have their counterparts in the world of nature.

One is reminded of Kant's discussion of natural laws in his *Prolegomena to Any Future Metaphysic,* where he asks, 'How is it that in this space, here, we can make judgments that we know with apodictic certainty will be valid in that space, there?' The answer, observes Joseph Campbell in one of his last works, 'is that the laws of space are known to the mind because they are *of* the mind.' In poetic fashion he goes on to say, 'In other words ... outer space is within us inasmuch as the laws of space are within us; outer and inner space are the same.' The coming together of these outer and inner realms in consciousness can be an experience of profound resonance. It was no mistake that the great romantic poet Novalis wrote, 'The seat of the soul is there, where the outer and the inner worlds meet.'

It would seem that there is more to the mind and brain than meets the eye. Globus, Vandervert, and Campbell are certainly not alone in this view. Indeed, how could anyone seriously question it? Our own lives each offer up a wealth of evidence. Who has not in a single day fallen into the depths of depression and soared to exquisite emotional heights, been transfixed by a striking work of art, or carried into a world of nostalgia by a forgotten poem found discarded on a bookshelf? Humanistic psychologist Abraham Maslow spent years studying certain deeply inspiring states of consciousness that he termed 'peak experiences,' which he believed to be the basis of both mysticism and religion.[14] Subsequent research has shown that these experiences are had by many, indeed, most ordinary people at one time or another during their lives.[15]

The question here, however, is whether even the most remarkable of such experiences are usefully explained as forward evolutionary leaps. I am inclined to think not, as I will explain below. But first let us attempt to put some order on to the vast range of experiences of which the human mind is capable. To this end it will be useful to recall the distinction between *states* and *structures* of consciousness, first introduced in Chapter 3. There we noted that a *structure* of consciousness is an entire framework for experiencing reality. In Gebser's model, the magic, mythic, and mental structures are examples of such frameworks. A *state* of consciousness, on the other hand, is a more or less fluid inflection on a structure. As such, states of consciousness are more mercurial, subject to rapid transmutation as the conditions that produce them change.[16] A few micrograms of LSD diffused throughout the nervous system, for example, can make a dramatic change in the state of one's consciousness, but are much less likely to alter its fundamental structure.[17] Structures are over-arching process patterns that can each support a variety of particular states, or attractors.

Another way to look at all this is to regard each structure as a very complex attractor basin in which states are particular regions, or wings. The latter is consistent with Ben Goertzel's cognitive equation, described in Chapter 3. These wings can also be thought of as positions on the periodic table of consciousness, but here we need to expand our metaphor to include separate pages, each representing a particular structure of consciousness and displaying a table of the states available to that structure. For Gebser, most people today experience the world through the mental structure of consciousness, with the integral structure moving on to the horizon.

Now, let us not throw out the baby with the bath water by forgetting Gebser's (and Wilber's) theory of the history of consciousness as a series of *structures of consciousness*. Without rehashing the entire rationale for this history, already presented in Chapters 5 and 6, I will simply note that it is both cogent and intellectually appealing. But most important, it will provide us with a practical foundation for an understanding of psychological and spiritual growth. The key is to recognize is that a considerable number of *states* of consciousness can be 'launched' from each single *structure* of consciousness.

I believe, in fact, that we are not dealing with a one-dimensional evolutionary map of human experience at all, but a two-dimensional map in which the Gebser-like *structures* of consciousness represent a historical sequence while the Vedantic levels represent *states* of consciousness. This point is very important, as it cuts between the evolutionary progression of *structures* and the immediate possibilities of *states.* The evidence of history and the great wisdom traditions seems to indicate that the Vedanta-like states are accessible to at least some degree from each of these, as represented in Table 4.[18]

The sheaths/koshas (Vedanta)				
Anandamaya (causal)	●	●	●	∧
Vijnanamaya (subtle)	●	●	∧	
Manomaya (mental)	●	∧		
Pranamaya (pranic)	●			
Evolutionary stages/structures: (Wilber/Gebser)	Archaic oroboric	Magic-typhonic	Mythic-member-ship	Mental-egoic

Table 4. Evolutionary stages, levels of being, and possible combinations.
Each ● *represents a potential state of consciousness achieved by moving into one of the sheaths as an attractor of consciousness from a grounding in one of the evolutionary structures. The arrows represent maximum ascensions achieved by rare individuals as suggested by Ken Wilber's work. The latter also suggests that certain individuals have achieved unconditional realization starting from the mental-egoic structure.*

Now let us again ask the question of whether spiritual growth follows an evolutionary course. It is now apparent that the answer depends on what is meant by spiritual growth. If it is simply experiencing or even identifying with the more subtle planes of being, then the answer is *no*. Contrary to Sri Aurobindo and Wilber, and in no way diminishing the wonderful elevation of some of these experiences, such experiences in and of themselves are simply not evolutionary. This is the case whether they are seen as metaphysical planes of being or simply as states of consciousness. If, on the other hand, such growth means to advance toward increasingly creative, dynamic, and expansive ways of living in and experiencing the world, then the answer is *yes,* and indeed this will be the topic of Chapter 11, where we will explore it at length.

The real connection between growth and evolution is found in principles and not in details. These are the principles that govern the growth and complexification complex self-organizing systems — systems such as the brain and the mind. They are the very principles that undergird the internal processes of the human being right down to the biochemical events that support life and sustain individual cells. They are also the same principles by which complex matter was originally formed, life was fashioned, and entire planetary ecologies find their process structures. Both the brain and the mind are complex autopoietic systems on the edge of chaos, systems that complexified over time through dramatic reorganizations. This complexification is witnessed in the historical progression of the Gebser-like structures of consciousness, each mutating (Gebser's word), or in modern terms bifurcating, into more sophisticated and complex forms, while continuing to carry the earlier forms nested within.

A brief look back

Let us finish with a brief look back to the notion, originally suggested by Wilber, that at various times in history certain individuals have penetrated to various depths into the subtle inner realms, opening their consciousness to higher octaves of experience. How would they explain such experiences to their contemporaries and, more importantly, to themselves? They would have available to them only the interpretive structures that had already evolved in their own time. For this reason we would expect their interpretations to be highly colored by their own historical and evolutionary settings.

Consider the shamans of the last ice age, when paintings were executed in the great cave sanctuaries of southern Europe. If Gebser is correct, this was a period steeped in magical consciousness, with the mythic structure just emerging. For this period we would expect any

penetration into non-ordinary realms of experience would be interpreted through a worldview of magic and myth. As we noted in
Chapter 5, the cave paintings themselves give testimony to this suggestion. Later, however, at the dawn of the neolithic farming revolution, we would expect a shift toward purely mythic interpretations of
non-ordinary experiences. It is of this era that Joseph Campbell
observed, for instance, 'the evidence is now before us of a late Stone
Age mythology in which the outstanding single figure is the Naked
Goddess.' Only later did the mental structure of consciousness become
sufficiently developed to provide interpretations of transcendental
states that were not entirely framed in mythic language. Here we find
the Buddha and Lao Tzu, for instance, offering descriptions of the
absolute that are not framed in images of gods and goddesses. There
also is evidence that Christ may have taught a mystical form of
Christianity that transcended images. This tradition seems to have been
carried primarily by the gnostics.[19]

Is it the case, as Wilber suggested, that the early shamans reached
only the lower subtle regions of the inner planes while later explorers
of inner space reached successively higher levels?[20] While it is not
possible to give a final answer, it is worth noting that the case for
modern shamans, at least, achieving virtually unlimited access to
alternative states of consciousness is fairly good. Psychologist Stanley
Krippner spent years studying and living with shamans throughout the
world, and based on his own observations as well as those of others,
makes a strong and detailed case that they are no less limited than
yogis or Zen masters.[21] The point here, however, is that no matter
what levels the early shamans may have reached, they would have
interpreted their experiences in terms of the noetic structures with
which they were familiar, whether those were magic, mythic, or
mental.

An interesting question presents itself at this point. Do spiritual
path-finders, such as those mentioned above, achieve greatness
through sheer penetration into the inner subtle realms, returning, as it
were, with the new insights obtained there, or is their greatness
founded, rather, on an evolutionary ability to interpret their experiences through noetic structures — structures of consciousness in
Gebser's terms — which are at the leading edge of their eras? I sus-

pect that it is the noetic structure itself that makes a spiritual genius, and not the depth of penetration into the subtle realms alone.

An individual's experiences, spiritual or otherwise, must be translated through the interpretive structures that he or she has available. We need only look around us today to see people translating religious experiences, and indeed reality as a whole, at virtually all of Gebser's levels. There are people still practicing Voodoo and other forms of magic. Much of the world's religion involves mythical concepts of gods and goddesses — and rightly so, for mythical consciousness is a wellspring of the spirit. At the same time, however, theologists discourse in mental-rational terms about ethics, the nature of God, and good and evil. Only to the *integral* mind are all these categories thrown aside in favor of the concrete and luminous reality of the moment.[22] It is in the language of the latter that the great ones seem to speak most clearly. The spiritual genius Shankara in the ninth century AD wrote:

> There is a self-existent Reality which is ... the witness of the three states of consciousness [waking, dreaming, and dreamless sleep], and is distinct from the five bodily coverings [sheaths or subtle planes] ... It is aware of the presence or absence of the mind and its functions. It is the Atman.
>
> That Reality sees everything in its own light. No one sees it. It gives intelligence to the mind and the intellect, but no one gives it light.
>
> That Reality pervades the universe, but no one penetrates it. It alone shines. The universe shines with its reflected light.

These words are reminiscent of the great German mystic, Meister Eckhart, who at almost the same time wrote:

> I have spoken at times of a light in the soul that is uncreated ... that little spark in the soul which neither space nor time touches. It is not satisfied with the Father, nor the Son, nor the Holy Spirit ... It wants to penetrate the simple

core, the still desert, into which no distinction ever crept ...
a simple stillness, which is unmoved itself but by whose
immobility all things are moved and all receive life.

Among spiritually sensitive people of each generation there can be
found individuals who translate their own experiences of transcendence in many different modes. Among the first generation of American astronauts, each returned to the Earth with his life somehow
modulated upward to a new level. Their explanations of this change
ranged from the deeply mystical, on the one hand, to fundamentalist
affirmations on the other, but they all had been to the same place. And
indeed, this is the way it must be with inner astronauts as well.

10. While the Mind is Utterly Indivisible

Unconscious thoughts

There is a great difference between the mind and the body, inasmuch as the body is by its very nature always divisible, while the mind is utterly indivisible.

René Descartes, 1641

Mind from an operational point of view does seem to be inherently holistic and not divisible into parts. Psychology, obviously has not yet come to grips with this problem.

Uttal, 1978

I have tried in this book to present a view of consciousness as an event that plots an exquisitely complex chaotic path through states of mind such as joy, sadness, elation, fatigue, nostalgia, daydreams, and night dreams, and within each, through the play of thought, imagination, and memory. This new conception of consciousness suggests revisions in the way we think about mind and experience. In line with this, the present chapter redrafts some traditional ideas about consciousness.

Unconscious thinking

One implication of the present view is to end the notion of the unconscious mind, at least as it is commonly understood. The idea of unconscious influences on the consciousness is ancient in Eastern thought, but relatively new to the West, especially in the form in which it was developed and popularized by Sigmund Freud and the psychoanalytic movement. The latter emphasized the notion of an active process beyond consciousness, one with a full set of dynamics of its own.

In Freud's time the topic of the unconscious was of lively interest in the philosophical circles of Europe.[1] During the decade following the publication of Eduard von Hartmann's enormously successful *Philosophy of the Unconscious* in 1868, no less than six books were published with the term *unconscious* appearing in their titles.[2] Much of this material dealt with the role of the unconscious in movement, perception, and thought, that is, in what came to be called 'unconscious inference.' Examples include the ability to walk down a flight of stairs without thinking about where to put one's feet. Or the *apperception* of visual wholes or *Gestalten*. In his 1890 *Principles of Psychology,* William James reviewed no less than ten 'proofs' of the unconscious, systematically dismissing each of them. Philosophers such as Schopenhauer and Nietzsche, on the other hand, expressed many seminal ideas about unconscious motivations, said to lie behind ordinary social behavior. Despite this attention, the fact is that the idea of an 'unconscious mind,' with its tacit implication of awareness behind ordinary awareness, was beset with problems from the beginning.

In the West, the notion of 'consciousness' dates essentially from René Descartes, who virtually 'discovered' it as a fundamental psychological fact.[3] His postulation of the *res cogitans,* or 'thing which thinks' as an elemental non-material reality emphasized consciousness as that which is apparent upon examining the content of one's own mind. The first person to use the word *consciousness* as an abstract concept, however, was John Locke, who in his 1690 *Essay concerning Human Understanding* defined it as 'the perception of what passes in a man's mind.' The notion of consciousness as the direct content of experience or awareness remained central in Western thought for two hundred years. So it is not surprising that when nineteenth-century thinkers first began to discuss the idea of 'unconscious inference' they were often received with blank stares. How could inference, indeed, any mental operation, be unconscious? The idea just made no sense. As contemporary philosopher John Searle has recently gone to pains to point out all over again, if it is *mind* it cannot be unconscious![4]

The modern fields of cognitive psychology and neurobiology have supplied considerable evidence that all sorts of computations occur in the human brain without apparent conscious participation.[5] Most if not all these, however, amount to more or less routine perceptual, motor, or judgmental processes that run along parallel to, but outside of, our ordinary attention. All this is fascinating, but does not require anything like a working mind, any more than my hand-held battery-powered spelling checker requires a cerebral cortex. The notion of an unconscious *mind,* with dynamics of its own, however, is a horse of a different color. According to psychoanalytic tradition this mind has fears and desires, preferences, anxieties, and complex motivations which can be quite different from, and independent of, those of the conscious ego. An active and dynamic mind that exists out of view of ordinary awareness is, indeed, so incredible that it is only the fact that we have grown up with it that allows us take it seriously to begin with.

Freud himself realized that such a concept had its difficulties. In particular, there was a seductive tendency to rectify the unconscious into something more solid and substantial than necessary to explain the facts of the consultation room, facts about hidden motives, selective forgetfulness, meaningful slips of the tongue ('Freudian slips'), and the like.[6] This problem has never been settled, and Freud, as well as modern psychoanalysts, continued on the whole to treat the unconscious as a 'mind below the mind.'

A vigorous criticism of the concept of the unconscious mind was mounted by the existential philosopher Jean-Paul Sartre. His argument is intricate and takes for granted a substantial knowledge of phenomenology, but in essence focuses on the inherent paradox of an unconscious *mental* process.[7] Sartre was particularly critical of the psychoanalytic treatment of repression, and the question of how a person can lie to him or herself. Suppose, for example, that I demonstrate by the content of my dreams, or by selectively forgetting certain passages from a poem, that I harbor a strong unconscious 'death wish' for my mother (an unconscious desire for her demise). Sartre would point out that resistance to experiencing or knowing such a death wish, the threat it poses to my conscious person, can in fact arise only if I am conscious of it! But wait a minute. If consciousness knows about the death wish then it isn't unconscious at all. We are left with the paradox of how consciousness apparently defends this condition of 'bad faith,' that is, of lying to itself.

Freud dealt with this paradox by postulating an independent third part of the personality, one separate from the conscious ego on the one hand, and the unconscious id on the other. This was the superego, or psychic censor, which serves the gate-keeper function of blocking threatening desires or memories from consciousness. However, for the censor to itself avoid the original paradox of knowing and not knowing at the same time, it must be placed outside the ego, more or less on its own. Sartre notes, though, that this does not solve the problem, because the superego can perform its function adequately only if it is conscious of the dreaded desire. In other words, we are now confronted with a superego that is itself in bad faith! In Sartre's words, 'psychoanalysis has not gained anything for us since, in order to overcome bad faith, it has established between the unconscious and consciousness an autonomous consciousness in bad faith.' To top it off, we now seem to be faced with two separate centers of consciousness within the personality, to say nothing of the original paradox of 'unconscious mind.' The whole affair puts a heavy strain on the credibility of the notion of unconscious desires such as the hypothetical death wish. In doing so, it also puts a heavy strain on Freud's entire concept of the unconscious, which is essentially composed of desires, memories, and impulses censored by the superego from entry into the light of ego consciousness.

Sartre's criticism of the psychoanalytic concept of the unconscious, based on the problematic and paradoxical character of 'the censor in bad faith,' is a powerful and celebrated argument. Sartre was preceded by several decades, however, by another French critic of the Freudian unconscious, one whose conclusions are very much in agreement with those of the modern sciences of complexity. This was Georges Politzer.[8]

Politzer actually had two criticisms of the Freudian unconsciousness, both of which fit together to make a total, and to my mind, very effective argument. The first concerns what Politzer termed *abstraction*. He observed that Freud's early work exhibited a freshness and intimacy that arose from a direct connection with the subjective lives of his clients. This intimacy was reflected in the originality of his interpretation of their dreams, clinical symptoms, and so on. As time went by, however, Freud began to rely increasingly on the abstract structure of his theory. His interpretations became dry and formal, disconnected from the immediate conscious experiences of his clients. Part of this change was due to the reification of concepts such as the id, ego, and superego, which in their original form had actually been processes. This was Politzer's second criticism, that of *realism,* and it applied especially to the notion of the unconscious mind. Politzer was particularly articulate when speaking of the supposed role of the unconscious in dreaming. According to Freud, each dream must be understood on two levels representing two different types of content. On the surface are the literal events of the dream, forming what Freud termed the *manifest content.* These in fact conceal the dream's true meaning, its *latent content,* which inevitably involves some form of wish fulfilment.

Suppose, for example, that a man dreams of a train rushing through a mountain tunnel and awakens to realize that he is sexually aroused. Or, he fights with his mother and later dreams that he is at a funeral where, strangely, no one seems sad. He asks who died. 'Your mother,' is the reply. We need not dig too deeply into the obscure symbolism for which Freud is so well known to discern the 'hidden' meanings — the latent content — behind the manifest events of these dreams.[9] In the first instance the train represents the erect phallus plunging through the symbolic vagina of the mountain tunnel.[10] In the second dream the death wish is expressed in a form that doesn't place direct blame on the dreamer, who appears only in third person and as an after-the-fact spectator to his mother's demise. Both dreams, however, enact wish fulfilments. According to psychoanalytic theory, both find their final symbolic (manifest) form through the influence of the superego, which packages the forbidden wishes in disguises that are minimally threatening to the conscious ego. Similar stories could be told of the psychic origins of clinical symptoms such as blindness, the loss of speech, of slips of the tongue, or failures of memory. Blindness, for example, could symbolically express a fear of sight, a desire never again to see some terrible truth. Such was the case with King Oedipus of Thebes who, in the ancient myth, blinded himself so as never again to see the terrible truth that he had murdered his own father and married his mother.

Returning to dreams, however, Politzer would agree with Freud that dreams may express desires in an unconventional form. But he would argue that this is no reason to postulate an entire unconscious mind. The problem, according to Politzer, seems to be an unwillingness on the part of Freud to allow the dream to speak its own language. Since the dream expresses wish fulfilment in a form other than the ordinary rational one, Freud supposed that there must be an ordinary expression of its meaning somewhere else. Somewhere there must be a linear narrative to account for the content of the dream.[11] Since such a linear narrative is not to be found in the manifest events of the dream, it must be hidden at a different level, namely at the level of the inferred latent content. It is this level that is associated with the unconscious mind. But wait a minute, if we would simply allow the dream to speak in its own terms there would be no need to postulate the nearby presence of a massive unconscious mind. In the words of the historian of the unconscious, David Archard, 'the purportedly unconscious wish ... is not absent from the narrated dream, only to be found at some distant place; it is present in, and immanent to, the dream, just as the rules of the game are present in a tennis match.' In other words, Freud was looking too hard for something hidden rather than allowing the dream simply to be itself.

These ideas are not at odds with modern criticisms of Freud. In a recent detailed review of scientific evidence relevant to psychoanalytic theory, Fisher and Greenberg conclude, 'there is no rationale for approaching a dream as if it were a container for a secret wish buried under layers of concealment.' In *The Dreaming Brain,* an exceptionally thorough book on the psychology and biology of dreams, neuropsychologist Allan Hobson comes to a similar conclusion. He writes:

> I differ from Freud in that I think that most dreams are neither obscure nor bowdlerized [censored], but rather that they are transparent and unedited. They reveal clearly meaningful, undisguised, and often highly conflictual themes worthy of note by the dreamer ... My position echoes Jung's notion of dreams as transparently meaningful and does away with any distinction between manifest and latent content.

Hobson places considerable stress on the creative aspects of dreaming, a point we will come back to. For the moment, let us note that he returns us to Politzer's original idea that the dream carries no excess baggage; the sleeping mind is not trying to conceal anything. This does not mean that dreams are easy to understand! As a matter of fact, however, the meaning of a dream (clinical symptom, slip of the tongue, etc.) is often less apparent to the subject than to others. Freud interpreted this as resistance generated by the psychic censor. Politzer and Sartre, on the other hand, point out that when it comes to understanding the meaning of our own dreams, as well as other expressions of our subjective lives, we are simply not in a privileged position. Let us examine what this means in terms of Sartre's notion of *thematization.*

Sartre argued that while consciousness perceives the entirety of its own content, it does not necessarily reflect on all facets of it. Certain elements of experience are not identified as themes in one's life. This means, for example, that I may be conscious of some desire, say, a hunger for sweets, but still not be able to tell anyone (including myself) that I have a sweet tooth. I just happen to eat sweets. Let us suppose that one day I notice I am gaining weight and on reflection realize that I've been feeding this sweet craving for several weeks. Now I have *thematized* my desire and may be able to act on it in an effective way, reducing my sweet intake or choosing less fattening sweets.

Even at this point I have not, in Sartre's terms, *conceptualized* the meaning of this craving in the broad context of my life. I might do this, for example, by coming to realize that it began with the breakup of a love relationship, and that such cravings have occurred in me before when romantic relationships were lost. It will probably take a shrewd objective observer, perhaps a psychotherapist, to see this clearly. When this is pointed out to me, I may find it difficult to accept. In time, however, I may come to understand where it began in my own personal history and to appreciate the full extent of its grip on my life.

The above example shows that we can discuss seemingly unconscious themes without appeal to unconscious motivations, much less to an unconscious mind. The entire matter can be reframed in terms of the thematization and conceptualization of aspects of our experience to which we simply do not attend. Furthermore, to argue that the failure to attend to these aspects is itself unconsciously motivated is to beg the question. The solution is to seek to thematize and finally conceptualize my sweet craving. I might recall, for example, that as a child my mother gave me sweets when I was upset. Rejecting the sweets was to invite her wrath. Today, I am still seeking solace in sweets, and still fear wrath if I reject them.

It is possible as well to be in love without knowing it. William James wrote:

> When I decide that I have, without knowing it, been for several weeks in love, I am simply giving a name to a state which previously *I have not named, but which was fully conscious.*

There is no need to conjure up an unconscious mind to account for what is missing in our own self-understanding.

Beyond the unconscious: complexity and creativity

What we seem to be faced with in trying to understand the human mind is a system of such exquisite complexity that at times it gives the appearance of several systems going at once. The depth of meaning that emerges from expressions such as dreams is so great, the content is so rich, that one is inclined to attribute metaphysical dimension to them. Both Freud and Jung drew heavily on a geological metaphor popular in the late nineteenth century, one of hidden strata. Plumbing the depths of the mind was like probing the depths of the earth, where deeper layers reveal increasing antiquity. While this metaphor has been very productive, it fractures the mental system into separate planes.

Looking at the exquisite moving arabesques created on the computer screen by chaos mathematics leads the eye to the impression of rich and changing depth. Reaching behind the screen to try to touch the source, however, would be to miss the point. The rich exfoliation of the mathematical expression that is programmed into the computer is sufficient alone to create the forms that please the eye. Moreover, in certain instances the results of programming a particular equation can be quite surprising. This is the case with fractal geometry, which must literally be explored as it unfolds, much as dreams must be explored as they unfold into consciousness.

In a complex and highly creative system the notion of an unconscious mind is metaphysical extra baggage. Beyond this, to attribute creativity — the creativity expressed in dreams, for instance — to an unconscious mind does not get us any closer to an understanding of it. It is true that dream images, like the imagination, enter consciousness through a border of Orphic liminality that surrounds awareness, but to conclude that they come from some other *place,* some other mind, adds nothing. It is the act of creation itself that we are experiencing, an act that emerges from the whole fabric of our conscious life. To shove it down into an unconscious mind doesn't explain it, and at the same time makes it gratuitously obscure.

Placing our emphasis, as does Hobson, on creativity, is very much in concert with Jung's notion that dreams express their meaning openly, though often through metaphor. I will not labor this point by reviewing the considerable literature that connects dreaming with creativity.[12] Let us simply note that dreams have often played a vital role in creativity, from Robert Louis Stevenson's conception of the plot for *Dr Jekyll and Mr Hyde,* to August von Kekulé's discovery of the chemical structure of the benzene ring. But the dream itself is its own greatest act of creation.

Jean Gebser was well aware of the natural human potential for creativity when he postulated the mythic structure of consciousness. As we have seen, this structure is characterized by the imagination and its ability to project the soul outward in the form of visual images. Let us not make the mistake, however, of solidifying this 'structure' of consciousness into a fragment of the inner person, separate from the rest. Its real significance is the human capacity to project creative and metaphoric narratives. Dreams are exactly this.

Karmic seeds and Jungian archetypes

Freud was not the only important theorist of the unconscious. I have focused on him so far because he developed a widely accepted model of a dynamic unconscious mind. There are, however, other conceptions of the unconscious that warrant our attention as well.

The notion that the mind is subject to influences from beyond the purview of consciousness is quite old in Eastern spiritual traditions. There, however, such ideas have rarely if ever have distilled into anything like the notion of a dynamic, organized mind. In Indian yogic philosophy, for instance, the unconsciousness is often viewed, at least in part, as a source of psychic noise, of emotional and mental perturbation. When one sits to meditate, for instance, one's mind is frequently filled by the raucous playback of thoughts and feelings from a busy outer life, much of which is presumably coming from impressions retained in the unconscious.

This view of the unconscious as a repository of impressions from the outer world is, in fact, very consistent with the complex systems view, in which we can imagine the mind as a self-creating system drawn into patterns of chaotic disorder by the demands and frustrations of the fast-track lives most of us live. Progress in spiritual work, on the other hand, generally requires that such patterns be abandoned so that we can overcome the internal noise so readily induced by the external disorder. Sri Aurobindo, for example, wrote:

> The first thing to do in the sadhana [spiritual work] is
> to get a settled peace and silence in the mind. Otherwise
> you may have experiences, but nothing will be permanent.
> It is in the silent mind that the true consciousness can be
> built.

On a deeper level, the unconscious in Eastern thought is often seen to be the repository of karmic 'seeds.' These are traces of thoughts and actions that are said to be carried forward from one lifetime to another, continuing to influence our thoughts and actions. They are the root source of karmic influences that draw us into certain situations or toward particular persons, and repel us from others. In some schools of Buddhism the layer of the mind that retains these seeds is referred to as *Alaya-vijnana,* literally 'storehouse consciousness.'[13] These seeds, which in systems theory we would refer to as control variables, are recognized as originating from beyond the boundaries of ordinary consciousness. But we find here no evidence of a dynamic unconscious mental process.

A Western concept reminiscent of the Eastern notion of the unconscious is Carl Jung's *collective unconscious.* Like the storehouse consciousness, it is a repository of influences which, when triggered by particular situations, come forward to deeply affect us. These influences are termed *archetypes.* Unlike the above seeds, however, they are not personal but universal, or *collective* — ideal themes and images that appear spontaneously in dreams and fantasies as well as in art, literature, and mythology.[14] Examples of archetypes include the hero, the earth goddess, the wise old man, the trickster, and many others. The Greek gods are virtually a study in archetypes, and the stories of their adventures are rife with archetypal motifs.[15] So are the tales of King Arthur and the knights of the Round Table. In the latter, Lancelot is the archetypal hero, Arthur the archetypal king, Merlin the archetypal wizard, and so on. Perhaps the most important feature of archetypes, however, is that we live them out in our day-to-day lives. Each of us plays the lover, the hero, the saint, and even the fool at some time or other. Indeed, participation in such themes would seem to be a vital part of living a deep and meaningful life.[16]

But just what are archetypes? According to Jung their roots penetrate down to the fundamental strata of reality itself, past even the distinctions between space, time, mind, and matter.[17] He believed that archetypes are built up from the accumulated experience of thousands of years of common, or collective human experience. For example, we might imagine that the presence of wise old men among tribal elders over many generations leads to the gradual imprinting of a familiarity with such persons, and ultimately to their crystalization in the human imagination.[18] Jung originally attributed this process to genetic memory, in other words to the gradual assimilation of common experiences over many generations into the genetic code.[19] These genetic changes ultimately found expression in the structure of the brain. In 1929 Jung wrote, 'the collective unconscious is simply the psychic expression of the identity of brain structure.'

From a neurological point of view this idea seems more than a little strained, and indeed has not generally been taken seriously. This, coupled with an absence of evidence in support of genetic memory, would seem to leave the notion of archetypes without a leg to stand on. Indeed, this has been a major point of criticism by hard-nosed scientists. Archetypes simply did not stand the acid test of the mechanistic science of Jung's day. Later in his life Jung himself seems to have more or less disregarded the notion of biological roots and came to treat archetypes simply as psychological realities.[20]

Ironically, today's science seems better suited to Jung's ideas than that of his own time. Sheldrake's morphic fields and Laszlo's psi-fields, as well as ideas from physics such as David Bohm's quantum potential, could provide a perfectly credible scientific foundation for archetypes. In Sheldrake's own words, 'morphic resonance theory would lead to a radical reaffirmation of Jung's concept of the collective unconscious,' that is, of archetypes. More recently Laszlo observed that:

> Jung's intuitive insight becomes clothed in the tangible
> substance of a [psi-field] theory that relates archetypes and
> the collective unconscious to the relationship between the
> living brain and the universe's basic energy field. This non-
> spatiotemporal field is the encoder and transmitter of all
> events in spacetime, including the neural network dynamics
> that underlie cognitive processes in human brains.

In Jung's psychology an understanding of the influence of archetypes, and thus of the collective unconscious, is important in understanding the deep structure of the inner person, or psyche. But we must ask, do such influences constitute an 'unconscious mind'? It would seem that what we have in the idea of archetypes is a nebulous array of influences that assert themselves in complex ways in the life of the individual. Jung himself wrote that 'the unconscious is not a second personality with organized and centralized functions but in all probability a decentralized congeries of psychic processes.'

Jung, however, did not consider archetypes to be passive. Far from it. They seem in fact to live lives of their own. In Jung's words:

> They form a species of singular beings whom one would like to endow with ego-consciousness; indeed, they almost seem capable of it. And yet this idea is not borne out by the facts ... They are masklike, wraithlike, without problems, lacking self-reflection, with no conflicts, no doubts, no sufferings; like gods, perhaps, who have no philosophy, such as the Brahma-gods of the *Samyutta-nikaya,* whose erroneous views needed correction by the Buddha. They evidently live and function in the deeper layers of the unconscious, especially ... the collective unconscious.

The apparently independent life of archetypes is seen both in dream material and in their influences on our waking lives. Dream characters, for example, are seen to change over periods of weeks, months, and even years. Less obvious but just as real are the gradual changes in waking life that reflect behind-the-scenes influences of archetypes. In my own opinion, however, these events do not require an explanation in terms of an independent unconscious mind. For example, the fact that archetypes as expressed through dreams seem to have a life of their own does not imply that they possess a degree of reality beyond that imparted to them by the wide realms of the imagination. Novelists tell us that characters about which they write can take on lives of their own. The writer may not know what the character will do from one scene to the next. We do not, however, assume such characters to be living independent lives in the writer's head, like figures moving in a fairy castle. Rather, we understand that writing is a creative process which allows the mysterious and unbounded play of the imagination.

Jung himself, as seen in the above quotation, was careful not to attribute ego consciousness to archetypes. Indeed, a careful reading of his work, and that of more recent Jungians, discloses, at least to my mind, that the apparent autonomous life of archetypes, though powerful, is more chimaeric than real. Their masklike, or wraithlike, projections appear on the screens of our rapidly changing lives giving the illusion of animation, when in fact it is *us,* the living, waking persons, that undergo dynamic growth and change.

I am not suggesting that the concept of archetypes is not useful, only that it does not require an 'unconscious mind.' Similarly, the influences of archetypes on the emotions and decisions of waking lives do not require the mediation of an unconscious. We short-change ourselves when we appeal to explanations which lie hidden beyond the creative dynamics of our being.

Archetypes as self-organizing fields

Given the previous discussions in this book, it is natural to wonder if archetypes fit in the overall plan of the perennial philosophy. At what level, if any, is their influence felt in terms of the traditional planes of being? Ken Wilber, for instance, refers to certain archetypes as 'highly advanced structures lying in the high-subtle and low-causal' planes. Wilber's archetypes, however, are not Jung's archetypes. Whereas Jung's archetypes are grounded in the evolutionary history of the species and are associated with the instinctual nature of the psyche, Wilber's archetypes are projections of the higher self, projections that can appear as beings in their own right when one achieves a state of identification with the higher subtle and lower causal planes. In his own words:

> It is a realm of higher presences, guides, angelic beings,
> ishtadevas, and dhyana-buddhas; all of which ... are simply
> high archetypal forms of one's own being (although they
> initially and necessarily appear 'other').

These observations are in perfect agreement with Sri Aurobindo, who, as we saw, noted that 'the beings native to the Overmind [causal plane] are gods.' Here, however, we have apparently left the domain of Jungian archetypes and entered into a discourse of phenomena native to the very highest forms of consciousness. Whatever the status of these appearances, they do not seem to be the archetypes that play a vital role in the psychology of day-to-day life in the ordinary world.

Returning to Jungian archetypes, let us note that the most credible modern explanation of them would seem to be in terms of something like Laszlo's psi-field or Sheldrake's morphic resonance. Could such fields exhibit the active qualities Jung often associated with archetypes? Such fields might, as Laszlo suggests, be formed by wavefunctions of the quantum potential type, built up into complex nested structures of a non-local nature.[21] For the sheer sake of speculation, let us imagine that such enormously complex structures might evolve semi-autonomous self-organizing dynamics of their own. In other words, that they are self-organizing systems, existing perhaps in a symbiotic relationship to the physical brain. Going this far, we might further suppose that they could even interact with each other.

These highly speculative thoughts evoke the specter of truly godlike forces acting in an all but eternal realm of their own. The magnitude and strangeness of such a vision staggers the imagination, but agrees surprisingly well with Jung's concept of archetypes. One is reminded of a science fiction motif that describes the spontaneous appearance of intelligence in the ultra-complex, self-organizing information structures of large computers or networks of computers. Novelist William Gibson, in *Count Zero,* creates a world in which godlike beings are auto-created in a future world-wide information network. He in fact gives them the names of Voodoo gods. Like true archetypes, they move in a nebulous, immaterial realm of the vast global network. And very much like Jungian archetypes, their appearance is often unexpected and charged with numinous power.

At present it is impossible to make even a preliminary guess as to the likelihood that complex nested psi-field structures could acquire an autonomous archetypal life of their own. So, to keep a modicum of credibility in this discussion I will not entertain the idea further. Thus, we are left with the basic question of the nature of psychological archetypes unanswered, though we have seen some intriguing candidates for this position. Let us now turn again to the issue of the unity of consciousness.

Divided states of consciousness

The greatest challenge to the unity of consciousness idea is not the unconscious mind, but certain exotic states in which consciousness itself seems to be divided. The turn-of-the-century French psychiatrist, Pierre Janet, for instance, visualized the mind not as a hierarchy of layered strata, but as a one-storied house with several rooms. The latter metaphor, today revised as *neodissociation theory* by the prominent American psychologist Ernest Hilgard, offers the possibility that consciousness can be in more than one room at the same time, or in other words that it can actually divide into separate but parallel streams.[22]

Janet had been a student of Jean-Martin Charcot, in Paris, with whom Freud himself studied as a young man. Charcot was famous for demonstrating that hysterical symptoms (nowadays called *conversion reactions)* such as blindness or the paralysis of a limb could be created and also temporarily cured when the patient was under hypnosis. In such demonstrations it became clear that hypnosis represents a state of mind distinct from ordinary consciousness. In fact, as early as 1870 it had become apparent to some observers that the hypnotic state is subjectively divided, 'as though the hypnotized part of the person was on stage, carrying out the behavior and having the subjective experience of the hypnotized person, while another part was as if in the wings, watching what was going on and ready to pull the actor off the stage.' Alfred Binet, creator of the first intelligence test, also commented on this aspect of the hypnotic experience in his 1889 book, *On Double Consciousness.*

The latter years of the last century saw a considerable interest in multiple personalities, in which an individual at different times exhibits two or more seemingly independent mental and behavioral patterns. It was in 1886 that the most famous story of all time about a multiple personality was written, the above-mentioned *Dr Jekyll and Mr Hyde.* Recent evidence indicates that persons with multiple personality disorders may even exhibit distinctive brain wave-patterns which correspond to each of their different personalities.

Multiple states of mind can be conceptualized in the complex systems framework as separate attractors.[23] Passing from one attractor to another amounts to a catastrophic bifurcation from one personality to another. In Figures 13 and 14 we see two hypothetical examples of such attractor patterns, the first representing two personalities and the second representing three. In each case consciousness tends to flow in one attractor till circumstances are appropriate for it to travel down the thin trajectory to another, where it remains till conditions there are right for a return trip to the original attractor or for a switch to yet a third one.[24]

An important question about multiple personality disorders is whether or not the two (or more) basins represent the fragmentation of a single previous attractor that existed some time earlier. In other words, did the person once have a unified personality? A view that is now receiving considerable attention is that, due to a disturbed childhood, a single well-defined attractor basin failed to form in the first place. One might imagine the infant personality as something like a cloud of processes that ordinarily congeal into a single structure. In the early stages of development, many potential or proto-personalities might even form, later to come together to make the final multifacetted personality.[25] A badly disturbed environment, however, could interrupt the final stage of this process, resulting in several separate personality systems, or a multiple personality.

A related situation is one in which two streams of consciousness appear to exist in parallel. William James discussed the existence of 'secondary personal selves' in cases of hysteria, post-hypnotic suggestion, and the like.[26] He reviewed a case reported by Pierre Janet involving a patient who suffered the hysterical loss of sensations to one hand. This symptom, common at the turn of the century, was known as *hand-in-glove* anaesthesia, because it presents a loss of sensation up to the wrist, as if the hand were covered by an anaesthetic glove. The condition corresponds to no known neurological disorder. James observed that:

> M. Janet caught the actual moment of [the creation of] one
> of these secondary personalities in his anaesthetic som-
> nambulist Lucie. He found that when this young woman's
> attention was absorbed in conversation with a third party,

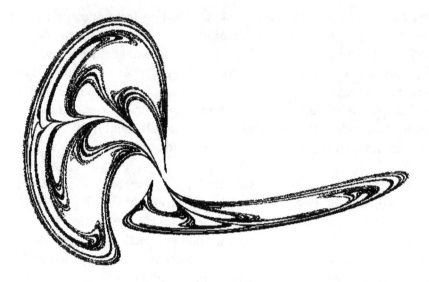

Figures 13 and 14. Three-dimensional phase portraits that suggest multiple personalities. Each chaotic attractor represents a single personality connected to the others by a thin trajectory.

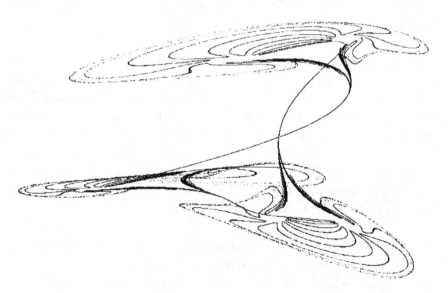

her anaesthetic hand would write simple answers to questions whispered to her by himself. 'Do you hear?' he asked. *'No,'* was the unconsciously written reply. 'But to answer you must hear.' *'Yes, quite so.'* 'Then how do you manage?' *'I don't know.'* 'There must be someone who hears me. *'Yes.'* 'Who?' *'Someone other than Lucie.'*

The conversation continued with Janet finally suggesting a name, 'Adrienne,' for this secondary personality. He observed that the personality grew into a 'more definite outline,' displaying an awareness of the sensations from the very anaesthetic arm that was excluded from the primary personality.

Hugh Lynn Cayce, psychic researcher and son of noted clairvoyant Edgar Cayce, described a dramatic case in which experimentation with a Ouija board led to what appears to be such a secondary personality.[27] It began when a young woman and her husband discovered that they could get interesting and sometimes apparently psychic answers from the Ouija board. Through the board the woman was soon told to take up automatic writing, which worked almost immediately for her. Such writing, by the way, can be produced by almost anyone simply by putting a pencil to a piece of paper and letting the hand move at random until eventually it begins to write of its own accord. I do not recommend it, however, for reasons obvious in this story. In fact, for this woman the automatic writing lasted only a short time until she began to hear a voice behind her left ear. It was at first soft and friendly, but in a few days became harsh and demanding, threatening to take her life by starvation. She soon found she could not eat without throwing up. At this point the situation was entirely out of hand and she was forced by desperation to seek professional help.

In cases such as these we seem to be confronted with a rare instance of two actual streams of consciousness proceeding simultaneously and independently of each other. Here, the models represented in Figures 13 and 14 must be modified to represent not a single system that periodically oscillates between two or more attractor basins, but systems which exist independently of each other, each in its own attractor basin as shown in Figure 15. In most instances it would appear that one system contains the bulk of the control structures we associate with a normal personality, while the other contains a limited set of functions that have been disconnected, or 'dissociated,' from the primary one. Janet believed that all such secondary personalities are abnormal, lurking, in James' words, 'in the background whilst the other appears on the surface as the only self the man or woman has.'

A recent and well known demonstration of parallel consciousness involves 'split-brain' patients, persons who have undergone a surgical disconnection of the two cerebral hemispheres. As early as the later eighteen hundreds Gustav Fechner — arguably the first experimental psychologist in history — stated that if the corpus callosum, the great fiber bundle that connects the two cerebral hemispheres, were to be severed, two entirely separate minds would result, each running its own independent course with its own thoughts.[28] In 1911 the prominent American psychologist William McDougall expressed the opposing view that consciousness must of necessity be unitary, even if the corpus callosum were severed. He went so far as to volunteer himself for such an operation in the event that he should ever contract a terminal illness! Happily for him, but not for posterity, he contracted no such illness and the question remained unanswered.

In the 1940s a series of operations severing the corpus callosum were performed to control cases of intractable epilepsy. The results were resoundingly uninteresting. Aside from dramatic improvements in the epilepsy itself the post-operative patients seemed perfectly normal — aside from various brain disorders that had been present to begin with and had probably contributed to the epilepsy. Not till the 1960s, when neurosurgeon Joseph Bogen teamed up with California Institute of Technology neurobiologist Roger Sperry on a similar series of operations, did the reality of divided consciousness in these patients become apparent. This was shown through ingenious experiments devised by Sperry. I will not review these in detail, or the subsequent debate as to whether or not split-brain subjects exhibit true intelligence in both hemispheres.[29] I will only note that in 1979 Sperry demonstrated beyond any doubt that the right brain as well as the left is capable of intelligence and self-conscious sensitivity, though its use of language is very limited. He did this by a very simple and decisive experiment. Without his patients' knowledge he obtained old familiar family photographs of them and their relatives. Part of the experiment

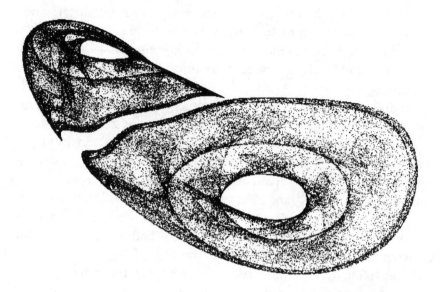

Figure 15. Here we have chaotic attractors that exist simultaneously and independently of each other, as in rare cases of multiple consciousness.

involved using a special procedure to present these photographs to each patient so that only his or her right hemisphere saw them, being sure that the left language hemisphere did not know their content. The response to these intimate, embarrassing, and touching photographs, though often more emotional than verbal, was so perfectly normal that there could no longer be any serious doubt that the right brain is intelligent and socially conscious. Since there has never been a question as to the presence of consciousness and intelligence in the left brain, it seems apparent that in 'split-brain' persons both hemispheres exhibit parallel and separate streams of consciousness.

A broad reading of the research on split-brain persons leaves one with the impression that these individuals exhibit a dual-consciousness which in some ways is reminiscent of Janet's primary and secondary personalities. The left hemisphere supports the primary personality, which retains ordinary language abilities, exhibits a strong sense of self, and exerts control over most of the person's behavior. The right hemisphere, on the other hand, supports the secondary personality, which in most people retains the lion's share of the person's abilities for holistic visual thinking, for art and music, and possibly for intuition and emotional expression. Both seem to have a normal degree of social awareness. Apparently, when the corpus callosum is cut the conscious mind itself is bisected creating two separate streams of experience.

The division created by split-brain surgery is inflicted on consciousness by an alteration of the brain itself. Janet's hysteric patients, on the other hand, exhibited a spontaneous dissociation of consciousness. Recently, Ernest Hilgard made a study of certain instances of dissociation that he was able to create in the laboratory.[30] He was not dealing with pathology as was Janet, but the removal of the sensation of pain under hypnosis. The pain was produced when a hypnotized volunteer placed his or her hand and lower arm into a bath of ice water while receiving the suggestion that no pain would be felt.

Hilgard found that while pain could be greatly reduced in the awareness of the hypnotized subject, a deeper and apparently dissociated part of the person — which Hilgard termed the 'hidden observer' — recorded the exact portion that was in this fashion omitted. In other words, if the hypnotized person reported only twenty percent of the equivalent waking pain the hidden observer was apparently experiencing the other eighty percent. This finding suggests, as did Janet's work a hundred years ago, that under unusual circumstances consciousness is capable of division into two separate streams. If this were not enough, psychologist Crabtree more recently has observed that in a single person different hypnotic states produce different hidden observers![31] Evidently where consciousness is concerned there is potential for systems nested within systems, and these parallel to yet other systems.

Being of a divided mind

At this point I would like to recall some thoughts on consciousness from Chapter 1. There I stuck my neck out and stated my opinion that, when all is said and done, consciousness is no more — and no less — than a *presence* that is *about* something. It is not thought, it is not imagination, nor is it memory or desire. It is not feelings or sensations. All of these are part of the landscape of consciousness; they are among the events of which we are aware. Thought, imagination, and memory reasonably fit the category of *mind,* while feelings and sensations are more rudimentary. Desire is somewhere in between. In plain English, however, consciousness is what it is to experience the world of thoughts, memories, desires, tastes, smells, textures, trees, clouds, rocks, frogs, shoes, and people — but it is itself none of them.

So what sense does it mean to speak of *divided consciousness?* Shoes come in pairs; they are already divided. Trees can be divided — with an axe. One can have conflicting desires, disparate opinions, and feel hot and cold at the same time. One can be of a divided mind. But what would one divide if one were to divide one's consciousness? The answer can only be that one would divide the objects of consciousness — what one is aware of. From this point of view fragmented consciousness is like moonlight shining on white clouds in an otherwise dark sky.

Attention, the dynamic aspect of consciousness, can easily be divided. Suppose that while I am reading a book a thrush starts singing outside my window. Let us further suppose I am so absorbed in my book that I do not notice it. Putting the book down, however, I find my mind turning to the song of the bird. But wait a minute. I was in fact reading at the time and not at all conscious of the song, while now recollection tells me plainly that I heard it, and what is more, was comforted by it! Probably such instances are common, happening to all of us virtually every day. We just do not often recall them later.

Many tasks seem to require some degree of divided attention. Suppose I am driving a car and carrying on a conversation at the same time. Under ordinary circumstances I can do this perfectly well, and even listen to the car radio. Each task gets part of my attention. If something occurs down the road that demands urgent action, however, I must stop my conversation and perhaps turn off the radio as well. Evidently I can attend to several things at once only if none of them is especially demanding. When one requires all my resources I give it my full attention and become conscious only of driving.

Now there is a fundamental difference between the above instance of hearing the thrush while reading, and the example of talking or listening to the radio while driving the car. In the latter I am know-ingly conscious of all I am doing — driving, talking, listening to the radio — while in the former — hearing the thrush — the part of me reading the book is totally unaware of the singing bird. They say one can have pain like this as well, never noticing it, and surely one can have psychological pain for years, never attending to it at all until it is somehow eased. Then one may cry with relief. These examples move ominously in the direction of Janet's 'secondary personal selves,' in which a significant piece of the apparatus of mind dissoci-ates itself from the rest of the personality. In all these instances, how-ever, it is the content of consciousness that is fractured, while con-sciousness itself, like the moonlight on the clouds, presents only the illusion of fragmentation. Itself, it is neither whole nor scattered. Freud made the mistake of treating consciousness as if it were a thing rather than an event, of making it a noun instead of a verb. This got him to an 'unconscious mind' that makes no sense. Let us not do the same.

Consciousness takes the form of its container. If the mind is mean, small, and self-centered, then consciousness is likewise limited. On the other hand, as the mind grows, opening itself to larger horizons both within and without, so consciousness bursts forth like light across an ever widening landscape. This will be the theme of the next chapter.

11. A Condition of Complete Simplicity

Conscious evolution and spiritual practice

*The soul goes ... through an evolution which leads it up to
the human state and evolves through it all a being that
supports the evolution and develops a physical, a vital, a
mental human consciousness ... All this is done from behind
a veil ... But a time comes when it is able to ... take
command and turn all the instrumental nature towards a
divine fulfilment. This is the beginning of a spiritual life.
The soul is able now to make itself ready for a higher
evolution of manifest consciousness.*

Sri Aurobindo

*Practice on ourselves, in the physical and spiritual sense, is
always of two kinds. It involves both the pulling-down of
everything that stands in the way of our contact with Divine
Being, and building-up of a 'form' which ... preserves this
contact and affirms it in every activity.*

Karlfried Graf Dürckheim

This chapter is about spiritual work, or the ways people have systematically approached the growth and transformation of consciousness.
Building on the foundations laid in previous chapters we will explore
certain technologies of the spirit, especially those practiced by the
perennial wisdom traditions of the world. In the process we will also
come to a richer understanding of ourselves.

At risk of putting the cart before the horse, I believe it will be
helpful here at the beginning of the chapter to have a rough notion of
where we are going, as well as an introduction to the map that will get
us there.

Two ancient orientations of the spirit

Two paradoxically disparate themes can be recognized as running throughout the history of human spirituality. These have dramatically different implications for the spiritual cultivation of consciousness. The first appeared in the Hindu *Rig Veda* roughly three thousand years ago, and holds that life in this world is essentially good. To eat, drink, make love, raise children, and share the joys and hardships of our families, are not to be avoided, but experienced in sacred fullness. The second appears in the Upanishads a few hundred years later. It is the idea that worldly life is not good, and that the wise person should seek escape from the whole vortex of earthly existence.[1]

Both views, which continue in one form or another to the present day, consider life *as ordinarily lived* to be inadequate, but the first aspires to a better, richer, earthly life, while the second seeks to escape corporeal life entirely. At its highest octave the first leads to the cultivation of an inner attitude of joy while overcoming pain at its root. This is not a hedonistic goal of sensual or even psychological gratification, but the inspiration to a rich life through wisdom and growth toward spiritual realization. The second view on the other hand emphasizes the unsatisfactory nature of life in this world and seeks release from it through complete absorption in the absolute.[2]

A parallel division is found in the history of Buddhism.[3] This polarity extends beyond wisdom traditions and into mysticism in general, where we find a dual movement toward affirming the world and, alternatively, withdrawing from it. Contemporary theologian Matthew Fox, for instance, distinguishes two kinds of mysticism in the history of Christianity. The first is introverted, emphasizing the mortification of the senses and a rejection of worldly life. The second is life-affirming and creation-centered, emphasizing the celebration of 'the primal sacrament, the primal mystery that is the universe.' It 'recognizes passion, the body, the senses, and sensuality as part of the divine gift, the original blessing that touches the depths of awe and gratitude in our lives.'

In the pages that follow we will find that these two attitudes have influenced the technologies of consciousness, either toward withdraw-

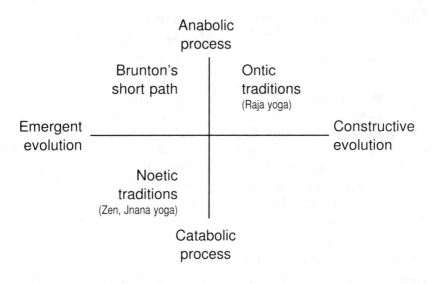

Figure 16. The coordinate system discussed in the text is presented here with two axes: emergent vs. constructive evolution, and anabolic vs. catabolic processes.

ing from the world and seeking realization in solitude and retreat from life, or alternatively toward seeking a rich and *realized* life in the world. It is the latter that will be of greatest interest here. This is because it seems more consistent with the realities of modern life, and because it represents an *integral* form of life and of consciousness — ideas to which we will return.

Now, about the map that will get us there.

The coordinate system

The intention of this map, actually a coordinate system, is not only to provide an overview of the technologies of consciousness that we will be looking at in detail as we continue, but at the same time to highlight the differences between these technologies. It will inject a degree of order into what appears on the surface to be a welter of practices, beliefs, and cultural biases. The system has three major axes, as represented in Figure 16. The first deals with how the practitioner of a given tradition is changed by that tradition — through rapid transformation or by gradual growth. The second deals with the tradition's goals and philosophy. The third deals with the mechanisms by which each practice works.

Axis one: Constructive versus emergent evolution

In Chapter 9 we examined three types of evolution. These were, first, *biological evolution,* for example of the Darwinian type, second, *historical evolution,* the broad informal notion of growth or change with the passage of time, and third, the *grand evolutionary synthesis* with its emphasis on complex self-organizing systems. Another way to think about evolution is in terms of whether it proceeds through the more or less gradual accumulation of individual changes, or advances by broad and sometimes swift transformations. The first type might be termed *constructive evolution* and the latter *emergent evolution.* Let me explain.

Now consider the growth and transformation of consciousness. One way these processes can occur is by the gradual accumulation, or piecing together, of individual elements. This is how a house is built. It is also the way intelligence develops during childhood, as we saw in Piaget's theory. An instance of this type of process among wisdom traditions is seen in Classical (Raja) Yoga, of which I will have much more to say below. On the other hand, certain conditions can lead to more abrupt transitions — the rapid emergence of complexity or the appearance of order where none existed before. We saw this in the formation of Bénard cells, in which hexagonal convection currents suddenly and spontaneously appear in water or air that is heated. Another instance occurs when lightning strikes sand. The sand is instantly fused into a complex glass structure that can resemble a large leaf. This is emergent evolution. A psychological example is the spontaneous emergence of deep insight during psychotherapy. Among spiritual traditions one thinks of the powerful restructuring of a Zen student's experience during koan practice. In the language of chaos theory such examples of emergent evolution are catastrophic bifurcations.[4]

Of the major thinkers we have examined, Vico, Hegel, Sri Aurobindo, Bergson, and Teilhard de Chardin espoused evolutionary theories of the constructive type. Gebser's theory, on the other hand, is about emergent evolution. It is for this reason that he chose to describe the appearance of each new structure of consciousness as a *mutation,* implying a radical bifurcation of structure. Wilber's theory seems likewise to deal essentially with emergent evolution. His highest stages of consciousness seem clearly to be best understood as emergent. He moors the early stages more tightly to actual historical epochs, however, than does Gebser, giving them a more historical or constructive flavor.

Axis two: Ontic versus noetic traditions

Certain wisdom traditions emphasize the realization of higher or more real levels of *being* while others emphasize the attainment of insight or *knowledge.* The first strives toward the *real* while the second strives toward the *true.* I will term these the *ontic* traditions (ontogenic or having to do with *being)* and the *noetic* traditions (having to do with knowing). Students of ontic traditions tend to progress by a constructive evolution while those of the noetic traditions progress by emergent evolution. Here I am drawing in broad strokes, but bear with me.

Not surprisingly, there is a tendency for ontic traditions to be concerned with the perennial subtle levels of being. Hinduism, which is founded in Vedanta and includes most forms of Indian yoga, follows an ontic progression through these subtle planes, leading toward the ultimate source of all being, absorption in *Brahman.* This progression is seen perhaps most clearly in Classical Yoga, with practices that lift the student step by step to ever more subtle realms of experience. In this progression illusion, or *maya,* finally falls away and one comes face to face with Reality. The yogin is then grounded in the Self (Atman), the true essence of his Being. In practical terms this concern with the subtle realms comes down to acquiring mastery of certain states of consciousness which are said to participate in these realms. The accessibility of these states depends on the extent to which the practitioner acquires physical and mental structures that will support them. Much of what is said below about the ontic traditions concerns the cultivation of such structures.[5]

Noetic traditions, on the other hand, tend not to be concerned with subtle realms of being, but work instead with cognitive structures. For instance most schools of Buddhism are committed to a noetic exploration of the human condition, in particular of the root cause of human suffering in individual ignorance, and so they emphasize mind and its role in the creation of the state of illusion and suffering in which we all live. The prominent Buddhist scholar Herbert Guenther comments that, 'The emphasis on mind/mentation ... is already present in early Buddhist thought,' and has remained central to it ever since.

Buddhism tends to see consciousness in an expansive cognitive framework which includes psychological processes in general. In its practices it encourages one to develop an accurate awareness of one's own experience, of the nature and content of one's own mind. This emphasis is seen, for example, in the style of meditation in which one simply and directly observes the content of consciousness. *Vipassana,* or Insight Meditation is an example of this, and could well be the single most widely practiced meditation in the world today. The emphasis on cognition or mentation is also seen in Zen Buddhism, in which the following story is typical:

> Two monks were arguing about a flag. One said: 'The flag is moving.'
> The other said: 'The wind is moving.'
> The sixth patriarch happened to be passing by. He told them: 'Not the wind, not the flag; mind is moving.'

Interestingly, the potential disorders or 'pathologies' that occur in connection with spiritual practices tend to be different in the ontic and the noetic traditions. Those of the ontic traditions may involve the awakening of subtle energies or powers before the student is adequately prepared to handle them. Wilber refers to these as *psychic disorders,* because they manifest at the pranic or, in his terms, psychic level of being. Pathologies of the noetic traditions, on the other hand, are often the product of frightening insights or misunderstandings. The so-called Zen sickness, for example, is the result of mistakenly identifying raptures and ecstasies of the subtle realm with ultimate realization itself.[6] A story is told of the student whose meditation was interrupted by a grand vision of a bodhisattva descending in glory, his body wrapped in halos of subtle flame. In great excitement the student ran to his master to tell him of the vision. The latter listened quietly then advised the student: 'Continue to concentrate on your breathing and it will go away!'

The ontic and the noetic paths may well ascend to something like a common ground. Many have argued that the 'final' forms of all authentic spiritual paths are, in fact, the same. There is increasing reason, however, to suspect that the final achievements of the diverse paths are not all the same, a point to which we will return below.[7]

Interestingly, there is a small but important class of traditions that seem to bridge the ontic-noetic division. These are exemplified by Indian Jnana Yoga, often called the yoga of knowledge or wisdom. This form of yoga springs straight from the Vedanta philosophy and its goal is direct identification with the Self. In other words, in Jnana Yoga one aims to consciously become nothing less than one's own true nature. This is achieved, however, not by the cultivation of the lower and intermediate levels of being, as in Classical Yoga, but in the Buddhist fashion of seeking direct intuitive penetration into the very essence of being. It departs, however, from the Buddhist bent toward overcoming illusion to stress, rather, the fulfilment of the ancient Hindu prayer, 'Lead me from the unreal to the Real.' In this sense it fulfils the ontic ideal of striving toward unity with ultimate reality. Jnana is often associated with the teaching of *neti, neti* ('not this, not this'). For example, to the question, 'Who am I?' the great Indian sage Ramana Maharshi, in a living demonstration of Jnana Yoga, answered: 'I am not the gross body, I am not the five senses, I am not my thoughts or emotions, I am not the subtle prana ...' And after negating all such answers, he said of that Awareness which alone remains: 'That I am.'

In the spirit of Jnana Yoga, one of the rare modern Western sages, also a student of Ramana Maharshi, Paul Brunton, described what he termed the *short path*. It is the habit of constantly reminding ourselves of our true nature. This leads to a form of practice that, in his own words, 'begins and ends with the goal itself':

The notion that we must wait and wait while we slowly
progress out of enslavement into liberation, out of ignorance

into knowledge, out of the present limitations into a future
union with the Divine, is only true if we let it be so. But we
need not. We can shift our identification from the ego to the
Overself [Self] in our habitual thinking, in our daily
reactions and attitudes, in our response to events and the
world ... By incessantly remembering what we really are,
here and now at this very moment, we set ourselves free.
Why wait for what already is?

Brunton, however, warns against taking up the short path without
plenty of preparation in the basics. 'The danger of the Short Path, and
of the 'As If' exercise, is to fall into deception of oneself, or even into
charlatanic deception of others.' Indeed, there are those who have not
only deluded themselves, but many others as well.[8]

Axis three: Anabolic versus catabolic practices

Returning to our coordinate system, the third distinction I want to
draw is between what I will term *anabolic* and *catabolic* practices. In
the language of chemistry, anabolic processes refer to constructive
metabolism — something is built. Catabolic processes, on the other
hand, refer to destructive metabolism — something is broken down or
taken apart.[9] The importance of these ideas to the present inquiry is
that most spiritual practices are either primarily anabolic or catabolic
in their impact on the mind and consciousness. Put in briefest com-
pass, what we find is that ontic paths tend to stress anabolic practices
leading to a constructive evolutionary development of the individual,
while noetic paths tend to stress catabolic practices that destabilize
ordinary consciousness, thus opening the way to catastrophic bifurcations which result in emergent evolution. Let us now put these ideas
to work.

The anabolic agenda: building from the bottom up
Some of the most revered wisdom traditions start the student off with
rules of conduct, attitude, diet, and exercise, all intended to lay a foundation on which the great work can later be built.[10] Classical or Raja
Yoga, as outlined in Patanjali's great *Yoga Sutra,* is a model instance

of an ontic path that cultivates the constructive evolution of the consciousness.[11] It involves eight 'limbs' arranged like a ladder of ascending phases of practice. The first two limbs lay a foundation of 'restraints' and 'observances' *(yamas* and *niyamas)*, which on the surface appear to be moral directives. In fact, they are guidelines for thought and behavior which establish a frame of mind conducive to advanced yogic practices. The restraints include the practice of non-violence in thought and action, an attitude of honesty, an absence of possessiveness, and so on. The observances include striving for purity of mind and heart, contentment (but not complacent satisfaction) with one's life, self-study, and surrender to a higher principle. As may already be apparent, if followed systematically and sincerely, these, or even any one of them, can amount to an entire practice in its own right.

In like fashion early schools of Buddhism such as the Sthavira, Vaibha-sika, and the Yogacara followers, developed amazingly sophisticated psychologies that emphasize those qualities of mind that promote a healthy outlook, as opposed to those which can 'pollute' one's psychological constitution.[12] These emphasize, for example, the cultivation of a general attitude of trust and confidence, at the same time overcoming irritability and conceit.

In his 1944 classic, *The Perennial Philosophy,* Aldous Huxley observed, 'In Buddhism, as in Vedanta and in all but the most recent forms of Christianity, right action is the means by which the mind is prepared for contemplation.' Psychiatrist Daniel Brown recently studied three meditation traditions, including Classical Yoga, the Tibetan Mahamudra, and Theravada Vipassana. He reports that each specifies principles of conduct and ethical practice that help set the stage for later work. In his words, these practices 'affect a complete psycho-behavioral transformation in order to prepare the beginner for formal meditation at some later point.'

Returning to the example of Raja Yoga again, the third limb of the yoga is the practice of *asanas,* or postures, importantly including meditative poses. Students also may practice various exercises popularly known as Hatha Yoga. This is helpful in creating a supple and healthy body, very useful for the more advanced work. Hatha can also be cultivated to the point of consciously working with the subtle energies of the body, though this is uncommon outside India. The fourth limb of Raja Yoga is the practice of breath control or *prana-yama.* Prana is associated with the breath and its practice brings the student into conscious contact with the subtle energies of the body. The final four limbs of Raja Yoga have to do with concentration, with meditation, and finally with several levels of *samadhi,* or absorption, leading finally to pure spiritual absorption. Thus, in the entire process of following the path of Classical Yoga the practitioner is led to successively subtler levels of being, and ultimately into the Absolute.[13]

Sri Aurobindo's *Integral Yoga,* described in Chapter 7, strives to transform the entire physical, mental, and spiritual being. While it does not prescribe particular diets or physical exercises, Sri Aurobindo and the Mother often emphasized the importance of exercise and physical as well as mental health in order to be prepared for the powerful subtle energies that are released later in the practice. Failure in this can lead to what Sri Aurobindo termed the 'yogic illness,' which evidently can include a variety of physical problems ranging from allergies to heart disorders as well as psychological problems.[14]

A survey of the literature of the wisdom traditions suggests, however, that psychological preparation is at least as important as work with the physical body, if not more so. Indeed, so widespread are the mandates for such preparation that they have sometimes been thought to be part and parcel with the perennial philosophy itself. Aldous Huxley, for example, wrote:

> The Perennial Philosophy is primarily concerned with the one, divine Reality substantial to the manifold world of things and lives and mind. But the nature of this one Reality is such that it cannot be directly and immediately apprehended except by those who have chosen to fulfil certain conditions, making themselves loving, pure in heart, and poor in spirit. Why should this be so? We do not know. It is just one of those facts which we have to accept, whether we like them or not and however implausible and unlikely they may seem.

Along related lines, it is the general consensus among transpersonal psychologists that a healthy ego is an important prerequisite for beginning the spiritual work.[15] Despite the fact that most traditions emphasize the ultimate transcendence of the ego in some form or other, the psychological stresses that are almost certain to occur during the early and middle stages of the work necessitate that the individual be well-organized in order to overcome them. It is likewise a mistake to throw oneself into spiritual disciplines as a way to solve personal problems, or as a substitute for psychotherapy. Such disciplines are *not* an answer to problems of immaturity, poor ego development, or poor adjustment in general. Indeed, engaging in them often makes one's problems actually become worse. Ken Wilber once commented in an interview:

> If you're doing meditation correctly, you're in for some
> very rough and frightening times. Meditation as a
> 'relaxation response' is a joke. Genuine meditation involves
> a whole series of deaths and rebirths; extraordinary conflicts
> and stresses come into play. All of this is just barely
> balanced by an equal growth in equanimity, compassion,
> understanding, awareness, and sensitivity, which makes the
> whole endeavor worthwhile.

Practices such as meditation can, for instance, bring up repressed anger and hostility that has previously been keep under wraps.[16] We have to deal with these. Otherwise we may, on the one hand, be overwhelmed by them, or on the other, find our lives degraded by subtle anger and depression of which we are largely in denial. This is not something to be taken lightly. For example, after years of intensive spiritual work the writer, teacher, activist, and translator of Eastern thought, Ram Dass, found himself face to face with episodes of serious emotional turbulence for which psychotherapy was quite helpful.[17] I personally believe it helpful for most students of wisdom traditions to engage in at least intermittent psychotherapy or analysis, say, of the Jungian variety, while continuing their spiritual work.[18]

The catabolic agenda: deconstructing ordinary consciousness
The practices prescribed by schools of perennial wisdom often seem to act as catabolic or corrosive agents against ordinary forms of mind,

while at the same time leading toward the (anabolic) construction of new ones. An example is meditation. Over the long term the practice of meditation seems to erode away at current states of consciousness and the structures that support them, while simultaneously shifting the practitioner toward new and more subtle ones. This erosion process can be understood as a dismantling of whatever psychological processes dominate at the moment. After surveying a variety of meditative traditions Brown came to the conclusion that:

> [the] underlying path is best conceptualized as a systematic deconstruction of the structures of ordinary waking consciousness ... As a result of dismantling the coordinates of ordinary perception, the meditator gains access to a non-ordinary, or extraordinary, structure of consciousness which does not operate by ordinary psychophysical laws. Deconstruction of even this deep state results in enlightenment.

Needless to say, the living effects of such deconstruction go well beyond shifts in awareness during meditation itself. They extend into one's daily life, often wreaking havoc on long-term emotional and behavioral patterns. Such effects are perhaps most prominent during the initial phases of the work, when old habits are first being eroded away and long term neurotic adjustments suddenly become no longer workable. In the same vein, the work itself is often most difficult in the early stages. It is during this period, for example, that the student is most easily distracted from the path. Continuing in the work, one eventually becomes 'established' and is less likely to lose balance. *The Gospel of Sri Ramakrishna* recounts a parable about this situation told by the master Sri Ramakrishna:

> Haven't you seen the trees on the footpath along a street? They are fenced around as long as they are very young; otherwise cattle destroy them. But there is no longer any need of fences when their trunks grow thick and strong. Then they won't break even if an elephant is tied to them. Just so, there will be no need for you to worry and fear if you make your mind as strong as a thick tree-trunk. First of

> all try to acquire discrimination. Break the jack-fruit open
> only after you have rubbed your hands with oil; then its
> sticky milk won't smear them.

For this reason it is recommended that in the early stages of the work
students limit their associations to others of like mind. Later, they can
chum with whoever they please!

Returning to the topic at hand, let us note that the catabolic processes in meditation operate across the whole range of states of consciousness, gradually deconstructing each as it emerges. At a finer
level of analysis, practices such as meditation exert a slow abrasive
effect on a multitude of negative personal dispositions which, taken *in
toto,* rob the mind of authentic intelligence and bar it from the state
of realization. These 'poisons' or 'pollutants'[19] are well-known in certain Buddhist traditions where over the years many lists of them have
been constructed. One of the most eloquent of these includes the
following: delusion-dullness, irritation-aversion, conceit-arrogance,
passion-addiction, and jealousy-envy.[20] Precisely speaking, the first of
these embraces all of the others, because they all derive from a dull
awareness that allows the rest to come into existence.

These pollutants are thought to operate by creating psychological
sedimentations such as anger, envy, guilt, jealousy, and a multitude of
other obsessions which lie dormant in the mind, waiting to be
triggered by the right situation. These are the 'seeds' of karma,
whether carried from lifetime to lifetime, or manifested from day to
day, month to month, or year to year, contaminating the purity of day-
to-day experience. Similar concepts are found in Hindu thinking,
where Patanjali gives the following list: ignorance, I-am-ness, attachment, aversion, and the will to live. These are said to produce karmic
'deposits,' or in other words sedimentations.[21]

The catabolic effect of meditation on such pollutants or sedimentations seems to be the natural consequence of focused awareness,
which in Tart's terms, operates on them as a *disrupting force.* Buddhist meditation methods such as Vipassana cultivate a direct awareness of the moment-to-moment content of consciousness. Others, such
as Zen meditation, instruct the student that the best way to deal with
potentially distracting thoughts and emotions is not to resist them, but

to let them flow through of their own accord. It is indeed rare in any tradition for meditation instructions to include active resistance of the subjective material that comes up during practice. Even in mantra meditation, typical in Classical Yoga, there is a constant peripheral awareness of the thoughts and feelings that enter and pass through consciousness, at least until one's practice becomes very advanced. In all these instances one eventually begins to *see* into the essence of one's experience. As the process continues, thoughts and feelings, even of emotional qualities and physical discomforts that occur during meditation begin to dissolve. Perhaps I should say one begins to see through them, and in so doing they seem to lose their power, as if the existential air were let out of them and they were only apparitions of what they had previously been. Such awareness works, in William Blake's famous phrase, in 'the infernal method, by corrosives, which in Hell are salutary and medicinal, melting apparent surfaces away, and displaying the infinite which was hid.'

Certain other methods of deconstruction are more direct, hitting the established mental structures with something like a psychological jack-hammer. One such jack-hammer is the Zen koan practice, character-istic of the Rinzai school of Zen. The koan is an enigmatic question such as, 'What was the appearance of your face before your parents conceived you?' The student rolls this over constantly in his or her mind in an effort to find the solution. But there is no rational solution to such a conundrum. The student simply bangs his head against it, shaking loose the hard structures by which he has previously organ-ized reality. In the koan practice, and sometimes by the whole manner in which he is treated, the Zen student is thrown into an intense search for meaning and clarity. But as the French existentialists have gone to such pains to point out, the world is silent. It offers no answers to the seeker. Thus, the student finds himself in a double bind. He yearns for a solution, but finds nothing. This is the situation of the existential *absurd*. The Zen student, however, will not be put off. He knows that there is such a thing as realization. Perhaps the Master is a person who has found it. He has come to study under this master for the very purpose of finding it himself. In his frustration we find the meaning of the ancient parable of the flea biting the iron bull: it is simply impossible.

Frustration builds until the student breaks under the strain of it. He gives up. The old structures crumble, clearing the way for the spontaneous emergence of a new order. At this instant the student achieves realization, or at least makes a quantal advance along his path. This is the point that the absurd man never reaches. Having affirmed the very contradiction in which he is caught, never wholeheartedly accepting the chaos which the world presents, he chooses to live in what the existential author Albert Camus called the 'desert of the absurd.'[22] For the Zen man, however, this desert is only a region through which he must pass on the road towards realization.

Another type of psychological jack-hammer comes in the form of the master who is a trickster, behaving in ways that utterly baffle or disarm the student, cracking open his or her shell of preconceived reality. A few rare masters have developed the style of the trickster as their own way of teaching, one that evidently grows out of their unique personality and training. Tales of such teachers are colorful and fascinating. Zen masters contribute more than a small part to this literature. The following example, for instance, is a Zen teaching story:

> Tokusan was studying Zen under Ryutan. One night he
> came to Ryutan and asked many questions. The teacher
> said, 'The night is getting cold. Why don't you retire?'
>
> So Tokusan bowed and opened the screen to go out,
> observing, 'It is very dark outside.'
>
> Ryutan offered Tokusan a lighted candle to find his way.
> Just as Tokusan received it, Ryutan blew it out. At that
> moment the mind of Tokusan was opened ...

Sufi tradition is also fond of teaching stories about wise but unpredictable individuals who appear as tricksters, or children, or some combination of the two. The mystic Persian poet Jelaluddin Rumi (1207–73), for instance, wrote in *The Sheikh Who Played with Children:*

> A certain young man was asking around,
> 'I need to find a wise person. I have a problem.'

A bystander said, 'There's no one with intelligence
in our town except that man over there
playing with the children,
             the one riding the stick-horse.'

[With some difficulty the seeker got the Sheikh to stop playing
with his stick-horse long enough to carry on a short conversation.
As the wisdom of the Sheikh was obvious, the seeker eventually
asked, 'Why do you hide your intelligence so?']

             'The people here
want to put me in charge. They want me to be
Judge, Magistrate, and Interpreter of all the texts.

The knowing I have doesn't want that. It wants to enjoy
      itself.
I am a plantation of sugarcane, and at the same time
I'm eating the sweetness.'
             Knowledge that is acquired
is not like this. Those who have it worry if
audiences like it or not.
             It's a bait for popularity ...

The construction of alternative forms of consciousness

In spiritual practices the deconstruction of ordinary consciousness is
usually paralleled by the active construction of non-ordinary forms of
consciousness. Catabolic processes are counterbalanced by anabolic
ones. In Tart's terms, disruptive forces are counterbalanced by positive
patterning forces.

One positive patterning force commonly used in many contemplative traditions is the development of a strong and stable posture for
meditation. Correct posture, which usually involves a solid sitting
position with the spine erect and straight, not only facilitates meditation, but gives one a sense of the nobility of the spirit. In the words
of the late Tibetan master, Chögyam Trungpa:

> In the practice of meditation, an upright posture is extremely
> important. Having an upright back is not an artificial
> posture. It is natural to the human body. When you slouch,
> that is unusual. You can't breathe properly when you
> slouch, and slouching also is a sign of giving in to neurosis.
> So when you sit erect, you are proclaiming to yourself and
> to the rest of the world that you are going to be a warrior, a
> fully human being.

This meditative posture moves the meditator toward a quiet and relaxed state of clarity. A frequently used metaphor for this state says that the ordinary mind is like a lake in which the water is muddy and turbulent. If it is allowed to become still, however, the mud settles out and the lake becomes clear and transparent. Virtually all of the subtle states of consciousness require this silent clarity, and only the most advanced practitioners can carry it outward into ordinary day-to-day living.

Perhaps the most central feature of meditation is that it inevitably involves attention. Cognitive psychologists have come to realize that attention, itself a strong patterning force, is perhaps the single most important factor in the activity of the mind. Sights, sounds, and textures are not acted upon unless we give them our attention. Attention is important in activating memories and emotion. Spiritual practices are full of references to attention. These range from the emphasis in Zen and in Gurdjieff work on simply attending to what we are doing from moment to moment while going about our daily business, to the highly concentrated attention that characterizes Indian Yogic meditation. In each instance, the very act of focusing the attention seems to bring an increased intensity and vitality to one's entire experience.

In the classic essay, *The Three Pillars of Zen,* Philip Kapleau tells the following story:

> One day a man of the people said to Zen Master Ikkyu:
> 'Master, will you please write for me some maxims of the
> highest wisdom?' Ikkyu immediately took his brush and
> wrote the word 'Attention.'

'Is that all?' asked the man. 'Will you add something more?' Ikkyu then wrote twice running: 'Attention. Attention.'

'Well,' remarked the man rather irritably, 'I really don't see much depth or subtlety in what you have just written.'

Then Ikkyu wrote the same word three times running: 'Attention. Attention. Attention.'

Half-angered, the man demanded: 'What does the word "Attention" mean anyway?' And Ikkyu answered gently: 'Attention means attention.'

Many sources speak of the importance of developing one-pointed attention. This means attention centered entirely on a single object or activity. Such attention may focus on the breath, as in Zazen, or on a word, such as a *mantra* (or *mantram*) — as in many forms of Indian and Tibetan meditation — or on a visual pattern *(yantra)*. It is said that many great artists and scientists have one-pointed attention when they are at their work.

John Lilly suggests that it is sometimes possible to move directly into a new state of consciousness by imaging it and simply leaping there![23] This is an application of attention as an energizer, in which one is able to actually activate an alternative state of consciousness by directing one's attention to it. Evidently some yogis are quite accomplished at making such transitions.[24] For most of us, however, other patterning forces, such as those activated during meditation, are necessary in order to create significant shifts in consciousness. In this connection, many wisdom traditions stress the importance of reading sacred texts as a complement to the practice of meditation, so the student does not drift through realms of experience without direction. Daniel Brown observes:

> In Buddhism, balance between scholarship and practice is considered necessary to avoid the extremes of intellectualism and directionless practice of meditation.

Such reading, and the thoughts that it inspires, provide an inner beacon for the student.

In mantra meditation, the mantra itself can become a strong patterning force for consciousness. First, it provides an object of concentration, as does the breath in Zazen. In some traditions the mantra also carries a particular meaning that further serves as a source of inspiration. Such a mantra might be carried beyond the meditation period and into one's daily life as a constant source of inner balance and guidance. A western example of this is the Greek Orthodox contemplative prayer, *Kyrie Eleison* ('Lord have mercy'), known as the prayer of the heart or the 'prayer that prays itself.'[25]

Mahatma Gandhi wrote:

> The mantram becomes one's staff of life, carries one
> through every ordeal. It is repeated not for the sake of
> repetition, but for the sake of purification, as an aid to effort
> ... It is no empty repetition. For each repetition has a new
> meaning, carrying you nearer and nearer to God.

Gandhi's own mantra was *Rama,* the name of the Lord. It is said that a mantra is not only a source of strength in life, but a bridge to cross through the shadows of death. In Easwaran's account:

> The person who has become established in the mantram,
> who has made the mantram an integral part of his or her
> consciousness, is prepared for death at all times. Mahatma
> Gandhi, explaining this state, said once that it would be
> easier for his life to stop than for his mantram *Rama* to
> cease reverberating in his consciousness. And this is indeed
> how it came to pass: when his body was pierced by the
> assassin's bullets, Gandhi blessed his attacker with folded
> hands and fell with *Rama* on his lips and in his heart.

Certain mantras are thought to have an intrinsic power of their own. Such mantras can be found especially in certain Tibetan Buddhist and Indian yogic traditions. Some of these mantras are chosen to resonate with particular cakras, the subtle energy centers of the body. Others seem to act as attractors for subtle states of consciousness. Perhaps there is something intrinsic in the resonant quality of the sound itself that gives these mantras their effectiveness. Perhaps, having been repeated virtually millions of times by yogis in deep states of meditation, they have taken on qualities best understood in terms of Sheldrake's morphic fields or Laszlo's psi-fields, gently nudging the consciousness of the meditator toward such states. Knowledge of these mantras is not widely accessible in the West.[26]

In fact, the simple uninterrupted repetition of virtually any sound would seem to have a potentially disruptive effect on the attractor of ordinary consciousness. The English poet Alfred, Lord Tennyson wrote of his own experience along these lines:

> I have never had any revelations through anaesthetics, but a kind of waking trance — this for lack of a better word — I have frequently had, quite up from boyhood, when I have been all alone. This has come upon me through repeating my own name to myself silently, till all at once, as it were out of the intensity of the consciousness of individuality, individuality itself seemed to dissolve and fade away into boundless being and this not a confused state but the clearest, the surest of the surest, utterly beyond words — where death was an almost laughable impossibility — the loss of personality (if so it were) seeming no extinction, but the only true life. I am ashamed of my description. Have I not said the state is utterly beyond words?

Tennyson seems to have achieved, all without training, a very subtle state of consciousness, one equivalent to some advanced form of *samadhi*.

Returning to the matter of patterning forces, one that is very important in virtually all wisdom traditions is the presence of an accomplished teacher. Without the guidance such an individual can provide it is very difficult to move to the most advanced stages of the work. Realistically, a teacher is a virtual necessity, at least at some point in our journey. If nothing else, the teacher is a social model for the student. He or she is a living representation of the fulfilment of the goals of the tradition. Beyond this, however, certain teachers have a special relationship with the student, similar to what in the West would be called a mentor, but emotionally and psychologically more intimate. This is the relationship of a guru.[27] Such a teacher provides highly individual instruction and direction for the student. Beyond this, sages often seem to operate at the subtle levels, as if creating a powerful field that acts as an attractor for the development of his students, and sometimes others as well. In India it is considered helpful simply to be present in this field. It is not unusual, for example, to make a pilgrimage simply to spend time in the presence of a great yogi, even if there is no opportunity to interact directly with him. Meditating with such an accomplished individual is considered very helpful to one's own growth.

In guru oriented wisdom traditions, the ability to influence the student at subtle levels is said to be an important aspect of the relation between the student and the guru. Some teachers have said that half of the responsibility for the student's growth lies with the guru — though this does not let the student off the hook in terms of his or her own practices. Many traditions, especially in India, also involve a direct 'transmission' from the teacher to the student, which quickens the spiritual awareness and may activate subtle energies that had previously remained dormant. If given too soon, however, the effect does not seem to last, so for this, and perhaps other reasons, it is usually given only to advanced students. *Shaktipata,* or the 'descent of power,' is such a transmission, often given by a tap on the head, but also sometimes by simply the guru's glance.

Other positive patterning forces could be explored, but we will leave the topic at this point. The essential point is that progress is made by the double-edged process of disrupting older forms of consciousness while introducing and strengthening new ones.

Being on the threshold

Liminality may perhaps be regarded as the Yea and Nay to all positive structural assertions, but [also] as in some sense the source of them all, and, more than that, as a realm of pure possibility whence novel configurations of ideas and relations may arise.

The life of spiritual commitment may be exhilarating at times, frightening at times, and depressing and discouraging at other times, but it is rarely boring. As we move forward, the corrosive aspect of the spiritual work tends to break down our accustomed habits, throwing us out from comfortable past patterns of thought, emotion, and behavior toward as yet indefinite futures. At such times we are out between attractors, floating in liminality. The word *limen* refers to a threshold. *Subliminal perception* refers to perceptions below the threshold, for instance, of hearing or sight. To be in a liminal state is to be at the threshold between two conditions, yet fully inhabiting neither. Liminality is experienced when we make transitions between periods in our lives, between states of consciousness, even between life and death.

Liminal states are often stressful and disorienting. The familiar is dissolving and a new place to stand has yet to be found. Such states often accompany the chaotic condition that sometimes occurs when a system is moving toward a bifurcation into a new pattern of organization. The events that bring about instability at such times may be external, such as the loss of a job or the death of a family member, forcing a person to seek new life adjustments. They may also be internal, developing over periods of time, and eventually up-ending the entire psychological order and forcing it to seek a new attractor basin. This is the case with the adolescent identity crisis, when changes in the mind and body eventually destroy the childhood identity and force a search for a new sense of self that is appropriate to adulthood. This is also the case in the mid-life crisis, when a previous style of living may suddenly seem empty and meaningless. It is the case at death, when the body itself takes its final plunge into disorder.

It is the flexibility inherent in liminal states that makes them rich ground for psychological and spiritual growth. It is their disorder, however, that may cause psychological disorientation, identity crises, and emotional upheavals. They are at the root of many of the psychological stresses referred to previously. Liminal states hold great possibilities and also real dangers, because in them we are bound by neither the past nor the future, and our fate is open-ended. At such times, when our personal boundaries and defenses are weakened, we may even be visited by the miraculous.

During periods of crisis, when our psychological limits are vague and our boundaries uncertain, we become available to insights about many things that were previously opaque to us. Aspects of our own personality may rise up to confront us in dreams, in our imagination, and in life itself. We may momentarily see ourselves with a degree of objectivity that we had not known before — all of this while experiencing a kind of vertigo. As we have no place to stand, we may also experience powerful emotions, both positive and negative, and the emergence of entire ecstatic as well as bleak existential landscapes which may stay with us for weeks, months, or even years.

In mythological terms, liminality is identified with tricksters. An example is the Greek god Hermes. One of the most ancient figures in the Greek pantheon, in his early days Hermes was associated with doorways and thresholds in general. He was also the patron god of travelers as well as of thieves. As Guide of Souls, he leads the way across the ultimate threshold into the underworld at death. Through his unique association with liminality he also served as gift bearer and messenger of Zeus, the king of the Olympian gods.

In the *Iliad,* Homer refers to Hermes as the friendliest of gods to humans, 'for you beyond all others it is dearest to be man's companion.' He also calls Hermes 'Bringer of Luck.' In his ability to cross boundaries, to lead souls, and to serve as the agent of the highest of the gods, Hermes, like other tricksters is associated with the sometimes miraculous appearance of those seemingly random but undeniably meaningful coincidences which Carl Jung referred to as *synchronicity.* Mark Holland and I have written on this topic in *Synchronicity: Science, Myth, and the Trickster.*[28] In that book we tried to show that when we follow our own genuine calling, the universe itself steps in at times to assist us along the path. This is luck from Olympus, brought to us by Hermes the trickster.

If your own calling is to follow a spiritual path, you should not be too surprised to find that at critical moments fate intervenes in the guise of lucky coincidence, helping you along your way. Moreover, we would expect to experience such boons — in so much as one can 'expect' them at any time — precisely during periods of transition, when we are crossing borders. These may be borders between stages in our own development, or borders between previously separated aspects of ourselves. In other words, we would expect them when we are in periods of growth.

Sri Aurobindo's partner, the Mother, a great yogi in her own right, once commented:

> If you have within you ... [an inner Being] ... sufficiently awake to watch over you, to prepare your path, it can draw towards you things which help you, draw people, books, circumstances, all sorts of little coincidences which come to you as though brought by some benevolent will and give you an indication, a help, a support to take decisions and turn you in the right direction. But once you have taken this decision, once you have decided to find the truth of your being, once you start sincerely on the road, then everything seems to conspire to help you in your advance.

A careful reading of the Mother's and Sri Aurobindo's writings suggests that this inner Being corresponds to Carl Jung's central aspect of the personality, the *self*. This is not the Indian *Self*, the Atman, but a downward reflection of it in the human personality. It also has much in common with the Western notion of the soul as an organizing principle (logos). In Sri Aurobindo's and the Mother's psychology this inner Being plays an increasingly important role in guiding spiritual growth as the individual progresses along the spiritual path.

Returning to ideas of transition and liminality, it would appear that these form part of a discernible cycle that often is seen in psychological as well as spiritual growth. In this cycle, growth tends to proceed through periods of stability that eventually deteriorate into intervals of instability and liminality. These lead to bifurcations, and on into new periods of stability. Put briefly, development often progresses through a series of stages marked off by bifurcations. This idea is reflected in many major theories of psychological growth and development, including Jean Piaget's theory of cognitive development, Laurence Kohlberg's theory of moral development, Erick Erikson's theory of personality development, and Daniel Levinson's findings on individual life patterns.[29] Others could be cited, but the point is simply to show the universality with which those who have studied individual development have discovered a pattern of plateaux separated by transitions.

Spiritual growth also seems often to follow a step-wise course comprised of stable periods interspersed with intervals of liminality. The positive patterning forces activated by practices such as mantra repetition, physical exercise, and correct posture, help to stabilize the student during periods of transition. So does the influence of a skilled teacher. I suspect that the 'dark night of the soul,' a significant period of depression, confusion, and deep desolation common in the lives of Christian mystics but relatively (though not entirely) unknown in the East, is due at least in part to the scarcity of systematic practices as well as accomplished teachers in the West.[30] It is hard to remain long in a state of drifting disorientation with a Zen master nearby to give you a sound crack on the head with his walking stick!

Quieting the turbulence within

Especially important in spiritual work are processes that quell internal disorder and affirm stability. Even aside from the risks incurred in growth-related bifurcations, many aspects of human experience conspire to lead us toward states of internal disorganization. The stressful lifestyles most of use are forced to endure tend to create and sustain a state of turbulence from which it is difficult to tune into the 'still small voice' of the subtle attractors associated with advanced forms of consciousness. Even aside from this, the constant agitations of an undisciplined mind, fed by the 'wild horses' of the senses, seem to sustain a continuous state of psychological turbulence.

From a complex systems point of view, one of the most effective ways to stabilize fluctuations is the use of what Tart terms feedback stabilization.[31] In engineering applications this begins with the creation of a signal that represents the state of the system. This signal is constantly fed back to a central control device, thus forming a cybernetic or control loop. A common cybernetic system involves the thermostat that regulates the room temperature of your home. It contains a thermometer which signals the air temperature to a circuit designed to activate the furnace when the room is found to be too cool, and to shut it off when the room is too warm. Like all cybernetic systems, the thermostat has a *set point* (in this case the temperature at which you set the thermostat) with which it compares the signal from the thermometer, thus deciding whether or not to turn on the heat.

Our nervous system uses more sophisticated feedback loops. One example is the system that regulates body weight. For each of us, our brain has a set point for total body fat. The actual amount of body fat at any given moment is evidently signaled by the insulin level in the cerebrospinal fluid.[32] If the amount of body fat, as communicated by this signal, falls below the set point, the brain causes us to become hungry, and so we eat more food and store more fat. Since the central set point changes only very slowly, a crash diet is typically followed by a crash weight gain.

Psychologists make use of cybernetic circuits when doing bio-feedback training to help persons gain control over their own internal processes.[33] A common application is to help a person reduce his or her stress level in frustrating situations by learning to relax physically. One way this can be done is by placing a couple of small electrodes on the forehead that signal electrical activity produced by the tension in the *frontalis* muscle. This signal is usually a gentle beeping tone or an easily read visual display. Now the frontalis muscle, like certain lower back muscles, tends to tighten up when we are under stress, and is thus a good rough gauge of the total stress level of the body, including the heart rate, blood pressure, and so on. The amazing part of it is that by watching the signal from the frontalis muscle, one can learn to allow it to relax, thus simultaneously relaxing the whole body. The goal of the bio-feedback training, then, is to learn to relax this single muscle at will, which in fact turns out to be relaxing the entire system.

The virtue of the bio-feedback machine itself is that it can make subtle physiological variables such as heart rate, blood pressure, or muscle tension, objective, even external, so that we can to find ways to regulate them. Indeed, it turns out to be considerably easier to focus one's attention on a meter or light that signals the level of contraction of the frontalis muscle, and learn to control that meter or light, than it is to control the frontalis muscle directly. One need only concentrate on changing the light or the meter reading to change one's own physiological reactions. Eventually, one learns to control these res-ponses directly and without the aid of a bio-feedback monitor. But in the early stages of training the monitor provides an essential ingredient that was previously missing, the clear and available signal of one's own physiological condition.

Now, it was pointed out some years ago by psychologist Elmer Green that entering into a cybernetic relationship with a system such as the heart, or the physiological stress mechanism of the body, not only tends to bring that system into stability, but also seems to center it to a more healthy set point. Thus, working with the stress reaction not only gives one some direct control over stress, but the stress res-ponse itself becomes more balanced and better behaved. Interestingly, it turns out that these are exactly the effects that contemplative prac-tices and especially meditation have on consciousness itself.

It seems that bio-feedback is effective because it focuses attention on some aspect of our bodily response, such as muscle tension, of which we were previously unaware. Some forms of meditation such as Vipassana focus attention directly on the content of consciousness, often beginning with physical sensations, and in some instances proceeding to the mental and emotional content of awareness. Anyone who has done mantra meditation, or practiced breath awareness, knows, however, that efforts to support a sustained concentration, no matter what its object, lead to a gradually increasing awareness of inner events such as thoughts and feelings. In this sense the practice of meditation creates a cybernetic circuit within awareness itself, resulting not only in an increased control over these inner processes, but a balancing and centering of them as well.

Part of this balancing involves a growing sense of detachment and objectivity toward our own mental and emotional reactions. Like physiological responses that are made objective by a light or meter on a bio-feedback instrument, we come to see our own mental activity from the perspective of an observer. I think it is a jarring but never-theless accurate observation that the thoughts and emotions of most people are as involuntary as their heart rate and blood pressure. They seem only aware of strong moods, and they have opinions which, in appropriate situations, they can report out. But these are perceived as facts of life, or states of the world, rather than arbitrary inner events.

Actually *observing* one's own process with a degree of objectivity is quite a different matter.

I once spent several hours in an allergy clinic watching people being tested for reactions to various chemical compounds. The procedure involved placing a minute quantity of the potentially offensive substance under the tongue and watching for reactions to it. The clients were told ahead of time that these substances could in some instances cause emotional reactions. The amazing thing to me was that a few minutes later, when emotional responses were actually produced, none of them displayed any insight into the cause of their condition. One woman became intoxicated for a short time, giggling and almost falling off her chair. A man grew depressed and moody, and another got angry and stormed out of the clinic, only to return apologetically an hour later. None gave any indication of being aware that their reactions were caused by the allergy tests, and some seemed unable to do anything with this information even when they were told it face to face.

The achievement of a significant degree of objectivity toward one's own inner process represents a major gain in self understanding and mastery. It is also an essential step in many if not all spiritual paths. In Sri Aurobindo's words:

> All developed mental men, those who get beyond the
> average, have in one way or other, or at least at certain
> times and for certain purposes, to separate the two parts of
> the mind, the active part, which is a factory of thoughts and
> the quiet masterful part which is at once a Witness and a
> Will, observing them, judging, rejecting, eliminating,
> accepting, ordering corrections and changes, the Master in
> the House of Mind.

Not only does the development of a degree of inner objectivity give us greater control and inner balance but, as indicated in the above words of Sri Aurobindo, it also elevates us to a higher perspective. No longer do we automatically identify with every passing thought and feeling that flows through the field of consciousness. We begin to establish a new platform from which to experience our landscape of existence. This platform is referred to above as the *Witness.* In Sri

Aurobindo's yoga, as the spiritual work proceeds the increasing elevation of this platform eventually carries it into the Atman itself.

As one might suspect from the above comments, when we begin to
free ourselves from the entanglements of uncontrolled and unbalanced
thought, and melodramatic and unregulated emotion, we begin to
experience a gradual clearing of the spirit that carries with it a new
sense of freedom and nobility. One is reminded of the words of the
great European esotericist, Frithjof Schuon:

> There is no knowledge without objectivity of the
> intelligence; there is no freedom without objectivity of the
> will; and there is no nobility without objectivity of the soul.

The achievement of an inner balance and the ability to stabilize the
ordinary fluctuations of mood and thought seems almost the hallmark of advanced stages of inner development. Individuals who have
reached such stages, whether they be Christian mystics, Buddhist
monks, or Indian yogis, often seem to possess an almost palpable
sense of personal peace, which communicates effortlessly to those
nearby.

A dramatic instance of this inner quiescence is demonstrated in a
story about Sri Aurobindo, told by the Mother. It seems that a great
storm was approaching the ashram in Pondicherry. The wind blew
violently, while she ran about closing windows and doors so that
papers and clothing would not be scattered everywhere. As she entered
Sri Aurobindo's study, however, she felt a palpable stillness that
seemed to surround him. He sat quietly writing at his desk, as was his
habit, with his windows wide open. But not a breath of air stirred in
the room! Perhaps you may feel that this was an exaggeration, but
whether it is literally true or not it demonstrates the profound degree
to which turbulence comes to rest in the presence of a sage.

Subtle states of consciousness, such as experienced in deep meditation, seem characterized by extremely low levels of within-system
turbulence. In fact, turbulence seems to vanish within them like waves
rolling on to dry absorbent sand. In this regard, such states approach
absolute point attractors in which consciousness settles into luminous
immobility.

The tendency to return to a quiet balance point, even after experiencing excitement or turmoil, seems to be a common quality of accomplished followers of many traditions. This is not to say that they never get excited or frustrated — far from it — but that they return quickly to a peaceful internal balance point, while most of us continue to spin around for hours, days, or even years. My own impression of such individuals is that they virtually never exhibit the kind of lobotomized daze of indifference suggested by popular images of total detachment. Rather, they display vigorous good will and humor, while appearing peaceful underneath. More than that, they can become quite animated, even angry, but it doesn't last for long.

It might be useful at this point to recall the role of the Witness, and its perspective on one's thoughts and feelings. This perspective amounts to a new hierarchical structure in the noetic organization of consciousness itself, one that surveys the passions, obsessions, and melodramas of the ordinary mind, granting, as we have seen, a degree of objectivity and detachment not possible as long as we continue to identify with them. From such a perspective it is possible to give up some of our neurotic and self-defeating habits, and thus to improve ourselves. What seems more important, however, is that even those personality traits so deeply ingrained that they are highly resistant to change begin to disturb us less and less. We begin to learn to live with ourselves, to accept ourselves for what we are and to get on to more important things. What I am saying here is that while spiritual work may in time bring about dramatic changes in who and what we are, in practical terms it is more likely to raise us above our less desirable qualities so that we need not take them so seriously, and in this we can allow others to take them less seriously as well.

Recapitulating

Before pushing on to investigate the actual state of realization, let us collect our thoughts by returning momentarily to the coordinate system introduced near the beginning of the chapter. This can be represented by process axes, as shown in Figure 16. These are, first, the polarity between emergent and constructive evolution and, second, the polarity between anabolic and catabolic practices. Here the third axis, the distinction between ontic and noetic traditions, is not drawn separately on the Figure, but discussed in relation to the other two.

Ontic traditions such as Raja Yoga are found in Figure 16 in the quadrant that represents the conjunction of constructive evolution and anabolic growth processes. These traditions work toward a gradual reordering of the entire human system, from the material body on through the most subtle levels of being. Many aspects of this work are described above in the discussion of Raja Yoga. Noetic traditions such as Zen Buddhism, on the other hand, are found in the quadrant that represents the conjunction of emergent evolution and catabolic growth processes. Though in reality work in these traditions may take as long as on the ontic paths, the goal is a radical shattering of old structures, especially those of the mental or noetic variety, allowing the spontaneous reformation of the vibrant living intelligence that characterizes realization.

It is important to realize that anabolic as well as catabolic practices play an important role in both the ontic and noetic traditions. The difference is in which is stressed in each tradition, and to some extent which is in the service of the other. The final thrust in the Rinzai school of Zen, for instance, amounts to an implosion of the old noetic structures, allowing the spontaneous emergence of *Original Mind* — though constructive practices have much to do with preparing the student for it. In Raja Yoga, on the other hand, the deconstruction of ordinary consciousness by meditation can be understood as a preparation for the construction of new and more subtle states. As we will see, however, there exists the possibility in yoga, as well as in the noetic traditions, of going beyond any special state of consciousness.

Jnana Yoga is shown in the quadrant of emergent evolution and catabolic processes. Though it seeks an ontic identity with the Self, it emphasizes the catabolic practice of *neti, neti* ('not this, not that'), directed straight at dissolving our identity with the mundane self in a fashion reminiscent of William Blake's 'infernal method' of corrosives. Paul Brunton's 'short path,' on the other hand, appears in the quadrant of emergent evolution and anabolic processes. It also seeks an ontic resolution, though unlike Jnana Yoga with which it has much in common, it does so by reaching toward a positive identity with the highest aspect of Being.

The liberated life

I suggested near the beginning of this chapter that there are two major themes that run throughout the history of human spirituality, and are reflected in two different modes of mystical experience. One is an active, outgoing, mysticism which finds its home in the worldly life. The other is a passive, introverted, mysticism that withdraws from the world. We now return to these, as they lead to different concepts of realization, one active and outgoing, and the other passive and introverted. We will first examine the introverted form, then move on to the extroverted or outgoing one.

The introverted traditions

These traditions are epitomized by the Hindu concept of *asam-prajnata-samadhi* in yoga philosophy, and its equivalent, *nirvikalpa-samadhi,* in Vedanta.[34] This samadhi is considered to be a state of ecstasy equally beyond pleasure and pain.[35] One Vedic philosopher, translated by great Indianologist, Ananda Coomaraswamy, wrote:

> In that rapt synthesis *(samadhi)* the Self has retained its
> primordial condition, 'as a man and a woman closely
> embraced,' and without awareness of any distinction of a
> within from a without. 'That Self art thou.'

During such rapture there is no movement, no questioning, no thought whatsoever.

This form of samadhi has much in common with the classical Buddhist concept of *nirvana.* Both represent states that are essentially ineffable, and both indicate an introverted withdrawal from the world. Both, in certain of their oldest conceptions, are perfectly achieved only after the death of the physical body. The language used to characterize nirvana tends to differ from that used to describe samadhi in that it emphasizes what it is not, or what it is beyond, rather than what it is. It is often said to be an escape from the cycle of birth and death, or more basically the absence of arising, subsisting, changing, and passing away. Such characterizations are not unknown to samadhi as well, which is said by Patanjali to be 'devoid of any content.' A broader characterization of nirvana is that it is a condition of 'oneness with the inexpressible reality that always exists, only not recognized.'

While both catabolic and anabolic processes are involved in the evolutionary events that finally achieve such forms of consciousness, once established such states seem to glow with an internal fire of their own. Samadhi, for instance, is said to 'burn' the seeds of karma, thus releasing the yogin from their burden. This is also a fire that evidently burns its own structural bridges. One highly respected text, the *Hatha Pradipika,* speaks of the highest state as 'that which remains after the lower mind has been dissolved through yogic practice.' Nirvana, which literally means *extinction,* is also called 'that which is not conditioned, not made up of parts,' and 'not being something that has been constructed.'

That these states remain stable after their structural supports have been burned or dissolved suggests that, once established, they become, in dynamical terms, self-creating (autopoietic) processes or self-sustaining attractors. An interdisciplinary group of anthropologists, Laughlin, McManus, and d'Aquili recently observed that such states have all the earmarks of coming into being through a catastrophic bifurcation, prior to which 'the period of actual structural transformation [of ordinary mind] at every level of hierarchic organization took months, and very likely years in each case,' suggesting in agreement with our present ideas, that the evolutionary preparation for this final leap took much time and effort.

The fire, energy, or simply *intensity* of the most advanced forms of consciousness is characteristic of not only the introverted modes of realization, but also of the outgoing modes as well. Speaking of the latter, Herbert Guenther quotes from one ancient Tibetan text:

> The difference between low-level cognitive intensity and originary awareness is as follows:
> Mind is like water, it gathers everything:
> Originary awareness is like the sun, it burns everything.
> Although water can gather rusty material
> It cannot burn it like fire can.

Water, even if as huge as the ocean with the nine
continents,
Is consumed by the fire at the end of time and dries up.

Here, the word *mind* refers to ordinary consciousness, and *originary awareness* refers to the condition of realization. Guenther's choice of the English word 'originary' in this translation is suggestive of Jean Gebser's concept of the *origin* as the essence that shines through the integral structure of consciousness.[36]

Laughlin, McManus, and d'Aquili, have systematically examined the role of energy or arousal of the physical body for a variety of non-ordinary states of consciousness. Their analysis focuses on two general configurations of physiological activity which they term the *ergotropic* and *trophotropic* systems. These correspond to the sympathetic and parasympathetic branches of the autonomic nervous system. In practical terms, the ergotropic system tends to prepare one for high levels of activity, in other words, for 'fight or flight.' It stimulates the release of adrenalin into the blood stream, accelerates the heart rhythm, causes blood to flow into the large muscles of the body and the brain, and activates an arousal condition in the brain wave pattern. The trophotropic system tends to have the opposite effect, conserving energy and putting one in a relaxed state in which the heart slows down, blood pressure drops, and the brain waves show signs of synchronization, indicating a passive state of mind.

The interesting point in all of this is that these authors argue that states such as advanced samadhi involve high levels of simultaneous activity in both the ergotropic and trophotropic systems at once. The point would seem to be that here, again, this time based largely on physiological analyses, we find evidence that such states involve considerable activation or energy. What is so remarkable is that this energy is couched in and supported by a profound background of relaxation. Here we have a physiological analog of certain ideas that we have already examined. These are, first, that advanced states of consciousness seem to be grounded in a profound and continuous state of global quiescence — in Sri Aurobindo's words, a 'settled peace ... in the mind' — and second, that they are marked by high energy or intensity.

The extroverted traditions

These traditions are characterized by the Vedanta ideal of *sahaja-samadhi* ('spontaneous samadhi'), meaning 'liberation while being alive.'[37] In the *Bhagavad Gita* and the medieval yogic classic, *Yoga-Vasishtha,* this goal is represented as *jivan-mukti:* ('living liberation'). The latter text provides us with several trenchant descriptions of this condition. Here is a sampling of them:

> [He is] wise, gracious, charming, suffused with his
> enlightenment, free from pressure and distress, an
> affectionate friend.

> [He behaves] as a boy among boys; an elder among
> elders; a sage among sages; a youth among youths,
> [and as] a sympathizer among the well-conducted
> afflicted.

> Remaining perfectly happy and experiencing enjoyment
> in all that is expected [of him], he performs all deeds,
> [ever] abandoning the misconception of doership.

Notions of active realization are in no way the exclusive province of Hindu thought. Similar concepts are found in many traditions, and are well articulated in Buddhism. Historically, the *Mahayana* Buddhist ideal of the *bodhisattva* brought with it an interest in active nirvana or liberation. Conceptions of this condition differ considerably from school to school, but all agree that it represents an active, outgoing, and compassionate involvement in the living world.

My understanding of the outgoing form of liberation owes much to the work of Buddhist scholar Herbert Guenther, who in his recent books has translated many of the concepts of the third and fourth century Buddhist *Yogacara* school, and particularly its rDzogs-chen ('supercompleteness') teachings, into thoroughly modern language.[38] These teachings, which we will examine carefully below, give us a process-oriented phenomenology of the outgoing, life-affirming, mode of illumination.

One approach to understanding this remarkable experience of the world is to see it as an upward inflection of the experience of meditation. In other words, a pattern of consciousness gradually takes shape in meditation which, at its highest octave, opens into the realm of active realization. Guenther makes a distinction between two types of meditation. The first involves a rigidly focused attention on the object of concentration. Such meditation, he suggests, is of limited value, though I would note that in certain traditions (for instance in Patanjali's *Yoga Sutra*) it is viewed as preparation for the second type, which Guenther terms bodhisattva meditation. The transition 'from the restrictive-control level to the [second type of meditation, or] opening-up level where creativity is given a chance, is marked by the dissolution of boundaries between subject (as controller) and object (as controlled).' The Buddhist text, *Rig-pa ran-shar,* states:

> Bodhisattva meditation is such that the mind does not exert subjective control. [Rather, this meditation] originates by its own dynamics ...

With the transition to bodhisattva meditation, consciousness enters into a configuration that Guenther characterizes as autopoietic. Such configurations are 'globally stable, but never static and resting ... They are expressive of a particular individuality within an environment comprising its cognitive domain.'

Guenther goes on to explain that by 'cognitive domains' he means 'spiritual levels' that form a hierarchical order in which each ascending level includes all lower levels. These are the perennial tiers of being as described in Vedanta, each of which is said to enclose all levels beneath it. The experience of each level 'brings new gestalt qualities of thought and specific ordering principles into play and thereby establishes a human individual as a creative being.' In this, Guenther points to the expanding realms of experience that we are already familiar with, for instance in Sri Aurobindo's hierarchy of minds where each sequential level is grounded in a progressively higher or more subtle plane of being. In agreement with our own observations, Guenther notes that, though we speak of such realms as higher levels reached in the pursuit of spiritual growth, 'the term "higher" should not be taken too literally ... Rather it must be understood as also pointing into dimensions of openness ...'

Put simply, we have here an understanding of meditation as a movement of consciousness toward a fluid autopoietic process opening to ever-widening realms of experience. While Guenther speaks of such realms in terms of cognitive domains, we could as well talk of them in terms of felt or intuitive realms, for the growth of inner sensitivity is also represented by feeling and intuition.[39] Guenther notes that such growth is also accompanied by the appearance of an inner calmness which constitutes an active force leading consciousness toward an increasing capacity to feel and appreciate life's dynamics. All this emerges from the self-organizing quality of consciousness as an autopoietic event. In his own words, 'The bodhisattva meditation is the total system's self-finding of optimal stability. It marks the ascendancy of pure experience over thematizing mind.' Such meditation gives birth to 'originary awareness' (Tibetan: *ye-shes)*, or the condition of realization.

Originary awareness

Guenther's description of originary awareness seems, on careful reading, to have a great deal in common with Gebser's idea of the integral structure of consciousness. Indeed, they both appear to be pointing toward the same reality. Gebser describes integral consciousness as diaphanous and suffused with the light of the origin. Guenther describes originary awareness as superdiaphanous and glowing with the inner radiance of being. Both point to an experience which, though diaphanous, yields to us the world in its immediate concreteness. Guenther speaks of going beyond the thematizing mind, Gebser of going beyond mental abstractions toward an experience of the immediate present. Both speak of the *intensity* of consciousness.

In coming to an understanding of originary awareness or integral consciousness it is well to recall our original concept of consciousness from the first chapter of this book. There I suggested that, in the final analysis, consciousness is essentially a subjective *presence.* This concept reminds us of the immediate and concrete nature of actual moment to moment experience, and avoids appeal to metaphysical constructions that amount to extra baggage in helping us appreciate the immediate nature of awareness. Here, we are interested in the qualities of experience itself, qualities which may seem paradoxical from a rational mode of understanding.

Preeminent in an appreciation of originary awareness or integral consciousness is the apparent paradox that it is concrete while being diaphanous. This is simply to say that objects and events are experienced in their immediate freshness, untrammeled by intellectual thematizations. At the same time, their undiluted immediacy, or 'concreteness,' does not solidify into a dense impenetrable mass, but remains self-luminous, translucent to the inner light of being. Thus, in another seeming paradox, originary awareness is not rooted in the abstract vagaries of the mind, but in the immediate reality of the physical body. Guenther, for example, comments that:

> Man's body is where perception happens, where interests
> are occasioned, and where action takes place. As such, the
> lived body is inseparable from 'mind' ...

Others, including Sri Aurobindo, have emphasized the importance of the body as the physical location and vehicle for the most advanced forms of experience. Zen teacher Karlfried Graf Dürckheim observes:

> The true man is he who is present in the world in the right
> way. Whether he be dense or transparent, withdrawn into
> himself or open to life, in form or out of form, centered or
> without center, he is all these things with his whole being,
> which is to say, also with his body!

Let us turn now to the theme of intensity as an essential aspect of originary awareness. Gebser views the final transition of consciousness to the integral structure as accompanied by a stepping up of the intensity of the origin itself. Guenther emphasizes the critical importance of the cognitive intensity of originary awareness. By this he gestures toward a vivid and penetrating experience of the present moment that cuts beneath mere intellectual conceptions of reality. The rDzogs-chen thinkers of Tibet went so far as to identify mental pollutants as nothing more than low intensity cognitive processes. These negative psychological dispositions, in fact, are exactly what drags consciousness down into its ordinary, 'normal,' low intensity condition. The sheer intensity of originary awareness, on the other hand, disrupts these dispositions, burning them away. In the introverted traditions, this is the meaning of the idea that *nirvikalpa-* or *asamprajnata-samadhi* burns away the seeds of karma. This is to say that psychological contaminants, no matter what their origin, present or past, are dissolved, catabolized, by the burning intensity, the penetrating light, of realized consciousness.

Another essential feature of originary awareness, or integral consciousness, is wholeness. Guenther observes that the term, *rDzogschen,* actually translates into English as 'ultimate completeness,' 'sublime wholeness,' or 'impeccable entirety.' His own choice, however, is to translate it as *supercompleteness.* The power of the supercompleteness of consciousness, and its relationship to intensity, are expressed in the translation of a Tibetan text which states that being (experienced in originary awareness):

> like the sun in the center of the sky, shines throughout its
> meaning-rich field; from its creative dynamics, like the
> sun's rays the whole universe comes into being with no
> segmentation.

Gebser's phrase, *integral consciousness,* carries the immediate implication of wholeness. This form of consciousness, as previously indicated, is not a 'structure' at all in the usual restrictive sense of Gebser's other structures (magical, mythical, etc.), each of which is exclusive of the others. It is, rather, a broader awareness, one in which these other structures can have their play. 'To live these structures together, commensurate with their respective degrees of conscious awareness,' comments Gebser, 'is to approach an integrated, integral life.' Likewise, Feuerstein notes that in the living liberation of *sahaja-samadhi,* 'the liberated yogin may experience a variety of states of consciousness.'

Integral consciousness is, in Guenther's words, 'globally stable, but never static and resting.' Its form is that of an autopoietic regime that transcends structure as we usually think of it. It is a structure only in the large sense of an entire *order* in which the Gebserian structures come and go at will. The idea of an *order* was developed by quantum physicist David Bohm,[40] though it was first suggested to him by an artist. It represents a basic pattern, agenda, or set of rules by which reality itself is organized. Thus, an order represents an inclusive field, as it were, in which particular structures constellate.

Here, let us note that the present discussion of integral conscious-ness and originary awareness contains little in the way of traditional religious or mystical language such as 'God,' the 'divine,' and so on. While such terms have played an important role in the understanding of mystical experiences for a great many people, Gebser would say that they show an 'indebtedness to the psychic-mythical structure' of consciousness. From the point of view of the perennial levels of being, such terms, as we have seen, seem to gain precedence at the causal level, retreating into the opened ground of experience at the level of pure originary awareness. This is certainly not to criticize the beatific level of experience, but rather to note that our business here, rather, is to come to grips with the form, or mode, of originary awareness itself.

A delightful quality of such awareness is its creativeness. Gebser states that 'creativity is of the origin.' Though each structure of con-sciousness is capable of its own forms of creativity, it is the brilliance and vibrancy of the origin itself shining through them that makes this possible. Psychologically, creativity is akin to spontaneity, which in turn is allied to freedom. Without the possibility of spontaneous free-dom at all levels of the human being there would be no true creativity. Feuerstein notes that in the term *sahaja-samadhi,* the prefix *sahaja* means 'spontaneous,' signifying the idea 'that freedom is not external to us but our very condition ... the true spontaneity of naturalness is an expression of [God or Being].'

Guenther observes that such spontaneity is an essential aspect of originary awareness. He likens it to the quantum state of an element-ary particle just prior to the moment at which an actual observation is made on it. The particle seems paradoxically to exist in several places at once, each representing, in the words of physicist Nick Herbert, 'unrealized tendencies for action, awaiting the magic moment of measurement that will grant one of these tendencies a more concrete style of being which we humans experience as actuality.' It is significant that Danah Zohar alludes to exactly this quantum phenomenon as a characteristic of consciousness itself.[41]

We are reminded that supercompleteness is not something alien to awareness as we ordinarily know it, but in fact is an intensification, an opening out and relaxing of consciousness in its original freshness. The world appears in *suchness,* to use the Buddhist term. Guenther speaks of the *autopresencing* dimension of being, suggesting a fullness of the experience of the present moment. Here, we again connect with the concrete quality of awareness in which the world is experienced, to use Gebser's phrase, as *the itself,* or in Guenther's words, 'in the immediacy of its abiding thereness.' All this is fancy language for the full appreciation of the moment and the mysteries it holds — the taste of tea, the fragrance of a rose, the soft touch of a word kindly spoken, the tearing edge of pain, the heat of desire. Zen texts state that the world comes to the realized person in its original, everyday, ordinariness. Nothing more is needed. It is an ordinariness that is fresh, clear, and bountiful.

> In my ten-foot bamboo hut this spring,
> There is nothing: there is everything.

> *Sodo*

It is:

> A condition of complete simplicity
> (Costing not less than everything).

> *T.S. Eliot*

12. Seeing into the Sun

True intelligence

Your intelligence is a camel-driver. You are the camel.
The Holy Ones are an Intelligence within your intellect.
Give your profoundest contemplation to this:
    Camel, camel-driver, the Sun ... Develop an eye
    that can see into the Sun ...
    And here it is, hidden in a speck of dirt!
      Like a lion somehow disguised
      in a fleece! Like an Ocean
      beneath a piece of straw!

Jelaluddin Rumi

What makes for an optimal realization of human nature? Here I do not mean the heroic achievement of great psychological or spiritual transformations, but simply a capable and graceful way of engaging the world. In this chapter I want to seek an understanding of what is commonly called *intelligence*. We will begin by pulling together some important notions from previous chapters.

Steps to an ecology of mind

To be human is to be a verb. We are not objects, but events. We are process beings, down to the cells that form our biological bodies and up through the elusive mental processes which articulate our thoughts, feelings, and emotions. Flux is our nature, but not random flux. Rather, we are intricate patterns of flow, hierarchical process structures rooted in the molecules, atoms, and even subatomic events that form our bodies, and ranging upward in steps through the complex processes of our cells, the myriad activities of our organs, and finally to realization of our bodies as whole events. The brain and mind are no different. We are heirs to an inner ecology of mind and spirit in which thoughts, memories, emotions, sense of self, and perceptions of others, are part of an exquisite fabric that shapes our personal lives and gives moment-to-moment substance to conscious experience.

I propose that our experiential lives are organized into at least three levels, each built in hierarchical fashion upon the one below (Figure 17). The first level might informally be called *states of mind.* These are conditions such as sadness, joy, melancholy, enthusiasm, and the like. They include the many moods and dispositions that take hold of us daily.[1] Second, and supporting these states of mind are *states of consciousness.* First clearly explored in systems theory terms by Charles Tart, these include experiential conditions such as dream and non-dream sleep, drug states, various states of deep meditation, hypnosis, shamanic trances, and ordinary awareness.

Tart believed that states of consciousness are formed by unique configurations of psychological functions such as thought, memory, emotion, perception of the external world, and perception of one's self. These functions differ from state to state, but combine in each to form a viable pattern. In modern terms such configurations can be thought of as attractors, which bring the functions together into a single dynamic process. Tart also suggested that in order to move from one state to another the forces that support the present state must be disrupted, while at the same time applying alternative patterning forces toward the desired state. For example, to go to sleep we put aside our daytime activities, change clothes into something loose and comfortable, and repose in a restful position.

The third, and most broad, of the levels of organization of our experiential lives are *structures of consciousness.* First described by Jean Gebser, these are entire overarching regimes that determine how the world is experienced and understood. Human history bears witness to a sequence of these, which Gebser termed the *archaic, magical, mythical, mental,* and presently emerging *integral* structures. Each is a unique way of knowing the world. For instance, magical conscious-ness sees natural events in terms of the operation of magical forces, while the mythical consciousness seeks explanations through grand images and stories of goddesses and gods. Mental consciousness searches for rational understandings. Integral consciousness allows the

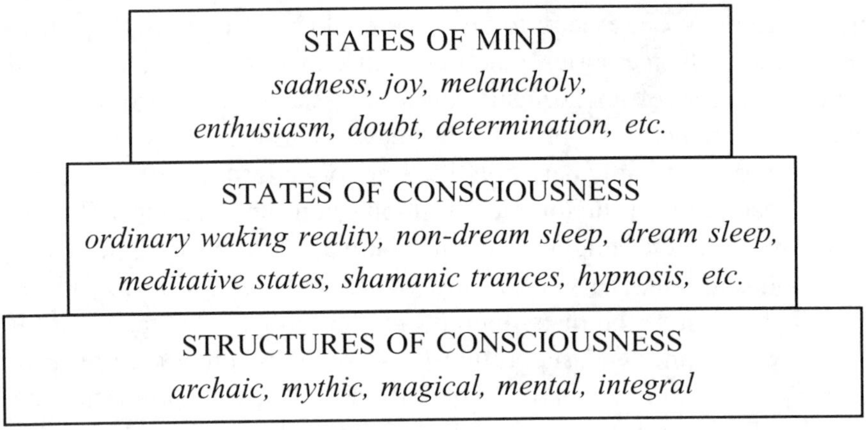

STATES OF MIND
sadness, joy, melancholy,
enthusiasm, doubt, determination, etc.

STATES OF CONSCIOUSNESS
ordinary waking reality, non-dream sleep, dream sleep,
meditative states, shamanic trances, hypnosis, etc.

STRUCTURES OF CONSCIOUSNESS
archaic, mythic, magical, mental, integral

Figure 17. The three levels of our experiential lives.

free expression of all the other structures without being captured by any of them. It yields a fluid perspective of reality in which time becomes a quality or essence and the self is no longer entrapped in a cartesian cage of spacial coordinates.

I believe that the events which structure our experience at all levels of organization are of a single kind. They are self-organizing, autopoietic processes, precisely analogous to the intricate events that create and sustain living cells, where complex metabolic reactions feed back on to themselves and on to each other in rich auto-catalytic and cross-catalytic interactions which create an intricate and self-sustaining fabric of the whole. Now, complex self-creating systems such as living cells, or the hierarchical structure of human experience, are by nature holistic. Every part, every reaction, every process is dependent on all others in a single flow of continual self-creation. As we saw in Chapters 2 and 3, these systems are often poised on the edge of chaos, moving back and forth between fixed and predictable cyclic patterns of activity, and chaotic patterns that assure flexibility in adjusting to the demands of a changing world.

An interesting feature of such systems is that they have no midpoint, but each point in them is a center in its own right. Thus, when pressure is applied at any location the entire system can be influenced. Applying patterning forces in order to transform consciousness from one state to another is an example of this principle.[2] The other side of this same coin is that even a small point in the system that has become immovable can sometimes tie the whole thing down. For example, a persistent emotional state can color one's entire psychological disposition, including thoughts, memories, and perceptions. Likewise, a psychoactive chemical such as a 'mood elevator,' operating on a particular subsystem of the brain, can exert a much wider influence than just making a person less depressed. He may find himself becoming more optimistic, generous in his disposition toward others, and liberal in his general outlook. I once read of an artist who through a rare brain dysfunction lost his ability to see colors. He had previously been fascinated by the daylight and the colors it disclosed his eyes. But now he became disenchanted entirely with the daytime, spending his waking hours at night, fascinated with its textures of light and darkness.[3]

It may seem that such a complex network of processes as gives form to our experience and understanding of reality, built of intricate arrangements of processes within processes, piled up in ascending hierarchies, would make for the most flimsy of constructions. In fact, nature itself tells us that such is not the case. Indeed this is the blueprint for all complex living matter. And though we rightfully concern ourselves with how fragile certain plants, animals, and ecologies can be, the fundamental fact of living matter is not its delicacy but, as biologist and writer Lewis Thomas observed, its tenacity. Grass grows from cracks in asphalt sidewalks, insects can live in high levels of atomic radiation; there are bacteria that thrive in tanks of jet fuel! Nevertheless there are limits. The highest levels of complexity and organization seem most vulnerable to stress and trauma, a fact seen as much in human psychology as in the world of plants and animals. And it is at these higher levels that true human intelligence is located.

The camel-driver

One way to understand intelligence is to view it in terms of flexible and adaptive process structures of the mind, brain, and consciousness. Such structures in turn yield flexible and broadly adaptive styles of behavior. We see an evolutionary thrust in this direction in the biological history of the nervous system itself.

Perhaps the oldest and most primitive method of regulating behavior is by genetic control. Most activities of invertebrates, such as the web weaving of spiders and the migrations of butterflies, are managed by mechanisms built into the nervous systems of these animals by their genetics. Much of the activity of fish and reptiles is the same. Genetically controlled behaviors can be quite complex and may appear to be intelligent, but for the most part are basically rigid and inflexible. Examples include the nest-building of certain fish, such as the stickleback, the mating rituals of birds, and the migrations of salmon back to their native waters to lay eggs and die.

Mammals, the evolutionary newcomers of the animal kingdom, depend to a much lesser extent on genetic wisdom, and to a greater degree on learning. Perhaps the oldest and most basic form of such learning is the stimulus-response variety technically called *conditioning.* There are at least two, and probably several, types of conditioning, but in each case a particular form of response becomes connected to a particular type of stimulus. A dog learns to paw at its owner's knee under the dinner table for scraps of food. A child learns to run away from yellow-striped insects that buzz. The odor of a particular food, eaten once when tainted, now brings a wave of nausea. The varieties are endless, but all involve more or less inflexible associations of responses with stimuli. In the nervous system these associations are evidently made, at least in part, in the older structures in the core of the forebrain. Such associations are adaptive, but always somewhat mechanical, and far from creative intelligence at its best.

Only when we come to the most recent evolutionary innovation of the mammalian brain, the *neocortex,* do we find the cognitive, that is *mental,* qualities of imagination, memory, creativity, and reason that we associate with true intelligence. The neocortex is the hallmark of modern mammals, and it is especially well developed in primates. In the human brain it shows special enlargement in the frontal lobe, associated with planning, projecting the future, and perhaps abstract thought, and in the language areas of the left hemisphere. The prominent neurologist, Sir John Eccles, refers to these areas as *neo-*

neocortex.[4] Their recent evolutionary advance, and the creative potentials they afford, finally bring us face to face with full human intelligence.

Exactly what is the nature of this fully human intelligence? Fortunately we are not alone in asking this question. Indeed, it has been the passion of some of the prominent psychologists of this century. One of the most important of these was Jean Piaget, whom we met in Chapter 3. As we saw there, his way of thinking about intelligence is entirely consistent with the systems approach used throughout this book. It is that intelligence is the fruit of complex and flexible systems built up of patterns of thought and behavior which he termed *schemata.*

Beginning in infancy, intelligence is constructed, level by level, by grafting new and flexible schemata on to the growing process of intelligence. With help from the parents, a child learns the basic concept of *numbers* by observing fingers, toes, toys, and other items that come in ones, twos, threes, and so on. This understanding in turn is the basis for learning to count, which is the successive assignment of numbers. The child is now ready to learn to count in a rapid shorthand procedure called *addition.* This, likewise, is the understanding upon which the skill of *multiplication* is built. Later, the child may continue to a knowledge of calculus, an even more complex skill that is based upon a flexible mastery of all the abilities above.

This surely is the general formula for the growth of intelligence from the infant mind all the way to the adult. Simple skills or concepts lead to more complex ones, which in turn lead in the direction of even more complexity. Schemata also interact with each other. For instance, mathematical concepts interact with growing linguistic skills to produce powerful mathematical deductions. In the field of art, recently acquired concepts of perspective interact with previously mastered skills in the use of color and shadow, to produce mature skills in painting and visual expression. The total effect of the growth and weaving together of diverse schemata leads toward powerful and flexible understandings of science, mathematics, art, law, and so on. Lawrence Kohlberg spent much of his life showing that similar ideas apply to the growth of the ability to make sound moral judgments. Again, we find that the child's abilities are not lost to the adult, but form a foundation upon which the more advanced moral judgments of the adult are built.

Studies of intellectual growth in college students tell a similar story. Psychologist W.G. Perry, who spent years studying students at Harvard, found an intellectual progression during the college years reminiscent of the growth of intelligence in children.[5] Students typically began with a very concrete attitude toward truth. For them, there was only one right answer to any question. Later they began to realize that there often can be more than one legitimate answer. For example, there can be several valid interpretations of Shakespeare's *Hamlet*. This was a transitional stage for the students, however, and they were likely to experience some confusion about the whole thing, feeling that somehow one of the interpretations must actually be the most correct. Only with full intellectual maturity did they come to realize that truth is a function of the entire context of a problem. Each historical epic can have its own perfectly legitimate interpretation of *Hamlet,* and indeed, can accommodate several of them. These might include existential, psychological, political, historical, poetic interpretations and more. The student that can understand this has developed a mature and flexible intelligence.

Whether we speak of Piaget, Kohlberg, Perry, or any of many other intelligence theorists, the result is the same. Intelligence is the outcome of a gradual construction of systems for interpreting and understanding reality, systems that gain power and flexibility as they mature and mutually interact.

The intelligence within your intellect

So far everything that has been mentioned could, at least in principle, be programmed into a computer. Let us ask if there is anything to intelligence not explained by building up of flexible and sophisticated structures of thought. Many would say there is not. Certainly, if you believe that the brain is essentially a computer or neural network,[6] you will find no difficulty with this notion. The other side of this coin is the idea that computers will eventually be truly intelligent, creative and conscious.

I have no desire to throw cold water on such ideas. Indeed, I only wish my desk-top computer were a little bit smarter. But there is something in me unwilling to give up the game to computers. Perhaps it is intuition, or even nostalgia, but something tells me that true intelligence is more mercurial, lyrical, and even impish, than anything that will ever come out of a machine. I don't intend to harangue this point. Indeed, I may well be wrong. But I would note that the predictions of coming machine intelligence have grown less and less optimistic as the years have passed since the days of the heady enthusiasm associated with the founding of 'artificial intelligence' in the 50s and 60s. In the late 60s, for instance, scenes of the sentient computer, HAL, in the film, *A Space Odyssey,* seemed at least conceivable for the then-distant year 2000.[7] Now that the time is nearly upon us the likelihood of a sophisticated talking computer seems much further away.[8]

Not everyone agrees with the idea that intelligence can be obtained by better programming. In fact there is a small but significant literature that argues for inherent limitations in machine intelligence.[9] Mathematician and Nobel laureate Roger Penrose has gone to great pains to demonstrate that intelligence simply cannot be programmed.[10] His arguments are long and intricate, even by mathematical standards, but represent a vigorous alternative point of view within the realm of formal scientific thought. He believes that consciousness itself plays a vital role in creativity and intelligence, noting that it is just those situations that require novel responses, ones in which routine behaviors are inadequate, that call on conscious attention. These are the moments when creative rather than stereotyped actions are needed. While mechanical or routinized thoughts and behaviors may play an important role in day-to-day activities such as driving the car, preparing breakfast, or brushing one's teeth, the appearance of a novel situation calls into play conscious attention to supply creative solutions.

The idea that there is something extra, some other dimension to intelligence, is consistent with many of the ideas in the previous pages. In Chapter 3 we noted chaos psychologist Larry Vandervert's notion that the brain itself is virtually a well of innate wisdom, out of which the mind ordinarily only partially partakes. He believes this inherent wisdom is due to an evolutionary similarity between the deep fractal-like structure of brain processes and similar patterns in the make-up of the external world. This is the source of the unaccountably good fit between mathematics, a product of the human mind, and the physics of the natural world. More than once in the previous pages we have come across ideas, such as Ervin Laszlo's theory of *psi-fields* and Rupert Sheldrake's notion of *morphic resonance,* which imply the presence of intelligent patterns in the cosmos itself, patterns that are perhaps sensed only through direct intuition. Such ideas suggest that wisdom is to be had from the very depths of our own being. They are reminiscent of the Greek notion that true knowledge is inherent in the soul at birth, but later forgotten.[11] Thus, Socrates would lead his followers to wisdom through dialogue, but not because he thought democratic conversation was the way to truth, but because it could bring forward the forgotten wisdom already within. Likewise, Plotinus would say that memory is only for those who have forgotten!

In this vein it is worth noting that there is an underground tradition in the West, running through the writings of Goethe, Schiller, Schelling, Hegel, Coleridge, and Emerson, and continuing in Rudolf Steiner and Carl Jung, which recognizes the importance of a contemplative approach to the discovery of knowledge in nature. For these thinkers the human mind was not separate from the natural world, as it was for Descartes, but a participating part of it. In the words of cultural historian Richard Tarnas:

> It is only when the human mind actively brings forth
> from within itself the full powers of a disciplined
> imagination and saturates its empirical observation with
> archetypal insight that the deeper reality of the world
> emerges.[12]

The basic idea, which can be traced all the way back to Plato, is that archetypal forms occur widely — for instance in the distributions of leaves on plant stems, the rudimentary bone structures of animal paws, and the spiral distributions of sunflower seeds and the stars of galaxies — and that these forms are best discovered, not by observation alone, but through observation coupled with introspective imagination. Other, more abstract patterns, may well occur in the human mind, experienced in dreams, stories, or works of art, as suggested by Jung's idea of psychological archetypes.

All this points to the presence of a spontaneous native intelligence fundamentally different from the sophisticated intelligence built up of acquired knowledge structures. Moreover, experience counsels that the only way to elicit this other form of intelligence is to let it flow naturally, or if we cannot do that, then to find a method that lets us get out of its way. A painter, for instance, may seek inspiration by drawing temporarily with his left hand. A writer may retreat to a particular room where ideas flow more easily, or move about from room to room trying to capture just the right feeling. Zen artists are renowned for capturing this sense of effortless spontaneity. For them, the act of painting itself is immediate and spontaneous, a spiritual exercise in which the painter must keep out of the way of his own creativity. The talent, however, does not come easily. As we saw in the last chapter, Zen training often emphasizes *catabolic* disciplines such as meditation, which work like Blake's 'infernal method, by corrosives.' In other words, they clean the mental system of the grit and impurities that block the spontaneous flow of creativity.

True intelligence, which might be called wisdom

In the last chapter we found two distinct themes in practices of wisdom traditions from throughout the world. One was the building of new and flexible structures within consciousness. The other was the dislodging of obstacles that impede the achievement of the highest goals. It is my belief that a similar dichotomy is useful in understanding the nature of intelligence.

On the one hand, a sophisticated and savvy understanding of the world requires the presence of complex and refined knowledge structures of the sort originally identified by Jean Piaget. Whether the skill in question pertains to art, science, mathematics, cooking, business, raising a child, or maintaining a rewarding relationship with a spouse, the story is the same. One must acquire the necessary skills. Without these even a natural talent will be limited. Casablanca was said to have been the greatest chess player of all time, but he never won a world class tournament because he did not bother to learn the complexities of the standard strategies for the opening game. These were simply too difficult to figure out in the heat of play, so he was defeated by the very opponents he had often beaten in casual play. Likewise, a musically talented individual can make considerable progress simply by playing an instrument for pleasure and without instruction, but will not achieve greatness without the discipline of acquiring a firm knowledge of the complex patterns taken for granted in formal composition.

On the other hand, the simple learning of skills, procedures, and protocols does not make a master. In most endeavors, especially those requiring creativity, a certain flexibility is also important, a relaxing of the usual constraints to allow for unique individual expression. Research indicates, for instance, that persons training to become psychotherapists, while learning new therapeutic procedures, actually lose some of their ability to interact with the warmth and spontaneity so important to therapy's success. Later, as they continue to use their newly formed skills, they recover these abilities and become better therapists than ever. Likewise, the self-taught musician loses a certain spontaneity by taking formal music lessons, but after the scales are learned and the difficult manipulations of the keys or strings are mastered, the combination of discipline and spontaneity returns at a new level of mastery.

It seems that in any area of competence it is necessary to learn the requisite skills, then to learn to relax them and regain communication with our own sensitivity and intuition. This relaxing does not come effortlessly. We cling to old habits as if they were personally handed down to us by the Almighty Himself. Something else is often needed to soften our defenses and limber up our tightly held patterns of thought and behavior. Fortunately the cosmos does not leave us wanting long, but provides exactly want we need — though not what we usually want — in what is called *the school of hard knocks*. Indeed, anyone who is awake and alive is regularly treated to demonstrations of the inadequacy of their formulas and protocols, whether these concern specific skills or life in general. Such formulas and protocols are learned from our parents during childhood, from school, religious training, and the like. They get us started but they do not lead us to wisdom.

For most of us, true intelligence — which might be called wisdom — is gained only as the reward of a rich life, born of the marriage of hard-earned sophistication with heartfelt intuition. For a few fortunate individuals, this marriage is nurtured by the personal influence of a spiritual teacher. Most of us, however, must rely on our own inner sense of what is right and compassionate; and ultimately all of us must do so.

Epilogue

Now that all is said and done I find myself at my own beginning, discovering consciousness as the illumination of each instant before it is obscured by its own content.

For as far back as I can remember, my own consciousness has seemed to me to be absolutely real and unwavering. I was fascinated by it, and that fascination eventually led to study and a career in the sciences of the mind and brain. As a student I learned to my amazement, however, that there were others who did not find it interesting or who denied its existence entirely.[1] Much has changed since those days, both in my own life and in science as well. The study of consciousness has since become not only legitimate but even fashionable. Nevertheless, conferences, professional meetings, and even popular books on consciousness often seem to entirely miss my original idea. They speak of behavior, they speak of cognitive networks, they frequently speak of neurons and the brain, but they too rarely speak of the simple crystalline reality that undergirds all experience — consciousness.

My personal search for an understanding of consciousness led me, like many in my generation, into a variety of philosophies, spiritual practices, and even martial arts. These included Taoist meditative practices, yogic disciplines, T'ai Chi, and Jungian analysis. My intellectual search has moved between mysticism, esotericism, the sciences of the mind and those of the brain. You have followed a model of this journey, cleaned up a bit and organized for this book.

One thing of value learned along the way is that spontaneous, natural intelligence shines effortlessly, like morning light bursting through an open window, when the mind is made clean and clear of the incrustations that life deposits upon it. This is the gift and genius of the wondering Taoist poet and of every child. Sophistication, however, must be constructed by building the lessons of life into a flexible dynamic mental system — an intelligent mind. Wisdom arises when these two mature and support each other.

Life is a passage from mystery to mystery. That is the wonder and the terror of being human. This book is my own story, my own truth. Each of us must finally write our own stories. If this tale of mine in some small way contributes to your own evolving story it would be my greatest honor.

Appendix I: Technical terms

Terms from dynamical systems theory

anabolic processes
Constructive processes that tend to move a SYSTEM toward a more complex structure. *Ana* (Gr.) means 'upward,' and *bolein* (Gr.) means 'to throw.'

attractor
In plain English, an attractor is a relatively stable configuration (or STATE) of a system. When the system finds itself in a nearby but different configuration, it tends to rebound back into that state. Speaking mathematically, an attractor is a configuration that the system approaches asymptotically as a limit. The approach itself is a TRANSIENT RESPONSE of the system. There are three known types of attractors: STATIC ATTRACTORS, PERIODIC ATTRACTORS, and CHAOTIC ATTRACTORS.

attractor basin
All the possible STATES of a system that lead it to a particular ATTRACTOR. On a STATE SPACE diagram the region representing these states can appear as a depression or basin.

autopoietic SYSTEM
A self-creating system. Maturana and Varela (1987) define an autopoietic system as a network of interconnected component-producing processes that create the same network that produces them. Organisms are prominent examples of such systems.

bifurcation
A significant change in a DYNAMICAL SYSTEM. There are three known types of bifurcation: SUBTLE BIFURCATIONS, EXPLOSIVE BIFURCATIONS, and CATASTROPHIC BIFURCATIONS.

catabolic processes
Processes that break down or deconstruct complex SYSTEMS into less complex configurations. *Kata* (Gr.) means 'down,' and *bolein* (Gr.) means 'to throw.'

catastrophic BIFURCATION
When, in a DYNAMICAL SYSTEM, an ATTRACTOR along with its ATTRACTOR BASIN abruptly appears or disappears.

chaotic ATTRACTOR (strange attractor)
Strictly speaking, this describes the pattern of a SYSTEM that is neither at rest

(STATIC ATTRACTOR) nor in a fixed cycle (PERIODIC ATTRACTOR), and so is 'strange.' When modelled by computer graphic methods such attractors are often found to reveal highly ordered geometric patterns. Speaking more casually, it is a common misconception to think that such attractors have no visible order at all. In fact, each is contained in its own ATTRACTOR BASIN, and may behave in a relatively systematic fashion, so that it is sometimes difficult to distinguish between an approximately PERIODIC ATTRACTOR such as the cardiac rhythm and a truly chaotic attractor such as described by weather patterns.

control variable (control parameter)
Variables or values that control the behavior of a system. The temperature of a chemical system, for example, is one variable that controls the rate of reactions.

cybernetic SYSTEM
A system that utilizes feed-back information about its own condition or behavior to regulate its output. Examples range from thermostats to living organisms.

disruptive force
An influence that tends to disrupt a STATE OF CONSCIOUSNESS. For example, loud noise tends to disrupt the state of sleep.

dissipative systems (dissipative structures)
SYSTEMS that retain energy, increasing their own internal order while dissipating disorder or entropy, usually in the form of heat. Prominent examples are living organisms.

dynamical system see SYSTEM, DYNAMICAL

emergent evolution
This concept is that of a relatively abrupt and spontaneous transition of a SYSTEM to a new or higher order of organization. This involves a quantal or CATA-STROPHIC BIFURCATION in the system's history.

explosive BIFURCATION
An ATTRACTOR undergoes an abrupt change, and possibly a change of type. For example, a STATIC ATTRACTOR rapidly becomes a large CHAOTIC ATTRACTOR.

fixed cycle attractor see PERIODIC ATTRACTOR

general theory of evolution
A systems-based understanding of evolution that emphasizes the development of DYNAMICAL SYSTEMS into complex hierarchical organizations.

grand evolutionary synthesis
Originally proposed by Ervin Laszlo (1987a) in reference to the GENERAL THEORY OF EVOLUTION in its broadest application. In this book it is taken to include the evolution of human consciousness toward its highest potentials.

historical evolution
This concept is that of a gradual development through time which involves the incremental accumulation of changes or BIFURCATIONS in a SYSTEM.

patterning force
An influence that tends to move consciousness toward a particular STATE. For example, fatigue tends to push consciousness in the direction of the state of sleep.

periodic ATTRACTOR (oscillations, fixed cycle attractor)
The system comes to a cyclic pattern as its limit (attractor). The rotation of the Earth around the sun describes a periodic attractor, as does (approximately) the rhythm of the human heart.

phase portrait
A topological diagram of the STATE SPACE of a system showing, usually with smooth arrows, the direction of change or 'flow' of the system from STATE to state.

saddle
If a STATE SPACE is drawn to represent the energy of the SYSTEM at each state, a saddle-shaped ridge (or saddle) may sometimes be seen to separate two distinct ATTRACTOR BASINS. In plain language a saddle is a type of threshold across which a dynamical system must move to come into the range of influence of a new ATTRACTOR BASIN.

separatrices
Elevated or peak regions of the STATE SPACE that separate two or more ATTRACTORS. In plain English this simply means that certain states of a system lie between attractors, and thus separate them. Such a state is that experienced halfway between sleeping and waking, from which one tends to slide back into sleep or forward into wakefulness.

state (of a SYSTEM)
An pattern of activity, or more broadly, a condition of a SYSTEM, the latter being organized into a particular STRUCTURE. A tuned violin is a system with a structure. It can be set into a number of states of resonant vibration or tones according to the values of the CONTROL VARIABLES supplied by the fingers of the violinist. Also see STATE OF CONSCIOUSNESS.

state of consciousness
A coherent pattern of psychological processes such as cognition, emotion, memory, body sense, and sense of identity. States of consciousness such as ordinary wakefulness, non-dream sleep, and dream sleep, each have distinct properties and are relatively stable compared to conditions such as momentary surprise or vertigo, but less stable than a STRUCTURE OF CONSCIOUSNESS.

state space
The topological representation of all possible STATES OF A SYSTEM.

static ATTRACTOR (rest point)
The SYSTEM comes to a resting state as its limit (attractor). For example, a cup set on a table at a slight angle rotates (TRANSIENT RESPONSE) until it comes to rest.

structure
A pattern of activity or configuration of a system that is relatively stable and may be capable of supporting a variety of STATES. Also see STRUCTURE OF CONSCIOUSNESS.

structure of consciousness
An entire experiential agenda. For example, Jean Gebser's structures of consciousness are noetic styles through which the world presents itself.

system
A set of processes that form a self-contained unit. A system can, however, be part or a larger system, if it retains its integrity. The processes of a living cell, for example, form such a unit, and at the same form a sub-unit within the larger organism.

system, dynamical (dynamical SYSTEM)
A system is understood to be dynamical when it has a 'rule of evolution,' in other words a rule according to which, for each possible STATE OF THE SYSTEM, the next future state is specified. Such a rule is usually mathematical. Indeed, conceptually the notion of dynamical systems is a mathematical one.

subtle BIFURCATION
A small change (BIFURCATION) in a dynamical system.

transient response (of a SYSTEM)
The temporary response of a system before it settles down into a stable pattern of behavior. Mathematically, it is the temporary response of a system that has been displaced from its nearest ATTRACTOR, or of a system that has just come into existence through a CATASTROPHIC BIFURCATION.

Terms from perennial philosophies

atman (SELF)
The essence of one's being, beyond qualifications and conditionality. The individual aspect of BRAHMAN.

Bhakti YOGA
A yogic tradition that stresses bhakti, or devotional practice.

Brahman
In Vedanta philosophy, the Absolute. The source from which flows all the diversity of the universe.

Buddha
From the ancient Pali language, literally 'awakened one.' The Indian word *bodhi* means 'awakening,' and the adjective *buddha* suggests 'spiritually awake.'

cakra ('wheel')
Seven subtle energy centers of the human body. In Indian philosophy these are often said to be located at (1) the base of the spine, between the genitals and the anus, (2) at the root of the genitals, (3) in the navel region, (4) in the heart region, (5) in the lower throat, (6) between the eyebrows, and (7) at the crown of the head. Each carries its own psychological significance.

Classical YOGA
A term commonly used to refer to the yogic path most thoroughly outlined in Patanjali's *Yoga Sutras*. It is also termed *RAJA YOGA*.

Hinayana Buddhism ('Small Vehicle')
Includes eighteen schools that developed out of the original historical Buddhist community. The only one that still exists is THERAVADA BUDDHISM.

Integral YOGA
This term has been used in a number of different ways, but in this book it refers to the yogic tradition started and developed by Sri Aurobindo. Also termed *Purna Yoga.*

jivan-mukti ('living liberation')
Described in some detail in *Bhagavad-Gita,* this is a state of active liberation. Also see *SAHAJA-SAMADHI.*

Jnana YOGA ('yoga of wisdom')
Closely associated with the philosophy of Vedanta, Jnana Yoga stresses cultivation of the ability to discriminate reality from unreality, and thus the realization of one's true nature, the SELF.

kaivalya ('aloneness')
This state has been variously described as the SELF's capacity for unbroken

apperception of the contents of consciousness (Patanjali), that which remains after the lower mind has been dissolved, and as 'a realization without the Lord.'

Karma YOGA

The yogic tradition that stresses progress through selfless work in the world. It is discussed at length in the *Bhagavad-Gita*. It is said that in some sense everyone is doing Karma Yoga (though not necessarily doing it well).

kundalini ('serpent power')

A form of SHAKTI, or subtle energy, said to reside at the base of the spine. When awakened, for example, by the practice of KUNDALINI YOGA, it may rise through a channel (the *sushumna)* at the center of the spinal cord, cleansing and activating the various CAKRAS.

Kundalini YOGA

A yogic tradition that emphasizes work with the KUNDALINI energy.

Mahayana Buddhism ('Great Vehicle')

One of the two major schools of Buddhism, along with HINAYANA BUDDHISM; it originally developed from the latter. In its multifaceted approaches to liberation it places less stress on monastic life and opens the way to the many.

moksha ('liberation')

Arising from the obliteration of all aspirations, liberation is said to be a state that transcends all duality. Also see *SAHAJA-SAMADHI* and *JIVAN-MUKTI.*

nirvana ('extinction')

The goal of all Buddhist traditions. In the older Buddhism it had two distinct meanings, one of a flame extinguished, and the other of a place or location. Since then it has taken on a considerable variety of meanings. These range from the absence in consciousness of arising, subsisting, changing, and passing away — and the departure from cycle of birth — to active liberation, as seen in Zen. In general, in Buddhist thought nirvana is 'oneness with the inexpressible reality that always exists, only not recognized' (Fischer-Schreiber, Ehrhard, Friedrichs, & Diener, 1989). The term is also used in Hinduism to refer to *TURIYA* and *NIRVIKALPA-SAMADHI.*

—*apratishthita-nirvana:* In MAHAYANA BUDDHISM, active liberation that is free from desire. The term probably derives from the idea of 'non-localizable' realization, as opposed to PRATISHTHITA-NIRVANA, which is 'localized.'

—*nirupadhishesha-nirvana:* In HINAYANA BUDDHISM, unconditional nirvana.

—*pratishthita-nirvana:* In MAHAYANA BUDDHISM, complete liberation attainable only after physical death; similar to NIRUPADHISHESHA-NIRVANA. The term suggests the idea of 'localized' liberation as opposed to APRATISHTHITA-NIRVANA.

—*sopadhishesha-nirvana:* In HINAYANA BUDDHISM, nirvana with a remainder of psychological conditionality.

originary awareness
This is Guenther's (1989) translation of the Tibetan *ye-shes,* where *ye* points to a beginning before there is any beginning in the usual Western sense. It is an anglicization of the French *originaire,* which is in turn a translation of the German *ursprünglich.* The latter word was also used by Gebser to describe integral consciousness, and is usually translated as 'originary awareness.'

prana ('life')
Life energy, said to circulate through the human body in subtle channels. It is particularly associated with the breath. In a broader sense, it is understood to be the elemental energy behind all energies of the universe. Also see PRANAYAMA.

pranayama
Yogic work with the breath as a vehicle for controlling the subtle energy of PRANA within the body.

Raja YOGA ('royal yoga')
Also see CLASSICAL YOGA. The YOGA involves eight 'limbs' or steps, beginning with ethical or psychological practices and leading through physical and subtle-energy disciplines, and on to the highest states of meditation.

samadhi
A state of spiritual absorption. Most literally it suggests a state of things falling into a pattern. The term takes on a considerable variety of meanings in both Hindu and Buddhist thought, ranging from 'one-pointed' attention in any activity, to complete absorption in the Absolute. Samadhi is the goal of virtually all forms of Indian YOGA. It is often translated as 'ecstasy' (Gk. *stasis,* stand + *ek,* outside) but Mircea Eliade (1973) suggests that a better term would be 'enstasy' (Gk. *stasis,* stand + *en,* in).
—*sahaja-samadhi ('spontaneous samadhi'):* Active liberation while being alive. In this condition, the liberated yogin can experience a variety of states of consciousness (Feuerstein, 1990a). Also see JIVAN-MUKTI.
—*savikalpa-* (Vedanta) or *samprajnata-* (Patanjali) *samadhi:* Absorption in the object of meditation, accompanied by higher thought forms. This form of samadhi is said to still contain traces of duality. It has been compared to the *visio Dei* of Christian mysticism.
—*nirvikalpa-* (Vedanta) or *asamprajnata-* (Patanjali) *samadhi:* Consciousness devoid of any content; identification with the SELF. This form of samadhi is said to go beyond all duality.

Self
In Vedanta philosophy, the Self is the essence of one's being, beyond all qualifications or conditionality. Also see ATMAN.

shakti ('power')
The divine subtle energy expressed in the mode of the feminine. In Indian thought often expressed as the Divine Shakti.

Theravada Buddhism
The only remaining school of HINAYANA BUDDHISM, it is widespread in Southeast Asia. Its approach is strongly analytical.

turiya
The fourth state of consciousness, beyond sleep, wakefulness, and dreaming.

turiya-atita
'That which transcends the fourth' state. The condition of living liberation. Also see *JIVAN-MUKTI*.

yoga ('to yoke, harness')
Meaning to harness oneself to the divine or to a spiritual endeavor. Stress is often placed on control of the mind or the senses, especially in CLASSICAL YOGA. Yoga philosophy as developed by Patanjali is considered to be one of the six classical schools of Hinduism.

Yogacara Buddhism ('application of YOGA')
Developed from MAHAYANA BUDDHISM and reaching ascendancy in the third and fourth century, it was a seminal influence on the sixth century Chinese Ch'an school, which in turn led to Zen around AD 1200. Especially in the form of the *rDzogs-chen* teachings, this school developed a dramatically process-oriented philosophy.

Sources

Abraham, A.H. (1987). Complex dynamics and the social sciences. *World Futures: The Journal of General Evolution*. 23, 1–10.

Abraham, A.H., & Shaw, C.D. (1984). *Dynamics — the geometry of behavior; Part I: Periodic behavior*. Santa Cruz, CA: Aerial Press.

Feuerstein, G. (1989b). *Yoga: the technology of ecstasy*. Los Angeles, CA: Jeremy P. Tarcher.

Feuerstein, G. (1990a). *Encyclopedic dictionary of yoga*. New York: Paragon House.

Fischer-Schreiber, I., Ehrhard, F., Friedrichs, K., & Diener, M.S. (Eds). (1989). *The encyclopedia of Eastern philosophy and religion*. Boston: Shambhala.

Guenther, H.V. (1990). Personal communication.

Appendix II: Transpersonal psychology in the work of Stanislav Grof and Michael Washburn

The field of transpersonal psychology has benefited from the contributions of many individuals, ranging from William James to Abraham Maslow to Carl Jung and others, to say nothing of those persons, both ancient and modern, discussed in this book. Two who have made substantial recent contributions, but whose work is not described in this book are Stanislav Grof and Michael Washburn. I include brief descriptions of their ideas here to round out the review of transpersonal psychologies presented in this book, which has a different agenda.

Stanislav Grof

Stanislav Grof has for many years been a leading researcher in the field of psychedelic drugs, specifically LSD, and their implications for self-exploration and the deep nature of the psyche.[1] More recently he has replaced LSD as a means of producing altered states of consciousness with *holotropic therapy,* which utilizes a variety of techniques including music, body work, and most notably a particular form of hyperventilation.[2] The structural model of the psyche that Grof has discovered in this work involves several successive levels, or spheres of experience, that are typically encountered sequentially as one engages in deep self-exploration using these methods. There are four such levels which we will examine below. They are *the sensory barrier, the individual unconscious,* the *perinatal level* or *the level of birth and death,* and *the transpersonal level.*

1. The sensory barrier

The sensory barrier is the first realm of experience typically encountered in LSD work or holotropic therapy. Many readers who have had even casual experiences with psychedelic drugs will recognize this realm. It is simply heightened sensory experience produced, for instance, in an LSD session, in which not only does the outer world take on altered qualities, but more importantly, with the eyes closed one may experience a kaleidoscopic variety of colors and geometric arabesques that are both dramatic and sometimes aesthetically pleasing. These can be symbolically evocative, such as mandala-like patterns that suggest Moslem mosques or the windows of Gothic cathedrals, though further examination rarely reveals profound meanings. While fascinating in its own right, this level of experience represents an obstacle to the deeper layers of self-exploration, and for this reason is termed the sensory 'barrier.'

2. The individual unconscious

Participants in self-exploratory LSD sessions and holotropic therapy eventually pass through the sensory barrier into what Grof refers to as a Freudian realm of personal biographical experiences. In other words, they begin to reconnect with and even relive significant past experiences from their lives. These may be un-available to ordinary consciousness, representing the content of the unconscious mind as it was originally conceived by Freud. They often differ, however, from material typically dealt with in classical psychoanalysis, with its emphasis on emotional psychological traumas, in that such experiences frequently center on physical traumas such as life-threatening illnesses, surgical procedures, or physical injuries.

In this work it is common for participants to reconnect with whole con-figurations of experiences that, in fact, may have occurred at quite different times in their lives. All that is necessary to bring them together is a common unifying physical or emotional theme such as a particular type of physical trauma or emotional pain. Such configurations can also draw on material from other levels of experience, such as what appear (in LSD sessions) to be memories of past lives. Grof was impressed with the frequency and importance of such constella-tions of experience for the individual. He refers to them as *systems of condensed experience* or *COEX* systems for short. Such systems are found at virtually all levels of self-exploration and, as indicated above, may transcend individual levels, bringing dynamic experiences from a variety of spheres of experience into a common nexus.

3. The perinatal level or the level of birth and death

Probing deeper into the psyche discloses an amazingly powerful and diverse range of experience that Grof characterizes broadly as related to the birth pro-cess. These realms of experience, for which he uses the term *perinatal,* contain intense experiences of pain as well as of joy and relief, and often involve the motif of death as well as that of birth. Grof finds these experiences to constellate into four basic categories that he terms *basic perinatal matrices (BPM),* and which in turn are associated with particular aspects of the birth experience. Thus, while the COEX systems represent unique constellations of a particular indivi-dual's feelings and memories, the BPM are generic categories of experience whose defining feature is their connection with the birth process. Thus, particular COEX systems may engage particular BPM. For example:

elements of important COEX systems dealing with physical abuse and violation, threat, separation, pain, or suffocation are closely related to specific aspects of BPM.

Grof identifies four categories of BPM. Each is associated with a vast sphere of actual experiences in the LSD or holotropic therapy session. Some are profoundly positive while many others are remarkably negative. Doing justice to them would require an entire book in itself. To provide some sense of what is implied, however, I will identify each briefly, below, and give some examples of experiences associated with them in LSD sessions.

The first BPM is connected with the original experience of symbiotic unity of the fetus with the mother during intrauterine existence. In the LSD session it may be identified with pleasant and apparently realistic recollections of intrauterine life, as well as with positive and even ecstatic experiences of nature, of cosmic unity, and of heaven and paradise. Negative intrauterine experiences such as produced by fetal crises, diseases, emotional turmoils of the mother, and attempted abortions, can yield feelings of universal threat and paranoia, the perception of demonic presences, as well as unpleasant physical sensations.

The second BPM is associated with the onset of delivery. This begins, for the fetus, as a series of alarming chemical signals followed by maternal muscle contractions. As this stage progresses, the fetus is convulsed by a series of periodic constrictions, though the still closed cervix offers no escape. Experiences connected to this BPM can include feelings of entrapment and encagement from which there is no escape. This BPM may evoke agonizing feelings of guilt or suffering, including visions of terror, the horrors of war and persecution, or the meaninglessness and absurdity of the human condition. This may be accompanied by physical sensations of compression, cardiac distress, or suffocation.

The third and perhaps most dramatic BPM is connected to the next stage of delivery. Now the cervix is dilated and the way through the birth canal is open. To move through the tunnel, however, requires an immense effort. In Grof's words, this experience involves:

> an enormous struggle for survival, crushing mechanical pressures, and often a high degree of anoxia and suffocation. In the terminal phases of the delivery, the fetus can experience intimate contact with such biological material as blood, mucus, fetal liquid, urine, and even feces.

Experiences activated by this BPM can intensify to cosmic visions of suffering. Powerful sadomasochistic passions, murders and sacrifices, sexual orgiastic feelings and more are connected with this crisis point in the birth process. Physical tremors, flashes of heat and cold, and nausea and vomiting, as well as cardiac distress, are among the physical symptoms sometimes experienced.

The final BPM brings the birth process to an end. The extreme discomfort of the final struggle ends with a tremendous relief and relaxation. This matrix is associated with visions of extended space, radiant colors and brotherly humanitarian feelings, as well as occasionally grandiose ones. These positive experiences can be interrupted by the *umbilical crisis,* which involves a sharp pain in the navel or fear of death or castration.

4. The transpersonal level

Somewhere in the process of deep self-exploration a transition is sometimes made into a realm of experience which does not appear to be contained within the individual at all, but seems to represent an ability of consciousness to reach beyond conventional limits of space and time. In this change inner experience paradoxically becomes outer experience.

> All we can say in this respect is that, somewhere in the process of perinatal unfolding, a strange qualitative Möbius-like leap seems to occur in which deep exploration of the individual unconscious turns into a process of experiential adventures in the universe-at-large, involving what can best be described as the superconscious mind.

A common feature of this rich and vastly diverse sphere of experience is the feeling that consciousness has expanded beyond the usual boundaries of the ego, transcending time and space. Examples include what appear to be authentic regressions to experiences of previous lives, or to earlier evolutionary stages of the human species. Sometimes under LSD these can retrace the entire history of organic life itself, or even the evolutionary history of the cosmos. A participant may feel his or her consciousness to be located in another person, as if behind that person's own consciousness, or may envision and experience the life of an animal, including its hunting or courtship rituals and so on. On later investigation, information from such experiences may prove accurate within the limits of available knowledge. (I should note here that Grof's use of the term 'transpersonal' differs somewhat in emphasis from its use in the body of this book, where it is restricted to spiritually quickened or ascendent experience.)

Other instances of transpersonal experiences may verge into the mythical realm, in which a person might relive an entire episode from an ancient Egyptian, Chinese, or Mayan myth, apparently without previous conscious knowledge of it. The gap between the level of the individual's previous education and the detail of the mythic experience, as represented for example in drawings made during LSD sessions, can be striking. Transpersonal experiences can also be of a dramatically mystical nature in which consciousness, for instance, might expand to identify with various levels of being or even the entire cosmos.

It is of interest to note that Grof takes the trouble to compare his own findings with Ken Wilber's theory. Viewing Wilber with high regard, he is nevertheless critical of the latter's apparent lack of 'a genuine appreciation of the paramount significance of birth and death,' as witnessed in the perinatal level of experience. He also criticizes Wilber's apparently linear model of development from the individual through the various transpersonal stages. Grof comments that:

> The psyche has a multidimensional, holographic nature, and using a linear model to describe it will produce distortions and inaccuracies ... My own observations suggest that, as conscious evolution proceeds ... it does not follow a linear trajectory, but in a sense infolds into itself.

I make no claim to settle this difference. I will, however, note that from the process perspective of the present book it is perhaps not entirely surprising that Grof and Wilber should come to different conclusions. They in fact seem to be observing different processes. Grof's work is based on the process of deep self-exploration, catalyzed by LSD or holotropic therapy. These procedures, as Grof himself observes, seem to act as an inner radar to pick up and magnify emotional psychological material especially of a traumatic nature, and apparently often lead to a reliving of such experiences and ultimately even to profound healing. It is apparent that these procedures also release tremendous creativity in the form of the imagination and, disrupting the ordinary bounds of experience, allow the development of a variety of psychic experiences. All of this may be cleansing, therapeutic, and growth inducing, but it is not the process that Wilber examines in his own writing.

Wilber is interested in the gradual and perhaps more permanent construction of structures or levels of consciousness as brought about by traditional spiritual practices, especially those derived from the various forms of the perennial wisdom. Since much of the present book deals with the same theme, I will not rehash Wilber's ideas here, or my own. I only note that it is useful in comparing Grof with Wilber to recall the distinction between a structure and a state of consciousness. Wilber is concerned with structures of consciousness and their construction, while Grof's work has dealt most directly with a variety of more or less mutable states of consciousness and the content available to them.

Michael Washburn

In 1988 Michael Washburn published a book titled *The Ego and the Dynamic Ground,* in which he set forth a theory of transpersonal growth which he further develops in his more recent, *Transpersonal Psychology in Psychoanalytic Perspective.* Here I will rely more on his first work, which lays out the broad terms of his theory in a very readable form. At first glance it is a relatively simple and

appealing theory of human psychological and spiritual development that starts
with infancy and progresses to the highest transpersonal realms of experience.
On closer examination, the theory is seen to have an elegance and subtlety that
renders it worthy of consideration in any discussion of transpersonal development.

Washburn characterizes his theory as *dynamic, triphasic,* and *dialectical.* By
dynamic, he means that the primary focus of the theory is with the relationship
of the ego to the 'dynamic life,' the source of which he terms the *Dynamic
Ground.* The focus,

> in the domain of psychology, [is] on the relation of the ego to the
> dynamic unconscious and, in the domain of spirituality, on the
> relation of the ego to possible religious (e.g., numinous, infused,
> charismatic, illuminated) experience.

The idea of the Dynamic Ground owes something to Freud's classical notion of
a dynamic unconscious, but owes more to Jung's collective unconscious. The latter is a wellspring of 'higher symbolic meanings and spiritual possibilities.'

Washburn criticizes Jung, however, for mixing up in a single broth both
spiritual and instinctual impulses, so that the prehuman, or animal nature, and the
transpersonal do not seem clearly distinguished. This is a problem that every
serious spiritually minded reader of Jung must sooner or later confront. The
concept of the Dynamical Ground is, in fact, itself very large, as it manifests at
times in the form of the Freudian unconscious, at other times as the Jungian
collective unconscious, and at still other times as the very essence of spirituality.
Washburn, however, takes care to explain, at least in broad terms, how these
different expressions come about.

Washburn conceptualizes the personality as a bipolar structure in which the
ego is one pole and the non-egoic process associated with the Dynamic Ground
is the other. Moreover, he refers to his theory as *triphasic,* because it postulates
that in the course of a lifetime the psychological make-up of an individual tends
to pass through three major phases or stages. Each of these stages is defined in
terms of a changing relationship between the two poles of the personality, the
ego and the Dynamic Ground. The first phase is the *pre-egoic stage,* which is
seen only during infancy and early childhood. In it the ego has not yet
established itself as an autonomous entity, and is still essentially engulfed in the
original non-egoic pole of the personality. During this period the ego begins for
the first time to differentiate itself from the non-egoic pole as a body-ego. Life
is charged with a primal numinosity, and the child is open to the outer world as
well as the deep source of life within.

In the *egoic stage* the ego establishes itself as an independent system, but only
at the cost of the *original repression* of the non-egoic pole of the personality.
During this stage the ego is primarily a mental identity which exists autono-

mously only by retaining a strong repression of the life-engendering forces of the Dynamic Ground. This is the condition in which most ordinary persons spend the greater part of their lives. Few grow beyond it.

Washburn's theory comes into its own when, as occurs in a small number of individuals, the original repression begins to break down, opening the way for further growth toward the *transegoic stage*. Thus begins a period of liminality, characterized by Washburn as 'regression in the service of transcendence.' This is a play on the Freudian notion of regression in the service of the ego, in which one temporarily abandons ego control, as in the passion of a sports contest, to actually further the ego's own goals. This initial interruption of the sovereignty of the ego is not usually a pleasant experience. The first signs of the weakening of the reign of the ego may include a growing sense of alienation. The world can appear flat and without meaning. This may lead to anxiety and fear of losing touch with reality, as well as a growing sense of dread. These are among the well known negative aspects of the existential experience.

As the egoic pole of the personality further weakens its repressive blockade on the non-egoic pole, powerful and threatening experiences may break through. These can include feelings of strangeness in an increasingly surreal world that now seems to contain hidden and sinister dimensions. Finally, one can fall prey to black depressions in which the ego is 'put in traction by the gravitational pull' of the Dynamic Ground. Here we find the roots of the long period of disorientation and depression termed the 'dark night of the soul,' experienced by so many Christian mystics. Surviving such experiences, one moves on to the transegoic stage proper. One is now elevated by the spirit, rather than being assailed by it.

In time, and if growth continues, the non-egoic pole of the personality comes to express itself in increasingly powerful and positive ways. The egoic pole at last gives up its sovereignty, but not its existence, to the rising tide of the Dynamic Ground. In the end a full working integration is achieved, one in which the ego continues to carry out its normal functions, but is informed at every step by the life-giving spirit of the Dynamic Ground. In this final sequence of growth, the individual may first find that the world acquires an enchanted quality. Ultimately it comes to present itself in hallowed resplendence.

Let us return now to the overall picture of Washburn's theory. An important aspect of his model of growth is that it is *dialectical*. This idea is expressed in the overall form of the developmental progression, as the ego moves from an initial condition of saturation by the basic potentials of life in the pre-egoic phase (the thesis), through the egoic phase in which the ego achieves autonomy at the expense of repression (the antithesis), and back again at the transegoic phase to a full embodiment of the life energies of the non-egoic pole of the personality (the synthesis). Washburn underscores this dialectical form of growth in which regression plays a central role, contrasting its cyclic quality with Wilber's model of an essentially sequential or linear form of development, one based on a hierarchical conception of the psyche in which growth progresses upwards from tier to tier.

One gets the impression, reading Washburn and Wilber side by side, that while both aim for a universally applicable model of transpersonal growth, Washburn draws most heavily on material from Western spirituality, while Wilber relies more on Eastern traditions. For instance, while both discuss negative experiences such as the dark night of the soul that seem particularly characteristic of Western mysticism, Washburn gives them a central position in his theory while Wilber does not. This is to be expected, given the former's stress on the importance of regression in service of transcendence.

Washburn (1990, 1994) has re-emphasized the distinction between his own dialectical model and Wilber's hierarchical one.[3] In doing so, he argues that Wilber's model is characteristic of Eastern modes of growth and development while the dialectical model is characteristic of Western ones. He asserts that the latter is more representative of both the psychology and the religion of the West, citing, for example, Carl Jung's work in the realm of psychology, and the fall and redemption tradition of Christianity.

To describe in detail Wilber's response to this 'criticism' would take us beyond our present purposes.[4] I will simply note that Wilber contends that his own model also allows for, and indeed includes, the dialectical process of which Washburn speaks.

It is my own opinion that Washburn's work has received less than its fair share of attention. For instance, its emphasis on the non-egoic pole of the personality and the idea of the Dynamic Ground seem quite compatible with the self-exploratory experiences reported by Grof's LSD and holotropic therapy participants. Many of these experiences clearly seem to exhibit the regressive qualities which Washburn emphasizes. Indeed, Grof himself stresses the non-linear character of human growth, as we have seen.

In completing this short review, I note that Washburn and Wilber both rely to a substantial extent on psychodynamic concepts, which stress unconscious forces, projections, and so on. (I did not emphasize this aspect of Wilber in my review of his theory, but it can be found in his major psychological works.)[5] In this respect at least, the approach of the present book departs widely from both of these theorists. Moreover, the approach here stresses the importance of process over structure, while Washburn and Wilber, though aware of process, tend rather to emphasize structures and the relationships between them. In the last analysis, all are narratives about human life in its many possibilities. The reader must choose that story which best fits his or her own experience.

Endnotes

Foreword

1. *Brahman* being the 'stuff' the universe is made of.

2. Speaking in terms of numbers, three and five as a centered four, play a significant role from a geometrical point of view in both Brahmanical and Buddhist thought. While seven and, more rarely, four, pertain to process and growth from a psychological point of view. But somehow and at some time the dynamic approach to reality was overshadowed or even cut short by the idea of a One — a beginning, even if this beginning was said to be no beginning in the strict sense of the word — which ultimately ended in a static cosmos.

3. Whenever the word 'Vedanta' — the end of knowledge as its gathering — is used, the non-theistic interpretation by Shankara (eighth century) is meant. All other interpretations have to be explicitly qualified by their authors' names such as the theist Ramanuja (twelfth century) or the dualist Madhva (thirteenth century) and others. Shankara whom the Indians quickly recognized as a 'cryptic Buddhist' *(prachanna-buddha)* was a disciple of Govinda, a Buddhist, who, in turn was a disciple of Gaudapada who blurred the distinction between the Buddhist notion of *advaya* 'non-duality' and the Brahmanical (Hinduist) notion of *advaita* 'one without a second.'

   Strictly speaking, what we call 'philosophy,' their seeking after wisdom and knowledge, is by the Indians themselves referred to either as a 'vision/perspective' *(darshana)*, or a 'belief-system/dogma' *(siddhanta)*, though not always clearly kept apart.

4. Although logic is one of the most reductive disciplines, its judicious use is of tremendous value and has always been recognized as such.

5. Due to his prolific literary output Sri Aurobindo's influence in the West was far greater than in India where his Integral Yoga was one among many other forms of yoga.

6. The earliest Samkhya teaching, mentioned in the writing of the physician Caraka, had spoken of the 'unmanifested' *(avyakta)* as an aspect of matter *(prakriti)*, which later separated into matter and a hypostatized *purusha* equated with the notion of the Atman. Other forms of the Samkhya systems recognized a plurality of *purushas*, but all agreed that it was the *prakriti* that underwent a series of transformations resulting in the physical world. One peculiar feature of this system was that what we would call the mental was one of the three strands *(guna)* that

constituted matter, the two others presenting the instinctual and the inert in an individual's make-up, respectively.

The *purusha* was conceived of as pure spirit or intelligence and as the enjoyer *(bhoktr)*, not as an actor *(kartr)*, of all activity, whether material-physical or mental, going on in the *prakriti*. This was a notion that had dire consequences for the social realm; the woman has to do all the work and the man has a good time. This may have been the reason for its appeal in spite of the fact that it is shot through and through with contradictions and fallacies. For while all Indian systems of thought insisted on some final emancipation *(moksa)*, how could this ever be realized since the everlasting presence of the *purusha,* one of the basic tenets of the Samkhya system, kept the *prakriti* busy and prevented a separation and with it annulling its presence.

7. One thinks of contemporary theorists such as Sri Aurobindo and Ken Wilber, and much implicit 'New Age' philosophy. (A. Combs)

Introduction

1. This brief story is taken from a similar one once told by Gregory Bateson. It was at a conference, and consistent with its message I have long since forgotten all but the story.

2. This is mentioned by Chögyam Trungpa in his 1975 translation of *The Tibetan Book of the Dead,* with F. Fremantle. The general principle, however, is widely apparent in Eastern thought. Concepts such as projection, repression, denial, and the unconscious are familiar in many Eastern traditions.

Chapter 1

1. The word *consciousness* takes many different meanings in the West alone. In this book I do not intend to occupy the reader with a lengthy discussion of this variegated topic. Such discussions are, however, available. I would particularly recommend the fine articles by Thomas Natsoulas (1978 & 1983) and David Rosenthal (1993), as well as Imants Baruss' book, *The Personal Nature of Notions of Consciousness.*

2. The notion that conscious thoughts, perceptions, feelings, and the like are always *about* something has been about in Western philosophy for a long time in one form or another, but was powerfully articulated by the late nineteenth-century philosopher and psychologist Franz Brentano, who was, incidentally, once an instructor of Sigmund Freud. Brentano's notion of *intentionality* became a foundation stone for Edmund Hus-

serl's phenomenology, which formed an important strain of European thought down through the writings of Jean-Paul Sartre.

3. It would seem that certain mystical and meditative states may be free of this focused aspect of consciousness. See, for example, Franklin Merrell-Wolf's classic book, *The Philosophy of Consciousness without an Object.* This type of consciousness has also been described by Zen master Hung Chih Cheng Chues, who wrote that it,

> ... consists in turning the *noesis* [or knowing function of consciousness] into a reality without coming in contact with things, and in bringing it all to light without objectifying it. (Toshihiko, p.192)

4. The field of psychology is increasingly recognizing the importance of attention in activating mental processes such as thought, memory, and decision-making. Without attention, mental events may still occur, but apparently only at a much diminished level (e.g., see Eysenck & Keane, 1990).

5. The mid-seventeenth-century *Meditations* of René Descartes were eminently philosophical but also conveniently political. They represented a deal cut with the papacy by which the Church could keep the soul — and thus the mind — if secular enquiry could have the body. The division was razor-sharp, thinking substance *(res cogitans)* on one side, and the physical world (extended substance or *res extensa)* on the other. These two realms were as different, one from the other, as the ideas in this book are from the material pages of which they are printed. Descartes never adequately explained just how these two levels of reality could interact, though he thought the pineal gland was involved. To this day metaphysical dualisms are plagued by the problem of how the two sides transact with each other.

6. William James, 1912.

7. My own view of the nature of consciousness is similar to that of Jean-Paul Sartre, who described it as a clear emptiness which discloses that which it contains. He likened it to the water of a clear stream, through which one sees the pebbles at the bottom. I also like the metaphor of light, which is not seen directly, but illuminates all that it touches.

Coming from the continental philosophical tradition, Sartre was also very much aware of the intentional nature of consciousness. Strangely, however, and contrary to my own inclinations, Sartre was a complete materialist. He felt, as did many of the existential philosophers, that speculations which range beyond the immediate givens of concrete experience are intellectually dishonest, failing in the courage to face reality in its immediate concrete starkness.

8. For example see Roger Sperry's article, *The Impact and Promise of the Cognitive Revolution,* or Daniel Dennett's popular book, *Consciousness Explained.*

9. In a delightful essay entitled *What is it like to be a bat?* philosopher Thomas Nagel puts forward a

devastatingly simple and straight-forward argument against material explanations of consciousness. This is simply that it is *like* something to be a living human being or even a brown bat, while on the other hand, it is not like anything to be a brick or a baseball bat! This is a strong way of pointing to the importance of the *subjectivity* of consciousness. Any explanation that ignores this aspect of consciousness denies the very thing it sets out to explain.

Coming from a different angle, philosopher John Searle develops a compelling argument against the common view in the cognitive sciences that consciousness is simply another way of talking about computational processes in the brain. This is the famous Chinese Room argument (1980, 1982). It suppo-ses that someone sits in a closed room translating Chinese docu-ments into English. Documents in Chinese are handed in to him and, after translating them, he hands them back out. Now, one might suppose that to do this job he would need to understand Chin-ese. But, a closer examination of the situation tells us that he, in fact, can do it simply by working from dictionaries that provide him with the rules of translation. In other words, the man in the Chin-ese room can operate mechanical-ly, as it were, from the rules with which he is provided, and need have no real understanding of the texts. In this sense he is like a Chinese translating computer.

Now here is the point. The claim that the essence of *understanding* — in this case the Chinese text —

is in the computations performed by the brain, mind, or a computer, is nonsense. The translator, in our case, understands not a word, though he translates perfectly. The further claim that the operation of a computational device such as a computer explains human under-standing also fails, for, as we see, the translator in the Chinese room understands nothing. The point of all this is that *meaning* is an essential aspect of consciousness and cannot be explained away as computation or any other mecha-nistic event.

10. See for example Herbert Guen-ther's work on Buddhism. Also, Indian theories of mind, though developed in the service of spi-ritual technologies such as yoga, likewise tend to place cognitive processes such as thought and memory in the foreground.

11. For a highly readable history of the cognitive sciences see Howard Gardener's book, *The Mind's New Science.* He devotes several pages to an examination of the parallels between classical rationalism and the cognitive sciences.

12. Varela, Thompson and Rosch, in their recent book, *The Embodied Mind: Cognitive Science and Hu-man Experience,* develop a con-cept of mind from a perspective that is both holistic and pheno-menological. They make an excel-lent case for a view of mind that is not an inner process at all, but an ongoing interaction between an organism and its environment that creates an experienced world. I think this is an important and for-ward-looking idea. At root it is

not inconsistent with the view of this book. Here, however, I emphasize the 'inner' aspect of mind for convenience's sake, since many parts of the book touch on traditional topics in psychology, all of which have conceived mental processes as something within the person. Also, I do not want to complicate an already complex subject with a new and perhaps unusual concept of mind.

13. William James began his masterful text, *The Principles of Psychology,* with the statement:

Psychology is the Science of Mental Life, both of its phenomena and of their conditions. The phenomena are such things as we call feelings, desires, cognitions, reasonings, decisions, and the like ... (1890/1981, p.15)

14. E.g., Dennett, 1991.

15. Cartwright, 1977.

16. For example, see Bernard Baars' excellent book, *A Cognitive Theory of Consciousness,* and Arthur Reber's article, *The Cognitive Unconsciousness,* for in depth treatments of the problem of mental processes as they occur within and outside of consciousness. The topic of the 'cognitive unconsciousness,' that is, ordinary mental processes that occur beyond the pale of consciousness, is of considerable interest to psychologists today.

Chapter 2

1. Technically, of course, Descartes' thinking substance *(res cogitans)* was to have equal reality status with the material world *(res extensa* or extended substance). It was, however, a metaphysical equivalence, and metaphysical notions, even if fortunate enough to be widely accepted in their own day, have a way of slipping off into history. This is what happened to the *res cogitans,* or in other words, the soul.

2. Watts & Huang, 1975.

3. Guenther, 1984, 1989, 1992, 1993.

4. By *subjective* I mean phenomenological, or dealing with the immediate givens of experience.

5. *General systems theory,* or just *systems theory,* is a big name for a simple but powerful concept. Essentially it is that any object or process that can be identified as existing more or less independent of its surroundings can be thought of as a system. Possibilities include lumps of coal, mushrooms, tadpoles, people, companies, whole societies of people, nation states, ecologies, solar systems, spiral galaxies, and just about anything else that can be recognized and discussed. Of course some systems, such as people, are more interesting to talk about than others (though there is no accounting for taste).

No system exists in isolation. Lumps of coal absorb heat from the environment and radiate it back when they cool off. Living organisms engage in complex interactions with their environments, taking in food and excreting waste material, just for starters. Further, they participate in complex exchanges with other organisms. A vital feature of the systems point of view is that systems, especially complex ones like organisms and ecologies, are dynamically engaged in matter, energy, and behavioral exchanges with their environments and with each other. A good review of these ideas is found in Ervin Laszlo's early book, *Introduction to Systems Philosophy: Toward a New Paradigm of Contemporary Thought.*

Another important feature of systems is their tendency to organize into hierarchies with smaller systems stacked, Chinese box fashion, inside larger ones. The cells of the human body, for instance, are systems in the major body organs, which themselves are part of the whole body. Less obvious but more pertinent to the present discussion, *processes* can also be systems. The metabolic cycles of individual cells contribute to larger organic processes such as physical growth or the expenditure of energy in behavioral activity. These ideas are developed in the main text. A good introduction to them, however, is found in Arthur Koestler's autobiography, *Janus: a Summing Up.* Koestler's allusion to the two-faced god, Janus, honors the dual tendency of systems to be complete in themselves and yet subunits in larger systems.

The term *cybernetics* comes from the Greek, *kybernetikos,* meaning 'good at steering.' Thus, cybernetics is concerned with guidance systems. One of the first sophisticated developments in cybernetic theory was Norbert Wiener's work on anti-aircraft weaponry during the Second World War, where it was necessary to take into account the trajectories of previous shots in selecting the best aim for the next round. From thermostats to organisms, cybernetic systems constantly monitor the consequences of their previous activities in selecting new trajectories, as it were, or new courses of action. This monitoring of the outcomes of one's own behavior is termed *feedback.*

As time went by it became increasingly apparent that virtually all dynamic systems, including human beings, societies, and entire ecologies, are involved in many levels of feedback. Gregory Bateson's early work with Margaret Mead on the Balinese character (1942) made early use of cybernetic thinking in the social sciences, as did his famous *double-bind* theory of schizophrenia. Today, cybernetic ideas are pretty much assumed when speaking of complex systems, though, as will be seen in the text, the notion of *feed-forward,* emphasizing the forward motion of systems into new states, has become an important concept as well.

6. Erich Jantsch, 1980; Ervin Laszlo, 1972.

7. Maturana, Varela, & Uribe, 1974.

8. The notion that human societies can be understood as self-creating systems is explored in a book I

recently coauthored with systems theorist Ervin Laszlo, historian Robert Artigiani, and ethologist Vilmos Csányi, titled, *The Evolution of Cognitive Maps: New Paradigms for the 21st Century.* The basic idea is that the knowledge, beliefs systems, and customs of a culture are created within it by artists, intellectuals, and spiritual pioneers, as well as by ordinary citizens, and are passed on from one generation to the next in an ongoing event of creation.

9. E.g., Abraham & Shaw, 1984; Briggs & Peat, 1989; Cambel, 1993; Gleick, 1987; Waldrop, 1992.

10. The terms *chaos theory* and *chaotic systems* have in recent years come to represent a broad range of complex processes which, as a whole, are not handled well by traditional Newtonian methods of analysis. For a broad view of the concepts often included under the topic of chaos theory see, for example, A.B. Cambel's excellent book, *Applied Chaos Theory: a Paradigm for Complexity.* Other surveys in all likelihood will continue to be published.

At this writing it seems likely that chaos theory will eventually become part of the larger category of *the sciences of complexity* (indicating the entire range of studies of complex systems from computers and artificial intelligence to complex systems theory and chaos, and often emphasizing the non-linear nature of such systems). If this happens, chaos theory disappears as a distinct field except in mathematics. On the other hand, it is possible that the sciences of complexity will in time all come to be called chaos theory. Perhaps the most likely outcome is that both chaos theory and the sciences of complexity will continue to be used in a very general way, each including parts of the other.

11. The breadth and variety of the applications of chaos theory are rapidly becoming too diverse to gather into a single book. And, unfortunately, no such book was assembled during the first years of chaos theory's growth. Crutchfield, Doyne, Packard, and Shaw's 1986 *Scientific American* article, *Chaos,* gives an excellent early survey of the field. On the other hand, informal books such as Mitchell Waldrop's, *Complexity: The Emerging Science at the Edge of Order and Chaos,* can be found on the shelves of many bookstores.

12. Abraham and Shaw, 1984; Ruelle, 1981.

13. The choice of velocity and position in these figures is arbitrary. We might, for example, have chosen velocity and acceleration, or even drawn a three dimensional portrait with position, velocity, and acceleration represented on separate axes.

14. Rossi, 1986; Werntz, Bickford, Bloom, & Shannahoff-Khalsa, 1982.

15. Combs, Winkler, & Daley, 1994.

16. Mathematically speaking, a chaotic attractor never repeats itself, and indeed its trajectories (plots) never actually cross each other (which requires that they be plot-

ted in at least three or more dimensions, unlike Figures 1 and 2). In other words, a chaotic attractor not only never follows the same temporal course twice through a cycle, but is never in exactly the same place twice. When viewed in cross-section chaotic attractors display a strange exquisite microstructure characterized by fractal geometry.

> If a system's attractor is strange,
> You will see its trajectory range
> Through every spot
> You can possibly plot
> In the state space of temporal change.
>
> *Ted Melnechuk, Amherst, MA*

17. Combs, Winkler, & Daley, 1994.
18. The circadian rhythm, in fact, displays a number of important features of chaotic attractors, and is thus clearly *chaotic-like*. For instance, its course is irregular though its overall pattern can be recognized and identified. It is unlikely it ever exactly repeats itself, i.e., that any two days will ever be precisely the same. Beyond this, the circadian rhythm, like a chaotic attractor, can be predicted in the short run with rough accuracy — for example on any given day we can make a good guess about when a person we know will go to bed — but it is not precisely predictable over long periods of time — for instance we cannot say at what time this individual will get up next Christmas morning.
19. There are serious limitations on the ability of the researcher to prove that a seemingly chaotic system in fact meets the mathe-

matical criteria for chaos. The most problematic but not the only one of these is that enormously large data sets are required for the analysis of chaotic behavior. For example, eight to ten thousand measurements on a single system would not be considered generous! In the meantime, if it is a human system under study, say, the human EEG pattern, then the original conditions that surrounded the experimental situation have in all likelihood changed between the first and last measurement, complicating matters considerably. See bio-mathematician Paul Rapp's 1993 paper for a discussion of some of these problems.

20. E.g., Kaufmann, 1993; Waldrop, 1992.
21. This figure is also known as the young woman and the old hag, and as the bride and the mother-in-law!
22. Abraham, 1994.
23. My own introduction to 'the sciences of complexity' was through H. Pagels' excellent book, *The Dreams of Reason: the Computer and the Rise of the Sciences of Complexity*. Since its publication a few years ago an increasing stream of books on the topic of have crossed the shelves of local bookstores and libraries. Some of the more recent include M. Mitchell Waldrop's previously mentioned *Complexity: the Emerging Science at the Edge of Order and Chaos,* and Murray Gell-Mann's, *The Quark and the Jaguar: Adventures in the Simple and the Complex*.
24. The psychological idea of *flow,*

for which Mihaly Csikszentmihalyi (1990) is well known, is that while engaging in challenging and rewarding activities, creative individuals become absorbed in a positive state of mind in which they forget themselves. They may also feel a sense of transcendence, becoming more than their ordinary selves. Csikszentmihalyi refers to persons who have developed this style of activity as a common part of their lives as *T-persons,* or *transcenders.*

25. Csikszentmihalyi, 1993.
26. Ronald Fox's book, *Energy and the Evolution of Life,* gives a clear but somewhat technical coverage of this matter.
27. Lynn Margulis, 1987, 1988; Margulis & Sagan, 1986.
28. Swenson, 1989.
29. Another highly readable introduction to these ideas is found in E. Chaisson's book, *The Life Era.*
30. Partial sketches of a psychology based on the grand synthesis have been presented in conference discussions and recently published in articles and book chapters (Combs, 1993a, 1993b, 1995a, 1995b, 1995c).

Chapter 3

1. Margulis & Sagan, 1986; Margulis, 1988.
2. It would take us too far afield to explore in detail the evolution of the brain. For those interested in serious reading in this area, I recommend Harry J. Jerison's classic, *The Evolution of the Brain and Intelligence,* as well as Sir John Eccles' book on the human brain, *Evolution of the Brain: Creation of the Mind.* This topic, along with the whole issue of human origins, however, is changing so rapidly that the best advice might simply be to see what is current at the time of your reading.
3. MacLean, 1958, 1970, 1990.
4. There is a curious correspondence between the three levels of the triune brain and certain aspects of human nature described by the Indian philosopher and sage, Sri Aurobindo, whose accounts of transpersonal dimensions of mind and consciousness will bring him to our attention in future chapters. Sri Aurobindo's description of *material consciousness* seems strikingly suggestive of MacLean's reptilian brain. Matching MacLean almost to the letter, Sri Aurobindo wrote:

> [The material mind] is mechanical, inertly moved by habits or by the forces of the lower nature. Always repeating the same unintelligent and unenlightened movements, it is attached to the routine and established rule of what already exists, unwilling to change ... Or, if it is willing, then it is unable. Or, if it is able, then it turns the action ... into a new mechanical routine and so takes out of it all soul and life. It is

obscure, stupid, indolent, full of ignorance and inertia, darkness and slowness. (Aurobindo, 1971, p. 1429).

Working to transform this mind 'is a monumental battle against habits going back thousands of years' (Satprem, 1982, p.68).

Sri Aurobindo's description of the *vital mind* seems similar to the paleomammalian brain. Like the latter, it is often occupied by social aspects of life, is unruly, and has a strong penchant for melodrama. It is the root of much pathology. Sri Aurobindo once commented that:

the psycho-analysis of Freud ... takes up a certain part, the darkest, the most perilous, the unhealthiest part of the nature — the lower vital subconscious layer, isolates some of its most morbid phenomena and attributes to it and them an action out of all proportion to its true role in the nature' (1971, p.1606).

Sri Aurobindo also described several levels of the thinking or rational mind, all of which seem to correspond to the neomammalian brain.

The evident similarity between MacLean's and Sri Aurobindo's descriptions suggests that these three aspects of mind may be ancient attractors for human consciousness.

5. Fodor, 1983.
6. Gazzaniga 1985, 1988.
7. E.g., Baars, 1988; Reber, 1992.
8. Gazzaniga, 1985, p. 87.
9. Baars, 1983, 1988.
10. Gazzaniga, 1985.

It is the case in all of us that objects or words seen in each half of the visual field are first registered on the opposite side of the brain, but in persons who have undergone the split-brain operation, which severs the corpus callosum, the main neural pathway connecting the two hemispheres, the message does not get communicated back to the other side. Thus, the individual is left with the information restricted to the hemisphere opposite the viewed object or words.

11. In a somewhat more complex situation, the young man was once presented with a variety of visual scenes, some to the left hemisphere and some to the right. They included a picture of a snow-covered farmhouse delivered to the right brain. Meanwhile, the left brain was treated to a drawing of the head of a chicken. Later when asked to choose between a variety of pictures by freely pointing with both hands, his left hand, controlled by the right hemisphere, went straight to a drawing of a snow shovel, while the right hand, controlled by the left hemisphere, pointed to a drawing of a chicken foot. He then was asked to explain why his left hand was pointing at the shovel. Since only the left brain had sufficient language ability to speak, and it had seen only the chicken head, in a perfect example of confabulation the young man exclaimed, 'To shovel the chicken shit!'

12. Cairns-Smith, 1990.
13. See Danah Zohar's book, *The Quantum Self,* for a readable re-

view of the whole matter of the relationship of consciousness to matter.

14. Nagel, 1974.

15. The presence of chaos in the brain as well as its possible role in memory, perception, consciousness, and other brain functions has recently become a common topic of discussion among neuroscientists. See, e.g., Basar, 1990; Kaufmann, 1993; Kelso, 1995; Pribram, 1994; and Waldrop, 1992.

16. Dreaming is seen in virtually all mammals, and is apparently experienced by the fetal infant before birth. These facts argue for a strong biological drive behind the dream state. This does not mean that dreaming has no psychological meaning. On the contrary, three thousand years of cultural history as well as modern psychiatry tell us that it does. An excellent resource on the biology of dreaming is Hobson's *The Dreaming Brain*.

17. Freeman, 1991, 1992, 1994.

18. We are again reminded of William James' conclusion in *The Principles of Psychology* that the same mental state can never occur twice because the brain itself is modified with experience (see also note 33 below).

19. Goertzel, 1994.

20. See Goertzel, 1994, 1993a, 1993b.

21. This book is *Chaotic Logic: Language, Mind and Reality, from the Perspective of Complex Systems Science,* now available from Plenum.

22. Kampis, 1991.

23. Ben Goertzel hardly disagrees with the notion of fundamental unpredictability, finding this aspect of Kampis' work unconvincing.

24. See Ulric Neisser's *Memory Observed* for a wonderful indictment of the reliability of ordinary memory, or Elizabeth Loftus's informal book, *Memory,* for a more systematic exploration of the assets and limitations of memory, including an excellent discussion of the difficulties these present for the reliability of eyewitness testimony.

25. Bower, 1981; Eich, 1980.

26. Dement, 1972.

27. Globus, 1986.

28. E.g., Kuhn, 1988; Flavell, 1963; Flavell, 1963; Gruber & Voneche, 1977.

29. E.g., Kohlberg, 1981.

30. Erikson, 1960; Maslow, 1968.

31. Grof, 1985, 1988; Grof & Bennett, 1992; Washburn, 1988, 1994; Wilber 1980, 1986b.

32. Gebser, 1949/1986.

33. William James took pains in *The Principles of Psychology* to point out that conscious experience never repeats itself. 'No state once gone can recur and be identical with what it was before' (1890/1981, p.224) The reason for this is plain; we are always acquiring new experiences which somehow, if ever so slightly, constantly modify us. We are never the same person we were at any time in the past, so cannot have the same experiences again.

Recently the renowned physiologist and chaos theorist, Walter Freeman (1994), came to the same conclusion based on his research into the nature of learning and the brain.

34. Blanck & Blanck, 1979; Erikson, 1960.
35. Wilber, 1986a.
36. Kellogg, 1969.
37. Ramana Maharshi, 1988.
38. Suzuki, 1952.
39. Vandervert, 1991, 1992, 1993, forthcoming.
40. I would include all subjective events in my idea of mind, what we ordinarily think of as the inner life including feelings, dreams, fantasies and so forth, while Vandervert emphasizes the cognitive aspect of mind with its social function of communication through pictures and symbol systems such as language. Moreover, in my own view consciousness does not structure anything, space and time included. That is why it is perfectly possible to have states of consciousness that lie outside of space and time.

    Interestingly, Ben Goertzel (1995) has developed a theory of consciousness in which he argues that 'randomness, if not the essence of consciousness, is at least the incarnation which consciousness assumes in the realm of regularities.' A very strange notion. But he makes an excellent case to the effect that it is the encounter of randomness with order, the 'collapse of the wave function,' that is most often associated with the appearance of consciousness. Moreover, the theory has the virtue of attributing no structure to consciousness itself, but leaving the latter for the mind, or in Goertzel's terms, the cognitive attractor.
41. Pribram, 1991.
42. For a fascinating treatment of the whole question of reality in the postmodern world see Walter Truett Anderson's, *Reality isn't What it Used to Be: Theatrical Politics, Ready-to-Wear Religion, Global Myths, Primitive Chic, and other Wonders of the Postmodern World*!
43. Bower, 1981.

Chapter 4

1. Patterson, 1987.
2. Ashe, 1992.
3. Vico, 1744/1984.
4. Vico's idea that history runs downhill has a certain following in the modern world. It seems to be embedded in James Joyce's *Finnegan's Wake,* and is the subject of a book by Norman O. Brown entitled *Closing Time,* a double reference to Joyce, suggesting the time of night when the pub closes and to the end of time itself. This title has recently appeared, as well, as a song by Leonard Cohen. Vico's writings have taken on a certain cult status in recent years, especially since they have been picked up and expanded by William Irwin Thompson.
5. The notion that organisms can benefit from the experiences of their ancestors never entirely disappeared. For example, it is at the root of the Jungian concept of archetypes, a notion which despite its continuing bad treatment at the

hands of hard nosed scientists has progressively gained acceptance over the past few decades. For a contemporary scientific look at archetypes see Anthony Stevens' *The Two Million-Year-Old Self.*

The whole idea of the presence of past influences is explored and defended in recent work by Rupert Sheldrake and Ervin Laszlo, of which I will have much more to say in Chapters 7 and 8.

6. Richards, 1987.
7. Bergson, 1907/1983.
8. From a biological point of view the idea of a goal-directed evolution, termed *finalism* by biologists, has serious difficulties. For one thing, it runs contrary to a whole tradition that sees evolutionary change as the result of random alterations in the genetic structure. Such alterations come about through random variations in the genetic code of each generation. In some instances these lead to improved adaptability and an increased likelihood of being passed on to future generations. This basic idea, thought to operate over the course of many generations of a particular species, is the heart of modern evolutionary theory.

Darwin himself knew nothing of genes, but postulated variation to occur in each new generation. In the early years of this century an emerging science of genetics gave a strong rationale for such variation in terms of the large number of traits represented in the gene pool of each species. This number was in time shown to be regularly supplemented by the appearance of new mutations. Thus, we come to the basic conception that is widely accepted today, one of variation and selection in which certain traits that appear in each generation are more adaptive than others, producing organisms more likely to thrive, reproduce, and pass them on.

9. Huxley, 1907/1983.
10. It is precisely such arguments that lend credibility to Rupert Sheldrake's (1981, 1988) notion of morphic resonance and Ervin Laszlo's (1987b, 1993) psi-field hypothesis, which postulate subtle lasting influences of form and process.
11. The neo-Darwinians were the evolutionists who during the first decades of this century demonstrated the mechanism for variation in each generation — which Darwin had originally postulated but did not explain — could be found in random genetic recombinations. To this, the additional feature of occasional mutations was eventually appended.
12. Schumacher, 1977.

Chapter 5

1. Nicholas of Cusa was an ancient analogue to David Bohm, both seeing the everyday world as the explication or 'unfolding' of a more basic implicate reality.
2. Eldredge & Gould, 1972.
3. Csányi, 1989.
4. Neumann, 1954/1973.

5. Coppens, 1981.

6. Interestingly, Duane Elgin in *Awakening Earth: Exploring the Evolution of Human Culture and Consciousness,* recently developed a view of the evolution of consciousness from a planetary and cultural perspective which he grounds in a dimensional analysis similar to Gebser's. The book is fascinating reading, a God's eye view of his vision of the evolution of human consciousness, reminiscent of Teilhard de Chardin. Gebser's work plays a prominent role in his discussion of correlated theories and resources at the end of the book.

7. Putman, 1988.

8. Eisler, 1987; Settegast, 1990.

9. Feuerstein, 1989a.

10. Campbell, 1988.

11. Eccles, 1989.

12. Jung, 1960/1973; Gebser, 1949/ 1986.

13. Eisler, 1987; Gimbutas, 1982.

14. Eisler, 1987; Thompson, 1981.

15. Kahler, 1956.

16. Brett, 1912/1921.

17. For example, see Emil Bock's study (1954/1993) of St Paul's spirituality.

18. It has been suggested that the absence of mirrors during the Middle Ages was in part due to the restriction against mirrors in monasteries, where many of the skilled workers were to be found as well.

19. Mickunas, 1990.

20. Behnke, 1987.

21. Behnke, 1987.

22. Feuerstein, 1987.

23. Behnke, 1987.

24. Cassirer, 1963.

25. Neoplatonism is usually dated from the writings of Plotinus in the third century Mediterranean world, but seems to have roots that extend back to the ancient Greek Pythagorean and Orphic mystery schools (Inge, 1918). Plotinus himself was the student of the enigmatic teacher Ammonius, in Alexandria, who did not write but directly taught a contemplative wisdom (Hixon, 1978).

Plotinus' writings named the eternal wellspring of existence as the One, which 'overflows' in its richness, making possible the multiple levels of being (Plotinus, 1930, 1992). The first beneath the One is the intellect or spirit, termed *nous,* not the intellect as we ordinarily know it, but a level of eternal being in which consciousness is completely at one with its object. This level in turn makes possible a multiplicity of living forms called souls, related at one end to the absolute, and at the other to the sensorial world. The soul embodies the principle of *logos,* or order. For example, the human soul sets the body and its elements into order. These three levels — the One, the *nous,* and the soul — are not separate, but are mutually enfolded within each other as different aspects of a single reality.

The One includes everything without any distinction. Intelligence [*nous*] contains all beings; but if they are distinct therein, they are nonetheless unified, and each of them contains all others potentially. In Soul, things tend to be distinguished from each other, until at the borderline they are dissipated and scattered into the sensible world. (E. Bréhier, 1958, p.46)

26. Bohm, 1980.

27. An in-depth exploration of emergence of the integral in today's world would be the object of a life-time's study, and in the case of Gebser it was almost just that. Much of *The Ever-Present Origin* is given over to an examination of the myriad expressions of the new integral awareness.

28. E.g., Anderson, 1990; Artigiani, 1990; Laszlo, Artigiani, Csányi & Combs, forthcoming.

29. The historical roots of deconstructionism as a kind of textual relativism can be found, in part at least, as early as Nietzsche.

30. In his exceptional book, *Reality isn't What it Used to Be,* Walter T. Anderson lucidly argues that the world today is made up of two kinds of people, those who believe in absolute values and a single reality and those who do not. The latter frighten the daylights out of the former, with their seemingly arbitrary play of ideas, art, morality, and so on. Anderson cogently asserts that this split is at the core of many if not most of the major value controversies that divide people today.

31. Duane Elgin's book, *Awakening Earth,* is in fact an entire speculative study of the future of the Earth in terms of consciousness and evolution (see also note 6 above).

Chapter 6

1. Wilber, 1977, 1979, 1980, 1981, 1983; Wilber, Engler, & Brown, 1986c.

2. Faivre & Needleman, 1992.

3. Smith, 1982; Wilber, 1983.

4. Many works describe the subtle sheaths of Vedanta. One that I frequently used was Rajmani Tigunait's *Seven Systems of Indian Philosophy.*

5. Wilber, 1973a, 1986b.

6. Actually there is more than one interpretation of Vedanta philosophy, of which the rendition by eighth-century sage and scholar Shankara is ordinarily assumed if others are not indicated. See Herbert Guenther's note 3 in his Foreword to this book.

7. Inge, 1918.

8. Among Ammonius' other students was Origen, the early Christian Church Father, who after his conversion to Christianity carried the influence of Neoplatonic ideas to the newly forming religion. One of these, for example, was a belief in the pre-existence of the soul prior to birth. It was a notion that is expressed in Plato's writings and was carried through to Neoplatonism. The Church, however, lost no time in declaring it a heresy after Origen's death.

9. Hixon, 1978.

10. Plotinus, 1930.

11. Becker, 1973, 1975; Brown, 1959, 1966; Neumann, 1954/1973.

12. E.g., Eisler 1987; Thompson, 1981.

13. Wilber, 1990.

Chapter 7

1. E.g., Satprem, 1970/1984, Aurobindo, 1972a.
2. Laszlo, 1987a, 1993; Sheldrake, 1981, 1982, 1988, 1991.
3. A recent collaboration between Rupert Sheldrake, chaos mathematician Ralph Abraham, and ethnopharmacologist Terence McKenna, *Trialogs on the Edge of the West,* contains considerable discussion of chaotic attractors.

   Indeed, in terms of brain activity if memories can be understood as chaotic attractors, then motor fields are potential attractor basins.
4. Koplowitz, 1983.
5. See Appendix I for a brief description of the seven *cakras* (also spelled 'chakras'), or centers of subtle energy that are associated with various points along the spinal cord and in the head. They are usually identified with Indian or Tibetan traditions, but seem to be virtually a universal constant in esoteric traditions throughout the world, and are symbolically represented in many traditional mythic forms as well.

   Perhaps the definitive modern work on these is Motoyama's *Theories of the Chakras: Bridge to Higher Consciousness.* For an excellent treatment of them from the point of view of traditional yoga see Swami Rama's *Path of Fire and Light: Advanced Practices of Yoga* and Swami Radha's *Kundalini: Yoga for the West.* And for a somewhat New Agey but well reviewed rendition, try *The Sevenfold Journey: Reclaiming Mind, Body, and Spirit through the Chakras,* by Anodea Judith and Selene Vega. If that isn't enough, the classic Western esoteric source is C.W. Leadbeater's *The Chakras,* a psychic's report which, as nearly as I can tell, has been more or less continuously in print from Theosophical Publishing since 1927!

Chapter 8

1. In the language of chaos theory, we might say that we would like to map the exquisitely complex and many-dimensional basin of the attractor of consciousness.
2. Bly, 1980.
3. Maturana & Varela, 1987.
4. Though Goertzel's cognitive equation was not originally conceived in terms of alternative states of consciousness, in principle it can be made to describe an individual's entire mental life, including all the states of consciousness he or she experiences or ever could experience.
5. Mountcastle, 1974.
6. Murphey & Donovan, 1988.
7. Volumes have been written on the myriad types of meditation recorded in the wisdom literature. An excellent resource is Daniel

Goldman's *The Meditative Mind: The Varieties of Meditative Experience*. A convenient division of practices, however, is made between concentrative types of meditation and observational or insight varieties. Most yogic meditation fits the former category and strives, at least in its early and intermediate stages, toward 'one pointed' concentration on a particular object such as a sound or mantra. Insight varieties, more common in Buddhism, open the participant to a continuous awareness of the changing content of experience. Vipassana and Zazen are examples of the latter.

While both types of meditation lead to a general slowing of the EEG rhythm, concentrative practices may lead the practitioner to successively deep trance states associated with experiences of the subtle planes of being and with remarkably slow rhythmic EEG patterns. For an extensive literature on the physiological effects of meditation, see Murphey and Donovan's *The Physical and Psychological Effects of Meditation: a Review of Contemporary Meditation Research with a Comprehensive Bibliography (1931–88)*.

8. Failure to develop an adequate physical vehicle before awakening the considerable energies involved in advanced yogic training can evidently result in what Sri Aurobindo termed 'yogic illness,' which includes a whole range of physical and mental disorders.

9. The failure, however, to make adequate preparations for the awakening of kundalini, or the spontaneous event of its unintentional arousal, can evidently hurl the mind-body system into what appear to be any of a variety of potentially chaotic attractor states. These may involve sensations of uncontrollable energy, intense psychological stress, and a considerable range of physical as well as mental pathological conditions (Sannella, 1987; Grof & Grof, 1990; Wilber, 1986a; White, 1979). Perhaps the most well-known instance of this type is that of Gopi Krishna, who managed to raise this energy entirely by his own efforts and as a result suffered years of physical and mental disorders. His story is chronicled in his autobiography, *Kundalini: The Evolutionary Energy in Man*.

10. Govinda, 1959; Liu, 1986.

11. One might suspect that in certain martial arts the goal of transforming the subtle energies is not so much directed toward personal transformation as to the mastery of self defense. Even here, however, many disciplines such as T'ai Chi, Aikido, and others are taken up in the broader context of contemplative self-discipline and transformation.

12. Laszlo, 1987b, 1993; Sheldrake, 1981, 1988.

13. Eccles, 1989.

14. Ervin Laszlo (1993) points out that chaotic systems are sensitive right down to the vacuum or quantum level. This is because of a quality called 'sensitivity to initial conditions.' In plain English it means that no influence is too small to have an effect, and indeed, given a short amount of

time any influence, however minute, can be just about as efficacious as any other. The motion of a butterfly wing can influence weather patterns over the North Sea as much as a bomb blast, given a few days for effects to increment naturally. (This example ignores possible thermal or chemical effects of the bomb!)

15. Sheldrake, 1983.
16. Bohm, 1982.
17. Green, 1977.
18. Smith, 1982.
19. Eliade, 1959.
20. Sri Aurobindo, 1971.

21. International Society for the Study of Subtle Energies and Energy Medicine, *Newsletter,* 1990.
22. Stevenson, 1974.
23. Roland, 1988.
24. Grof & Halifax, 1977.
25. Da Free John, 1978a.
26. Murphey & Donovan, 1988.
27. The idea of a continuum of matter and spirit is consistent with many mystical traditions including Vedanta, Neoplatonism, and Sri Aurobindo's yoga philosophy.
28. Fischer-Schreiber, Ehrhard, Friedrichs, & Diener, 1989; Feuerstein, 1990.

Chapter 9

1. Dissipative systems are ones that absorb energy and use it to increase their degree of organization or complexity. Examples include living organisms, ecologies, and the Earth with all its rich web of life. Much of this energy is released in a less organized form. For instance the Earth radiates heat into space and living organisms expel waste products. Thus they are called 'dissipative' systems. The notion is closely related to the concepts of 'self-organizing' and 'autopoietic' systems.

2. For a fascinating account of the variety of early evolutionary theories concerned not with the selection of biological species but with the evolution of mind and behavior, both human and otherwise, see J.R. Richards' *Darwin and the Emergence of Evolutionary Theories of Mind and Behavior.*

   Unfortunately, the theories of economic and social evolution typical of those days only slightly concealed a political agenda according to which the white male European industrialist was at the peak of the evolutionary ascent, thus providing an explicit justification for European colonialism (e.g., Thompson, 1989).

3. Under the rubric of *biological evolution,* I informally include classical Darwinian evolution, neo-Darwinian ideas, punctuated equilibrium, and so on — the whole discussion of how gene pools change with time and species evolve.

4. At this time there is much discussion and theory generation going on concerning the relationship between energy and complexity in self-organizing systems, and how these in turn can be understood in terms of information. For an excellent review of all these

ideas, and more too, see Sally Goerner's recent *Chaos and the Evolving Ecological Universe*. A good source for a more technical treatment is A.B. Cambel's *Applied Chaos Theory*.

5. Though Teilhard de Chardin wrote highly regarded books about spiritual and moral matters.

6. Also see Herbert Guenther's comments on Sri Aurobindo in the notes to the Foreword.

7. Wilber, 1995.

8. Wilber's work has not gone uncriticized, including his depiction of human evolution. Anthropologists have contended that his views on early humankind are essentially Victorian (e.g., Stanford, 1882; Winkelman, 1990). In the late nineteenth century it was fashionable to view primary cultures, including those of our own ancestors, as simple and childlike in comparison with ourselves. Today the pendulum is at the opposite apogee and it is fashionable to consider them to have been just as intellectually advanced as ourselves, but different. The difficulty here is not just in the interpretation of artefacts from ancient cultures, but exactly what it means to be intellectually advanced. For instance, is the older analogic mode of thought (characteristic of mythic consciousness) less 'advanced' than the modern rational one? These are difficult questions, and not entirely value-free. Certainly they are unlikely to be solved in the near future.

9. E.g., Flavell, 1963; Kohlberg, 1981; Piaget, 1977; or just about any formal work on psychological stage theories.

10. A 'softer' version of this line of thought would propose that these gifted individuals did not actually leap ahead, but represent a rapid ascent of the evolutionary pathway. This presumes a predestined evolution, like climbing the rungs of a ladder.

11. Da Love-Ananda (1977). Da Avabhasa has previously called himself Da Love-Ananda and Da Free John.

12. Globus, 1986, 1987.
The term *holonomic* is often used to refer to a holographic-like process, for example in the brain, but with the intention of avoiding the implication that it must be constructed like a mechanical hologram.

13. Vandervert, 1991, 1992, 1993, forthcoming.

14. Maslow, 1962/1968.

15. Greeley & McCready, 1975.

16. It is very likely, however, that states of consciousness, like structures, are constrained by the same kinds of inherent limitations that Goodwin points out as characteristic of all complex self-organizing systems.

17. Actually, it seems to me that under the right circumstances a drug may move the mind in the direction of new structures, but of itself does not often produce them. For instance, a psychedelic drug used in conjunction with psychotherapy or shamanic training might have a more profound effect on the undergirding structure of consciousness than the same drug taken recreationally.

18. It is significant that none of the highest states in Wilber's system, those representing the Vedantic levels of being, have yet been achieved for extended periods by more than a few rare individuals. That is to say, they have been achieved only in what Wilber views as the 'advanced' form of consciousness for each of the lower evolutionary stages — in other words by leaping evolutionary steps. A simpler explanation is that each of the dominant historical structures of consciousness holds possibilities which have been fully explored by only a few rare individuals — the shamans, saints, and sages or our past and present.

    For a fascinating idea different from my own, but representing a similar way of thinking, see Sean Kelly's article (1996). Kelly, at the University of Ottawa, speculates that Wilber's transpersonal levels lie behind the personal ones in an implicate to explicate relationship (suggestive of David Bohm's implicate and explicate orders). for example, the *causal level* is the implicate order beneath the *mental egoic level* (the explicate order), and so on.

19. Pagels, 1979.

20. Despite his high regard for the apparent achievements of paleolithic shamans, Wilber (1981) clearly does not consider shamanism a refined practice, commenting that, 'There is, however, no doubt that even true shamanistic religion is extremely crude, very unrefined, and not highly evolved ...' (p.75).

21. Krippner's recent article, *Shamanism and 'Higher' States of Consciousness* (forthcoming) points out that, like other practitioners of consciousness, shamans range individually in ability and accomplishment. Moreover, since they often use their skills primarily for the good of the community, they present quite a different figure than the contemplative monk of Buddhism, or the meditative yogin. Thus it is easy to mistake their more community-oriented activities for a less refined degree of achievement.

    In this article, Krippner goes on to develop a detailed critique of Wilber's evolutionary model, which includes the feminist criticism that it stresses the masculine value of solitary achievement over the more feminine values of community and nurturance. Krippner also points out the problem that it seems to suggest that non-Western cultures are less advanced than our own.

22. Remember, though, that the integral structure is capable of appreciating all the structures of consciousness, so that a mythic image of a god or goddess, for example, might be celebrated as a focus for the religious life, but not held too rigidly.

Chapter 10

1. Archard, 1984.
2. Whyte, 1960/1979.

   The notion of a hidden or dark side to the personality, as embodied in the concept of the unconsciousness mind, was perfectly consistent with the Victorian temperament (Baumeister, 1987). For the first time in history it became fashionable to examine the human character for hidden flaws. Victorian mannerisms were genteel to the limit, and dress was dark and concealing. All this, of course, led to a fascination with scandal, a fascination that Freud cashed in on greatly by showing that even the most respectable facade concealed a seething dark sexual interior.
3. Recall Gebser's history of the structures of consciousness. The ancients spoke of logic, insight, intuition, and dreams, indeed all the elements of the inner life, but did not have a unified concept of 'consciousness.'
4. Searle, 1992, 1993.
5. E.g., Baars, 1988; Gazzaniga, 1985; Lashley, 1956; Reber, 1992.
6. One can even dispute the validity of Freud's interpretation of such phenomena as indicative of unconsciousness motivation at all. For example Timpanaro's thoughtful book, *The Freudian Slip: Psychoanalysis and Textual Criticism,* represents a small but cogent literature that deconstructs Freud's interpretations, leaving little of logical substance standing. But to follow up this line of thought would take a chapter in and of itself. My own impression is that it is convincing when taken in detail, but unsatisfying in the larger sense. That is, it casts substantial doubt on many of Freud's particular interpretations of words spoken in the consultation room, but fails to provide an alternative account of the larger issues with which Freud grappled.
7. Sartre, 1957, 1962.
8. Politzer, 1928/1974.
9. Freud, 1900/1955.
10. While this example may seem to us today to be exaggerated, the early annals of psychoanalysis contain many instances of dreams of no less subtlety than this one — women entwined by snakes, and so on!
11. Here we see the strong Newtonian underpinnings of Freud's thinking. If a linear-rational process was not visible in the manifest productions of the mind then they must be hidden somewhere within it. In Gebser's terms, Freud was operating entirely in the perspectival mode, and trying to make the psyche do the same. Jung was much more comfortable with the a-rational aspects of the mind, but for other reasons believed in a dynamic unconscious mind.
12. E.g., Rothenberg, 1979; Ghiselin, 1955.
13. Kapleau, 1965; Fischer-Schreiber, Ehrhard, Friedrichs, & Diener, 1989.
14. E.g., Storr, 1983.
15. There is nothing exclusive about the Greek pantheon. Indeed, the Norse gods and goddesses could

as well be chosen for study, as could the mythic stories of India, Africa, China, Japan, Meso-America, and so on. All have received attention, but the long and continuing influence of Greek culture on Western civilization has led to a particular familiarity with things Greek. Beyond this, Jung himself believed that archetypes are tied to ancestry, so to some extent at least one would be best advised to pursue the study of those myths nearest one's own roots.

16. E.g., Feinstein & Krippner, 1988; Pearson, 1989.

17. E.g., Jung, 1965.

18. For a modern scientific examination of Jungian archetypes see Stevens' excellent book, *The Million-Year-Old Self.*

19. Freud believed in genetic memory as well.

20. Archetypes, however, are clearly more than *merely* psychological. Their influence is too pervasive, and can border on the super-normal as demonstrated by their influence in synchronicity (Combs & Holland, 1990; Jung, 1973). For this reason archetypes have sometimes been discussed as metaphysical entities, comparable perhaps to Alfred North Whitehead's *eternal objects.* Roughly speaking, the latter are process analogues of Plato's eternal forms. For an introduction to this line of thinking see Ray Griffin's collection of papers, *Archetypal Process: Self and Divine in Whitehead, Jung and Hill-man.*

21. Laszlo, 1993.

22. Hilgard, 1977, 1987.

23. E.g., Abraham, 1994.

24. Each of these hypothetical dual-personality systems could alternatively be viewed as a single complex attractor with more than one basin. Consistent with this idea the examples in Figures 13 and 14 were in fact each generated by a single equation.

25. Psychologist and systems theorist Robin Robertson (1987) once observed, 'Every conscious part of the human personality begins as a crude, almost mechanical, figure with few defined qualities, but eventually develops into a multifaceted part of consciousness.'

26. James, 1890/1981.

27. Cayce, 1964.

28. Zangwill, 1974.

29. Several prominent neuroscientists, including Michael Gazzaniga and Sir John Eccles, argued that only the left hemisphere retains anything like normal intelligence and consciousness. For Gazzaniga this came largely from observations made when one or the other hemisphere was anesthetized prior to or during brain surgery. For Eccles it was related to his strong belief in the importance of language, a dominantly left brain function, for both intelligence and consciousness.

30. Hilgard, 1977.

31. Crabtree, 1985.

Chapter 11

1. O'Flaherty, 1984.
2. This ideal state of absorption is referred to as *asamprajnata-samadhi* (absorption in the Self; see the Technical Appendix for more about *samadhi* in its various forms, as well as other terms from Eastern traditions) leading to *kaivalya* ('aloneness'), a state of pure presence, or pure awareness. In the Classical Yoga of Patanjali, this samadhi is fully achieved only with the 'dropping of the body' in death.
3. Buddhist traditions yield a parallel division. Buddhism is fundamentally concerned with the problem of suffering. Virtually all forms of Buddhism seek a solution to this problem in the state or condition of *nirvana* ('extinction' like a flame going out; see *nirvana* in the Technical Appendix for more). The meaning of nirvana changes dramatically, however, in different traditions. Though there were exceptions, the oldest major branch of Buddhism, the *Hinayana* tradition, tended to hold as its central goal the complete release of consciousness from the world process. This is the ideal of the *Arhat*, still seen today in *Theravada* Buddhism, the only Hinayana school still in existence. The latter is widespread in Southeast Asia, and of growing interest in the West. In this view nirvana represents a release from the cycle of birth. It is a condition of salvation — the absence of arising, subsisting, changing, and passing away.

   The later *Mahayana* tradition developed the compassionate ideal of the *bodhisattva,* the advanced being who puts off unconditional nirvana to work toward bringing all beings that suffer into the light. The schools within the Mahayana tradition tend to stress forms of nirvana that represent active liberation and freedom from desire. (E.g., *apratishthita-nirvana,* as opposed to total release, *pratishthita-nirvana*. Schools differ greatly here also.)
4. Actually, emergent evolution need not occur quickly according to clock time. The important thing is its spontaneous and self-organizing nature.
5. The American yogi and trickster, Da Avabhasa (previously Da Love Ananda and before that Da Free John; 1977), offers a three-part division of the wisdom traditions, terming these the path of yogis, the path of saints, and the path of sages. The path of yogis dwells intensively on physical and subtle energies. It includes, for example, the practice of Kundalini Yoga. Raja Yoga cultivates these levels as well, but passes beyond them toward the unconditional reality of the Atman. Kundalini Yoga, in its highest forms, does the same. Meditative and contemplative traditions that focus on beatific images of the divine, as well as those that dwell on certain inner sounds, fall, on the other hand, into Da Avabhasa's second category, the path of saints. This path seems to lead to the subtle realms (Wilber, 1980).

Evidently, particular individuals on this path may move beyond this level, as did Meister Eckhart when he went beyond images of a divine creator to the experience of the unconditional ground. Such a transition is not always welcome. The great Indian sage, Sri Ramakrishna, believed in a formless god, but preferred the guise of a deity, saying 'I would rather eat sugar than be sugar' (Nikhilananda, 1977). He loved the worship of the divine Mother. His guru, who he referred to as 'the naked one' would give him no rest, though, until he finally gave up his attachment to form.

Da Avabhasa's path of sages seems to step over the lower and intermediate subtle levels, stretching directly toward ultimate realization. Examples of this path include Zen Buddhism and Jnana Yoga, the yoga of wisdom.

6. Suzuki, 1952; Wilber, 1986a, 1986c.

7. E.g., Feuerstein, 1974; Brown, 1986.

8. Carl Jung would say that such individuals have made the fatal error of actually identifying with the archetype of the god-man, or mana-man as he called it — the ideal of god incarnate. This brings about a powerful 'inflation' of the personality, so that the person seems to become bigger than life. From contact with the archetype, such people may gain considerable charisma, like a huge static electrical charge picked up from contact with a generator. They may attract large numbers of followers at much risk to themselves and everyone concerned.

9. *Ana* (Gr.) means 'upward,' and *bolein* (Gr.) means 'to throw'; in other words, anabolic processes throw the system upward toward a more complex structure. In doing so, they often use up free energy to bind together separate particles or subsystems, as is the case with dissipative systems in general. *Kata* (Gr.), on the other hand, means 'down,' so catabolic processes throw the system down to a less complex configuration. In other words, they break down or deconstruct complex systems into elemental parts, often releasing free energy that was previously bound up in the original system.

10. Brown, 1986.

The importance of building an adequate foundation is not restricted to the ontic traditions alone. The noetic traditions likewise need to lay a firm foundation, one that will support emergent transitions that will be triggered by their spiritual practices (Brown, 1986). These traditions, however, often focus more on right thinking and conduct, preparing the practitioner psychologically for the transitions in consciousness that will follow. They do not often systematically cultivate the physical and subtle levels of the student.

11. E.g., Feuerstein, 1974/1989b.

12. Guenther, 1989.

13. Failure to build an adequate foundation in the spiritual work can lead to consequences that range from the profound to the absurd. Justin Stone (1977), for instance, notes that stomach problems are common in Zen monasteries,

where monks have the habit of sitting for long meditations shortly after eating. Evidently the characteristically Zen noetic emphasis on mental clarity sometimes overlooks certain basic facts of physiology. An Indian yogin, for example, would not be caught dead meditating on a full stomach! In a more serious vein, Wilber (1986a) has catalogued a variety of pathologies reported by students of traditional disciplines which evidently result from less than adequate attention to basic preparations. For example, the awakening of powerful subtle energies such as kundalini without preliminary work can lead to disastrous consequences (Grof & Grof, 1990; Sannella, 1987; White, 1979).

14. Wilber, 1986a.
15. Wilber, 1986a, 1986c, and many others.
16. E.g., Walsh, 1979.
17. R. Alpert/Ram Dass, 1982.
18. It is possible that the need to do psychological work, for instance in psychotherapy, may be more characteristic of Western than of Eastern students. There is reason to suspect that the typical Westerner develops an ego structure that is more rigid and less permeable than is typical in Eastern cultural traditions (Roland, 1988). To my thinking, what this means is that Westerners may have to work harder to achieve results similar to those experienced by Easterners (also see Feuerstein, 1974, 1987), and that they are likely to accumulate larger amounts of negative emotional material in general, which remains repressed or

simply not dealt with. On the other hand, Sri Aurobindo (1971) observed that while Eastern students tend to submit to the rigors of spiritual disciplines more readily than Westerners, the latter often retain a more critical intellectual faculty, which can be extremely valuable, especially during the early phases of the work before the development of a deeper intuitive guidance.

19. They are termed *visa* in Pali, for poisons, and *kilesa* in Pali as well as *klesa* in Sanskrit, for pollutants.
20. Guenther, 1989, p. 225.
21. Feuerstein, 1990a.
22. Camus, 1955.
23. Lilly, 1976.
24. Green & Green, 1977.
25. Bacovcin, 1978.
26. E.g., Arya, 1981.
27. The term *guru* literally means 'heavy one,' one who is 'weighty' (to which Tibetan tradition adds 'vastness' of vision); but has also been taken to mean 'one who dispels darkness' (Rama, 1978).
28. Combs & Holland, 1990.
29. Erikson, 1960; Flavell, 1963; Kohlberg, 1981; Levinson, 1978, 1986.
30. Underhill, 1911/1961.
    Friend and Indianologist Georg Feuerstein could not disagree with me more about this!
31. Tart, 1975.
32. Bloom & Lazerson, 1988.
33. Green & Green, 1977.
34. Patanjali, for instance, describes a number of stages of *samadhi,* or absorption, through which the student passes in his or her ascent to perfect absorption in *Brahman.*
35. Ecstasy means literally to stand (Gk. *stasis)* outside (Gk. *ek)* of

something, in this case the mind — in other words, to be outside of one's ordinary mind. Since, however, samadhi usually represents an inward turning of consciousness, Feuerstein (1974) prefers the term *enstasy*, originally suggested by Mircea Eliade (1973), which means to stand in (Gk. *en)* or inside of something — in other words, to be in one's essential consciousness.

36. *Originary awareness* is Herbert Guenther's (1989) translation of the Tibetan *ye-shes,* in which *ye* implies a beginning before any beginning. It is an anglicization of the French *originaire,* which is in turn a translation of the German *ursprünglich.* The latter word was also used by Gebser to describe integral consciousness, and is usually translated as 'originary awareness.'

37. Feuerstein, 1990a.

38. Herbert Guenther's recent works include, *From Reductionism to Creativity; Matrix of Mystery; The Ecstasy of Spontaneity;* and *Meditation Differently.*

39. Welwood, 1977; Gendlin, 1978.

40. Bohm, 1980.

41. Zohar, 1990.

Chapter 12

1. This is in fact the common meaning of the phrase, *states of mind,* as used in philosophy.

2. It is worth reminding ourselves, however, that only certain states of consciousness are viable. As shown by Brian Goodwin's (1994) work on the dynamics of biological systems, discussed in Chapter 9, certain configurations, or attractors, are stable and self-perpetuating, while others are not.

3. The effect of a fixed point in an otherwise fluid process was demonstrated some years ago in terms of belief systems. This was an informal study in which hypnotized volunteers were told they did not like the state of Nebraska. After being instructed not to remember having been so directed, they were awakened and questioned about which states they liked and which they did not. It was no surprise, despite their previous preferences, that they now did not like Nebraska. The striking thing was that they had good and ready reasons for this feeling! They recalled bad experiences had there by relatives, unpleasant things heard about people from Nebraska, problems with the weather there, and so on. Most insisted that they had *never* liked the place and probably never would. All this from the one fixed point of information, 'you don't like Nebraska,' planted hypnotically. In Chapter 3, we saw examples of the lengths to which brain injured patients will sometimes go to make their world congruent with some fixed and immobile idea which they have somehow acquired. For instance, recall the woman who believed herself to be at home in Freeport Maine, while in reality she was in a hospital bed in New York City.

She interpreted everything around her, even to the large elevator doors just outside her room as ordinary parts of her home. In such cases we see illustrated dramatically the principle that a fixed point in the mind, an unmovable idea, perception, or memory, can make itself a center around which the entire mind holistically reorganizes itself.

4. See Sir John Eccles' excellent book, *The Evolution of the Brain.*
5. Perry, 1970.
6. Neural networks, or *connection machines,* are the most recent and optimistic candidate for a mechanism, essentially a type of computer, that can at least model, and possibly explain, the brain.
7. At a recent conference on science and reductionism, neurologist Oliver Sacks commented:

   I remember the excitement with which I read Norbert Wiener's *Cybernetics* when it came out in the 1940s. And then, in the early 1950s, reading the work of Wiener's younger colleagues at MIT — a galaxy of some of the finest minds in America, including Warren McCulloch, Walter Pitts, and John von Neumann; reading about their pioneer explorations of logical autonama and nerve nets, I thought, as many of us did, that we were on the verge of computer translation, perception, cognition; a brave new world in which ever more powerful computers would be capable to mimic, and even take over, the chief functions of the brain. (1995, p. 101)

8. Despite the popularity of Data, the intelligent and likeable robot (but completely human character) in the *Star Trek* television series.
9. For example, see Dreyfus' *What Computers Can't Do.*
10. Penrose, 1989, 1994.

    In somewhat more formal terms, Penrose's argument is that intelligence cannot be the product of an *algorithm,* or pre-programmed sequence of operations.
11. Mircea Eliade's *Myth and Reality.*
12. See Richard Tarnas' excellent book *The Passion of the Western Mind,* for a brief description of this tradition. This quote is from page 434.

Epilogue

1. The behaviorists and logical positivists of the 50s and 60s. As an undergraduate I was advised by one philosopher not to bother with Bergson but to spend my time with Wittgenstein.

Appendix II

1. Grof, 1975.
2. Grof, 1985, 1988; Grof & Grof 1990; Grof & Bennett, 1992.
3. Washburn, 1990, 1994.
4. Wilber, 1990.
5. Wilber, 1980, 1986a, 1986b, 1986c.

Quotation sources

Foreword

So desperate is our dependence ... Erich Jantsch, 1975, p.194.

Introduction

Rather than discrete things ... Ervin Laszlo, 1993.

Chapter 1

The faculty of voluntarily bringing back ... William James, 1890/1981, p.401; *no activity of mind* ... Karl Lashley, 1956.

Chapter 2

And all shall be well ... T.S Eliot, from *Four Quartets,* 1971; *built up from other cells* ... Margulis, 1987, p.109; *In the penultimate decade* ... Laszlo, 1987a, p.18.

Chapter 3

In fact, the brain is ... D.Zohar, 1990, p.65; *Our nerve cells are the outcome* ... Margulis, 1988, p.46; *If we feel possessed of several minds* ... Margulis, 1988, p.47; *programs stereotyped behaviors* ... MacLean, 1970, p.339; *nature's attempt to provide* ... MacLean, 1970, p.339; *I argue that the human brain* ... Gazzaniga, 1985, p.4; *conscious experience involves* ... Baars, 1988, p.43; *The causal power attributed to* ... Sperry, 1977, p.101; *underlies the ability* ... Freeman, 1991, p.78; *The brain, like other* ... Goertzel, 1994, p.157; *a unique, dynamic pattern* ... Tart, 1975, p.5; *consciousness continuously constructs* ... Vandervert, 1993, p.11; *How far experience and reality* ... Comfort, 1984, p.82; *The simplest intuitive description* ... Jerison, 1973, p.429; *The belief system which we call* ... Goertzel, 1994, p.214.

Chapter 4

Here and elsewhere ... Aristotle, 1947; *Earth, untroubled, unhurried* ... Ovid, 1955, p.6; *Because our culture* ... Thompson, 1981, p.7; *An evolutionary process* ... Richards, 1987, p.5; *Consciousness, even in the most* ... Bergson, 1907/1983, p.179; *The more complicated the brain* ... Bergson, 1907/1983, p.80; *Oh, my Bergson* ... Gunter, 1983, p.xvii; *a highly perfected arrangement* ... Teilhard de Chardin, 1959/1961, p.65; *towards ever greater complexity* ... Teilhard de Chardin, 1959/1961, p.65; *The exterior world* ... Teilhard de Chardin, 1959/1961, p.72; *Whatever instance* ... Teilhard de Chardin, 1959/1961, p.72; *Dead matter seems* ... Popper & Eccles, 1977, p.11; *have the advantage* ... Nagel, 1979, p.184; *the mental and and the material* ... Bohm, 1986, p.129; *I think our consciousness* ... Dyson, 1979, p.249; *at the heart of life* ... Teilhard de Chardin, 1959/1961, p.148; *Love alone is capable* ... Teilhard de Chardin 1959/1961, p.265; *easily recognized* ... Teilhard de Chardin, 1959/1961, p.264.

Chapter 5

Behold! It is the eve ... Gebser, 1949/1986, p.102; *his shadow falls* ... Wilber, 1981; *The chimpanzee* ... Travis, 1976, p.v; *Origin is ever-present* ... Gebser, 1949/1986, p.xxvii; *How far back we wish* ... Gebser, 1949/1986, p.51; *self-possessed, all-enclosing* ... Wilber, 1981, p.22; *Dreamlessly the true men* ... Gebser,1949/1986, p.44; *It is akin, if not* ... Gebser,1949/1986, p.43; *In the Congo jungle* ... Gebser, 1949/1986, p.47; *The evidence is* ... Campbell, 1988, p.73; *a "galaxy" of female* ... Campbell, 1962/1976, pp.36f; *not to a new theory* ... Campbell, 1962/1976, p.47; *The mythic consciousness* ... Feuerstein, 1987, pp.85f; *renders the soul* ... Gebser, 1949/1986, p.67; *Poetic wisdom* ... Vico, 1744/1984, p.116; *Humanity embarked* ... Feuerstein, 1987, pp.76f; *Periods of strong* ... Berman, 1989, p.45; *Mirrors became* ... Berman, 1989, p.46; *Ratio must not be interpreted* ... Gebser, 1949/1986, p.95; *Compelled to emphasize* ... Gebser, 1949/1986, p.94; *Isolation is visible everywhere* ... Gebser, 1949/1986, p.95; *accompanied by an increasing* ... Gebser, 1949/1986, p.117; *The pretemporal becomes* ... Gebser, 1949/1986, p.543; *The future will definitely* ... Gebser, 1949/1986, p.297; *If mankind can endure* ... Gebser, 1949/1986, p.297; *No (mythical) world-view* ... Feuerstein, 1987, p.150; *no awakening of consciousness* ... Gebser, 1949/1986, pp.194, 203; *can be realized only out of* ... Gebser, 1949/1986, p.132.

Chapter 6

The subconsciousness ... Wilber, 1981, p.8; *Philosophia perennis* ... Huxley, 1944, p.vii; *The conception of* ... Lovejoy, 1936, p.26, 56; *The One includes everything* ... Bréhier, 1958, p.46; *Evolution, then* ... Wilber, 1980, pp.174f; *It is only language* ... Jaynes, 1976; *It is, I think, this* ... Wilber, 1981, p.93.; *Gold became new immortality* ... Becker, 1975, cited in Wilber, 1981, p.101; *I once remember* ... Serrano, 1966/1968, pp.54f; *The old conservative* ... Thompson, 1981, p.198; *Fixing my gaze upon* ... Wilber, 1980, p.68; *There is now perfect release* ... Wilber, 1980, p.73; *original Condition and Suchness* ... Wilber, 1980, pp.73f; *He has forgotten* ... von Franz, 1979, p.83; *The higher modes* ... Wilber, 1980, pp.174f; *as we separate ourselves* ... Wilber, 1990, p.125.

Chapter 7

They climb Indra like a ladder ... Sri Aurobindo, 1970; *neither you nor anyone* ... Sri Aurobindo, 1972a, p.vi; *Before there could be* ... Aurobindo, *The Hour of God*, p.18; *Evolution is nothing but* ... Sri Aurobindo, *The Hour of God*, p.41; *All evolution is* ... Sri Aurobindo, *The Hour of God*, p.41; *We are in respect to* ... Sri Aurobindo, 1970, p.55; *It lends substance* ... Laszlo, 1987b, p.21; *Personal growth and development* ... Laszlo, 1987b, p.21; *In my explanation* ... Sri Aurobindo, 1972b, p.47; *It is necessary to lay stress* ... Sri Aurobindo, 1971, p.887; *instrument of understanding* ... Sri Aurobindo, 1971, p.1266; *Never in the field* ... Ghiselin, 1955, p.36; *One evening, contrary* ... Ghiselin, 1955, p.36; *simply higher mind* ... Sri Aurobindo, 1971, p.264; *like a man who* ... Sri Aurobindo, 1972b, pp.458f; *he believes that* ... Clark, 1939, p.25; *I never grope* ... Clark, 1939, p.21; *The beings native to* ... Sri Aurobindo, 1974, p.288; *...in the overmind* ... Sri Aurobindo, 1971, pp.283f; *I live in the woods* ... Clark, 1939, pp.22; *When I touch* ... Clark, 1939, pp.39; *When the thought* ... Koplowitz, 1983a, pp.38f; *The archetypes of melody* ... Thompson, 1978, p.176; *Keeps from us* ... Sri Aurobindo, 1971, p.243; *into the One and stand* ... Sri Aurobindo, 1971, pp.283f; *If supermind were to* ... Sri Aurobindo, 1971, p.243.

Chapter 8

On a visit to Leningrad ... E.F. Schumacher, 1978, p.1; *there is neither* ... Rama, 1982, p.53; *Daylight has got* ... Bly, 1980, p.49; *They wish to inculcate* ... Head & Cranston, 1977, p.222; *The ancients* ... Head & Cranston, 1977, p.222; *Purusha is the shining* ... Mundaka Upanishad, Shearer & Russell (Trans.), 1978, p.31.

Chapter 9

Complexity provides a benchmark ... Csikszentmihalyi, 1993, p.159; *And we can only stand* ... Wilber, 1981, p.71; *Our normal waking consciousness* ... James, 1902/1929, pp.378; *the brain in its unsurpassed* ... Globus, 1986; *In other words* ... Campbell, 1986, pp.27f; *the evidence is now before us* ... Campbell, 1988. p.73; *There is a self-existent Reality* ... Isherwood, 1947, p.52; *I have spoken at times* ... Meister Eckhart, 1941, p.147.

Chapter 10

There is a great difference ... Descartes, 1641/1951, p.86; *Mind from an operational point of view* ... Uttal, 1978, p.208; *psychoanalysis has not gained* ... Sartre, 1957, p.53; *the purportedly unconscious wish* ... Archard, 1984, p.39; *there is no rationale* ... Fisher and Greenberg, 1977, p.68; *I differ from Freud* ...

Hobson, 1988, p.12; *When I decide that* ... James, 1890/1981, p.175; *The first thing to do* ... Sri Aurobindo, 1971, p.635; *morphic resonance theory* ... Sheldrake, 1987, p.12; *Jung's intuitive insight* ... Laszlo, 1993, p.192; *the unconscious is not* ... Jung, 1939, p.494; *They form a species* ... Jung, 1939, p.501; *highly advanced structures* ... Wilber, 1985, p.85; *It is a realm of higher presences* ... Wilber, 1980, p.68; *the beings native to* ... Sri Aurobindo, 1974, p.288; *as though the hypnotized* ... Hilgard, 1987, p.302; *M. Janet caught the actual moment* ... James, 1890/1981, p.222; *in the background whilst* ... James, 1890/1981, p.222.

Chapter 11

The soul goes ... Sri Aurobindo, 1971; *Practice on ourselves* ... Dürckheim, 1971/1988; *the primal sacrament* ... Fox, 1988, p.39; *The emphasis on mind/-mentation* ... Guenther, 1989; *Two monks were arguing* ... Reps, 1961, p.114; *That I am* ... Ramana Maharshi, 1988, p.3; *The notion that we must wait* ... Brunton, 1988, p.3; *The danger of the Short Path* ... Brunton, 1988, p.31; *In Buddhism, as in Vedanta* ... Huxley, 1944, p.295; *affect a complete psycho-behavioral* ... Brown, 1986, p.226; *The Perennial Philosophy* ... Huxley, 1944, p.viii; *If you're doing meditation* ... Wilber, 1987, p.43; *underlying path is best* ... Brown, 1986, p.263f; *Haven't you seen* ... Nikhilananda, 1977, p.327; *the infernal method* ... Blake, 1953, pp.128f; *Tokusan was studying Zen* ... Reps, 1961, p.112; *A certain young man* ... Rumi, 1988, p.3; *In the practice of meditation* ... Chögyam Trungpa, 1984, pp.37–39; *One day a man of the people* ... Kapleau, 1975, pp.9f; *In Buddhism* ... Brown, 1986, p.221; *The mantram becomes* ... Easwaran, 1977, p.42; *The person who has* ... Easwaran, 1977, p.179f; *I have never had any revelations* ... Quoted by James, 1902/1929, p.374; *Liminality may perhaps* ... Turner, 1967, p.7; *If you have within* ... The Mother, 1972, p.233; *All developed mental men* ... Sri Aurobindo, 1972a, p.83; *There is no knowledge* ... Schuon, 1981, p.15; *In that rapt synthesis* ... Coomaraswamy, 1943, p.24; *oneness with the inexpressible* ... Fischer-Schreiber, Ehrhard, Friedrichs, & Diener, 1989; *that which remains* ... Kingsland & Kingsland, 1977, IV. 62; *that which is not conditioned* ... Guenther, 1989; *the period of actual* ... Laughlin, McManus, & d'Aquili, 1990, p.323; *The difference between* ... Guenther, 1989, p.226; *[He is] wise, gracious* ... Feuerstein, 1974, p.167f; *from the restrictive-control* ... Guenther, 1989, p.83; *Bodhisattva meditation* ... Guenther, 1989, p.83; *globally stable, but never* ... Guenther, 1989, p.84; *brings new gestalt* ... Guenther, 1989, p.84; *the term 'higher'* ... Guenther, 1989, p.85; *The bodhisattva meditation* ... Guenther, 1989, p.86; *Man's body is where* ... Guenther, 1989, p.211; *The true man* ... Dürckheim, 1971/1988, p.25; *like the sun* ... Guenther, 1989, p.241; *To live these structures* ... Gebser, 1949/1986, p.272; *the liberated yogin* ... Feuerstein, 1990a, p.297; *indebtedness to* ... Gebser, 1949/1986, p.134; *creativity is of* ... Gebser, 1949/1986, p.313; *that freedom is*

... Feuerstein, 1990a, p.297; *unrealized tendencies* ... Herbert, 1987, p.195; *in the immediacy* ... Guenther, 1989, p.230.

Chapter 12

Your intelligence is a camel-driver ... J. Rumi, in R.A. Nicholson (1925–40), *The* Mathnawi *of Jelaluddin Rumi,* Book I, pp. 2492ff. London: Luzac and Co.

Appendix II

elements of important COEX ... Grof, 1985, p.101; *an enormous struggle* ... Grof, 1985, p.116; *All we can say* ... Grof, 1985, p.127; *The psyche has a multidimensional* ... Grof, 1985, p.137; *in the domain of* ... Washburn, 1988, p.4; *higher symbolic meanings* ... Washburn, 1988, p.13.

Bibliography

Abraham, F.D. (1989). Toward a dynamical theory of the psyche: Archetypal patterns of self-reflection and self-organization. *Psychological Perspectives*, 20, (1), pp.156–67.

—, (1991). *A visual introduction to dynamical systems theory for psychology.* Santa Cruz, CA: Aerial Press.

Abraham, R. (1987). Complex dynamics and the social sciences. *World Futures: The Journal of General Evolution*, 23, pp.1–10.

—, (1992). Mathematical Cooperation. In A.L. Combs (Ed.), *Cooperation: beyond the age of competition.* (pp.68–74). New York & London: Gordon & Breach.

—, (1994). Erodynamics and the dischaotic personality. In F.D. Abraham & A.B. Gilgen (Eds.), *Chaos theory in psychology.* Westport, Connecticut: Greenwood.

—, & Shaw, C.D. (1984). *Dynamics — the geometry of behavior; Part I: Periodic behavior.* Santa Cruz, CA: Aerial Press.

—, Sheldrake, R., & McKenna, T. (1992). *Trialogs on the edge of the West.* Bear & Co.

Alpert, R./Ram Dass. (1982). A ten-year perspective. *Journal of Transpersonal Psychology*, 14, (2), pp.171–83. *(See also* Ram Dass.)

Anderson, W.T. (1990). *Reality isn't what it used to be: theatrical politics, ready-to-wear religion, global myths, primitive chic, and other wonders of the postmodern world.* New York: Harper & Row.

Apuleius (1951/1988). *The Golden Ass.* (R. Graves, trans.); In D. Gochberg (Ed.), *Classics of western thought: The ancient world.* (Vol. 4, pp.521–36). New York: Harcourt Brace Jovanovich.

Archard, D. (1984). *Consciousness and the unconscious.* La Salle, Illinois: Open Court.

Aristotle (1947). *De anima.* In C.R. McKeon (Ed.), *Introduction to Aristotle*, pp.145–240. New York: Modern Library.

Artigiani, R. (1990). Post-modernism and social evolution: An enquiry. *World Futures: The Journal of General Evolution*, 30, (3–4), pp.237–81.

Arya, U. (1978). *Superconscious meditation.* Honesdale, PA: Himalayan Publishers.

Arya, U. (1981). *Mantra and meditation.* Honesdale, PA: Himalayan Publishers.

Ashe, G. (1992). *Dawn behind the dawn: a search for the Earthly paradise.* New York: Henry Holt.

Aurobindo Ghose, Sri (1958). *On yoga II; Tome 2.* Pondicherry, India: Sri Aurobindo Ashram Press.

—, (1970). *The life divine.* Pondicherry, India: Sri Aurobindo Ashram Press.

—, (1971). *Letters on yoga* (Vols. 1–3). Pondicherry, India: All India Press.

—, (1972a). *On himself.* Pondicherry, India: All India Press.

—, (1972b). *The synthesis of yoga.* Pondicherry, India: All India Press.

—, (1974). *Guidance from Sri Aurobindo* (Vol. 1). Pondicherry, India.

—, (1982). *The Mother with letters on the Mother and translations of prayers and meditations.* Pondicherry, India: Sri Aurobindo Ashram Press.

—, *The Hour of God.* Pondicherry, India: Sri Aurobindo Ashram Press.

Baars, J.B. (1983). Conscious contents provide the nervous system with coherent, global information. In R. Davidson, G. Schwartz, & D. Shapiro (Eds.), *Consciousness and self regulation* (Vol.III, pp.45–76). New York: Plenum.

—, (1988). *A cognitive theory of consciousness.* Cambridge, England: Cambridge University Press.

Bacovcin, H. (1978). *The way of a pilgrim.* Garden City, New York: Doubleday.

Barks, C., & Moyne, J. (Eds./trans.), (1988). *This longing: poetry, teaching stories, and letters of Rumi.* Putney, Vermont: Threshold Books.

Baruss, I. (1990). *The personal nature of notions of consciousness.* Lanham, Maryland: University Press of America.

Basar E. (Ed.). (1990). *Chaos in brain function.* Berlin: Springer-Verlag.

Bateson, G. (1979). *Mind and nature: a necessary unity.* New York: Dutton.

—, & Mead, M. (1942). *Balinese character: a Photographic analysis.* New York: New York Academy of Sciences.

Baumeister, R. F. (1987). How the self became a problem: A psychological review of historical research. *Journal of Personality and Social Psychology,* 52, (1), pp.163–76.

Becker, E. (1973). *The denial of death.* New York: Free Press.

—, (1975). *Escape from evil.* New York: Free Press.

Behnke, E. A. (1987). How we shout into the woods is how the echo will sound: Remarks on the reintegrations of projections. In E. A. Behnke (Ed.), *Toward integral consciousness for an integral world; Gebser studies* (Vol. 1; pp.59–144). Felton, California: California Center for Jean Gebser Studies.

Bergson, H. (1907/1983). *Creative evolution.* (A. Mitchell, trans.). Lanham, MD: University Press of America.

Berman, M. (1986). The cybernetic dream of the twenty-first century. *Journal of Humanistic Psychology,* 26, 2, pp.24–51.

—, (1989). *Coming to our senses: body and spirit in the hidden history of the West.* New York: Simon & Schuster.

Berry, T. (1988). *The dream of the Earth.* San Francisco: Sierra Club Books.

Binet. A. (1889). *On double consciousness.* Chicago: Open Court

Blake, W. (1953). The marriage of heaven and hell. In, *Poetry and prose of William Blake.* New York: Modern Library.

Blanck, G., & Blanck, R. (1979). *Ego psychology: Theory and practice.* New York: Columbia University Press.

Bloom, F.E., & Lazerson, A. (1988). *Brain, mind, and behavior.* (2nd ed.). New York: W.H. Freeman.

Bly, R. (1980). *News of the universe: poems of twofold consciousness.* San Francisco: Sierra Club.

Bock, E. (1954/1993). *St Paul: life, epistles and teaching.* (Maria St Goar, trans.) Edinburgh: Floris.

Bohm, D. (1980). *Wholeness and the implicate order.* Boston: Routledge and Kegan Paul.

—, (1982). Nature as creativity: a conversation with David Bohm. *ReVision,* 5, (2) pp.35–40.

—, (1986). A new theory of the relationship of mind and matter. *Journal of the American Society of Psychical Research,* 80 (2).

Bower, G.H. (1981). Mood and memory. *American Psychologist,* 36, pp.129–48.

Bréhier, E. (1958). *The philosophy of Plotinus.* (J. Thomas, trans.). Chicago: University of Chicago Press.

Brett, G. S. (1912/1921). *A history of psychology.* 2 vols. London: George Allen and Unwin, I:302.

Briggs, J., & Peat, D. (1989). *Turbulent mirror: An illustrated guide to chaos theory and the science of wholeness.* New York: Harper & Row.

Brown, D. P. (1986). The stages of meditation in cross-cultural perspective. In K. Wilber, J. Engler, and D. P. Brown (Eds.), (1986), pp.191–218.

Brown, N.O. (1959). *Life against death.* Middletown, Conn.: Wesleyan University Press.

—, (1966). *Love's body.* New York: Vintage.

Brunton, P. (1988). *The notebooks of Paul Brunton* (Vol.15), *Advanced contemplation/The peace within you.* Burdett, New York: Larson Publications.

Cade, C.M., & Coxhead, N. (1979). *The awakened mind: bio-feedback and the development of higher states of awareness.* New York: Delacorte.

Cairns-Smith, A.G. (February, 1990). *Evolution and consciousness.* Paper presented at the First International Conference on the Study of Consciousness in Science; San Francisco.

Cambel, A.B. (1993). *Applied chaos theory: a paradigm for complexity.* New York: Academic Press.

Campbell, J. (1962/1976). *The masks of god* (Vol.2), *Oriental mythology.* New York: Penguin.

—, (1964). *The masks of god* (Vol.3), *Occidental mythology.* New York: Penguin.

—, (1986). *The inner reaches of outer space: metaphor as myth and religion.* New York: Alfred van der Marck.

—, (1988). *Historical atlas of world mythology* (Vol.I), *The way of the animal powers; Part 1: Mythologies of the primitive hunters and gathers.* New York: Harper & Row.

Camus, A. (1955). *The myth of Sisyphus.* (J. O'Brien, trans.). New York: Random House.

Cartwright, R.D. (1977). *Night life: explorations in dreaming.* Englewood Cliffs, New Jersey: Prentice-Hall.

Cassirer, E. (1963). *The individual and the cosmos in Renaissance philosophy.* (M. Domandi, trans.). Oxford.

Cary, S. (1985). Are children fundamentally different kinds of thinkers and learners than adults? In S.F. Chipman, J.W. Segal, & R. Glaser (Eds.), *Thinking and learning skills: current research and opened questions* (Vol.2). Hillsdale, New Jersey: Erlbaum.

Cayce, H.L. (1964). *Venture inward*. New York: Harper & Row.

Chaisson, E. (1987). *The life era*. New York: Atlantic Monthly Press.

Chi, M.T.H., & Koeske, R.D. (1983). Network representation of a child's dinosaur knowledge. *Developmental Psychology*, 19, pp.29–39.

Clark, G. (1939). *The man who talked with the flowers*. Saint Paul: Macalester Park.

Combs, A. (February, 1990). *Concepts of consciousness: a historical survey*. Paper presented at the First International Conference on the Study of Consciousness in Science; San Francisco.

—, (1993a, June). *A naturalist's process phenomenology of the human mind*. Paper presented at The First Brandenburg Colloquium on Evolutionary Thought, Potsdam, Germany.

—, (1993b). The evolution of consciousness: a theory of historical and personal transformation. *World Futures: the Journal of General Evolution*. 38, pp.43–62.

—, (1995a). Consciousness: chaotic and strangely attractive. *PsychoScience*, 2, 1, pp.50–58.

—, (1995b). Psychology, chaos, and the process nature of consciousness. In F. Abraham and A. Gilgen, *Chaos Theory in Psychology*. Westport, CT: Greenwood Pub.

—, (1995c). Consciousness as a system near the edge of chaos. In S. Hameroff & A. Kaszniak (Eds.), *Toward a scientific basis for consciousness: Proceedings*. Cambridge, Mass. MIT Press.

—, & Holland, M. (1990). *Synchronicity: science, myth, and the trickster*. New York: Paragon House.

—, Winkler, M., & Daley, C. (1994). A chaotic systems analysis of circadian rhythms in feeling states. *The Psychological Record*, 44, pp.359–68.

Comfort, A. (1984). *Reality and empathy: physics, mind, and science in the 21st century*. Albany, New York: State University of New York Press.

Coomaraswamy, A.K. (1943/1971). *Hinduism and Buddhism*. Westport, Connecticut: Greenwood Press.

Coppens, Y. (1981). *Exposé sur le cerveau: le cerveau des hommes fossilés*. Paris: Institut de France, Académie des Sciences.

Crabtree, A. (1985). *Multiple man*. Ontario: Collins.

Crutchfield, J., Doyne, F., Packard, N., and Shaw, R. (1986). Chaos. *Scientific American*, (Dec.), pp.46–57.

Csányi, V. (1989). *Evolutionary systems and society: a general theory of life, mind, and culture*. Durham, North Carolina: Duke University Press.

Csikszentmihalyi, M. (1990). *Flow: the psychology of optimal experience*. New York: Harper & Row.

—, (1993). *The evolving self: a psychology for the third millennium*. New York: HarperCollins.

Da Free John (1977). *The paradox of instruction.* San Francisco: Dawn Horse Press.

—, (1978a). The way of sacrifice and the super-physics of divine evolution. *ReVision,* 1, (2) pp.33–42.

—, (1978b). *The enlightenment of the whole body.* San Francisco: Dawn Horse Press.

Descartes, R. (1641/1951). *Meditations on first philosophy.* (L.J. Lafleur, trans.). New York: Bobbs-Merrill.

Dement, W.C. (1972). *Some must watch while some must sleep: exploring the world of sleep.* New York: W.W. Norton.

Dennett, D. (1991). *Consciousness explained.* Boston: Little, Brown.

Dreyfus, H.D. (1972). *What computers can't do.* New York: Harper & Row.

Dürckheim, K.G. (1971/1988). *The way of transformation: daily life as spiritual exercise.* London: Unwin Hyman.

Dyson, F. (1979). *Disturbing the universe.* New York: Harper & Row.

Easwaran, E. (1977). *The mantram handbook.* Berkeley, California: Nilgiri Press.

Eccles, J.C. (1970). *Facing reality: philosophical adventures by a brain scientist.* New York: Springer-Verlag.

—, (1989). *Evolution of the brain: creation of the mind.* New York: Routledge.

Eckhart, Meister (1941). *Meister Eckhart: a modern translation.* (R.B. Blakney, trans.). New York: Harper & Row.

Eich, J.E. (1980). The cue-dependent nature of state-dependent retention. *Memory and Cognition,* 8, pp.157–73.

Eisler, R. (1987). *The chalice and the blade: our history, our future.* San Francisco: Harper & Row.

—, & Loye, D. (1990). *The partnership way: new tools for living and learning, healing our families, our communities, and our world.* San Francisco: Harper Collins.

Eldredge, N., & Gould, S.J. (1972). Punctuated equilibria: an alternative to phyletic gradualism. In T.J.M. Schopf (Ed.), *Models in paleobiology.* San Francisco: Freeman.

Elgin, D. (1993). *Awakening Earth: exploring the evolution of human culture and consciousness.* New York: William Morrow.

Eliade, M. (1959). *The sacred and the profane: the nature of religion.* (W.R. Trask, trans.). New York: Harper & Row.

—, (1963). *Myth and reality.* New York: Harper & Row.

—, (1973). *Yoga: immortality and freedom.* Princeton, New Jersey: Princeton University Press.

Eliot, T.S. (1971). *The complete poems and plays: 1909–1950.* New York: Harcourt, Brace, & World.

Erikson, E.H. (1960). *Childhood and society* (2nd ed.). New York: Norton.

Eysenck, M.W., & Keane, M.T. (1990). *Cognitive psychology: a student's handbook.* London: Lawrence Erlbaum.

Evens-Wentz, W.Y. (1935). *Tibetan yoga and secret doctrines.* London: Oxford University Press.

Faivre, A., & Needleman, J. (Eds.), (1992). *Modern esoteric spirituality.* New York: Crossroad.

Fedotov, G. P. (1977). *A treasury of Russian spirituality.* London: Sheed & Ward.

Feinstein, D., & Krippner, S. (1988). *Personal mythology: the psychology of your evolving self.* Los Angeles: Jeremy Tarcher.

Feuerstein, G. (1974). *The essence of yoga: a contribution to the psychohistory of Indian civilization.* New York: Grove Press.

—, (trans.; 1979/1989). *The yoga-sutra of Patanjali: a new translation and commentary.* Rochester, Vermont: Inner Traditions.

—, (1987). *Structures of consciousness: the genius of Jean Gebser.* Lower Lake, California: Integral Publishing.

—, (1989a). *Jean Gebser: What color is your consciousness?* Mill Valley, California: Robert Briggs Associates.

—, (1989b). *Yoga: the technology of ecstasy.* Los Angeles, CA: Jeremy P. Tarcher.

—, (1990a). *Encyclopedic dictionary of yoga.* New York: Paragon House.

—, (1990b). *Holy madness: the outer limits of religion and morality.* New York: Paragon House.

Fischer-Schreiber, I., Ehrhard, F., Friedrichs, K., & Diener, M.S. (Eds.), (1989). *The encyclopedia of Eastern philosophy and religion.* Boston: Shambhala.

Fisher, S. & Greenberg, R.P. (1977). *The scientific credibility of Freud's theories and therapy.* New York: Basic Books.

Flavell, J. H. (1963). *The developmental psychology of Jean Piaget.* New York: Van Nostrand.

Fodor, J.A. (1983). *The modularity of mind: An essay on faculty psychology.* Cambridge, MA: MIT Press.

Fox, M. (1988). *The coming of the cosmic Christ: the healing of mother earth and the birth of global renaissance.* San Francisco: Harper & Row.

Fox, R. (1988). *Energy and the evolution of life.* San Francisco: Freeman.

Freeman, W.J. (February, 1991). The physiology of perception. *Scientific American.* pp.78–85.

—, (1992). Tutorial in neurobiology: From single neurons to brain chaos. *International Journal of Bifurcation and Chaos,* 2, pp.451–82.

—, (April, 1994). Some category confusions in studies of the psychology of consciousness. Paper given at the conference, *Toward a scientific basis for consciousness.* Tucson, Arizona.

Fremantle, F., & Trungpa, C. (trans.) (1975). *The Tibetan book of the dead.* Berkeley: Shambhala.

Freud, S. (1900/1955). *The interpretation of dreams.* New York: Basic Books.

Frobenius, L. (1905). *Kulturgeschichte Afrikas.* Vienna: Phaidon.

Gardener, H. (1985/1987). *The mind's new science: a history of the cognitive revolution.* New York: Basic Books.

Gazzaniga, M.S., LeDoux, J.E. (1978). *The integrated mind.* New York: Plenum Press.

—, (1985). *The social brain: discovering the networks of the mind.* New York: Basic Books.

—, (1988). *Mind matters: how mind and brain interact to create our conscious lives.* Boston: Houghton Mifflin.

Gebser, J. (1949/1986). *The ever-present origin.* (N. Barstad and A. Mickunas, trans.). Athens, Ohio: Ohio University Press.

Gell-Mann, M. (1994). *The quark and the jaguar: adventures in the simple and the complex.* New York: W.H. Freeman.

Gendlin, E.T. (1978). *Focusing.* New York: Everest House.

Ghiselin, B. (1955). *The creative process: a symposium.* New York: New American Library.

Gibson, W. (1986). *Count zero.* New York: Ace Science Fiction.

Gimbutas, M. (1982). *The goddesses and gods of Old Europe.* Los Angeles: University of California Press.

Glaser, R. (1984). Education and thinking: The role of knowledge. *American Psychologist,* 39, (2), pp.93–104.

Gleick, J. (1987). *Chaos, making a new science.* New York: Viking.

Globus, G. (1986). Three holonomic approaches to the brain. In B. Hiley and D. Peat (Eds.), *David Bohm: physics and beyond.* London: Routledge & Kegan Paul.

—, (1987). *Dream life, wake life: the human condition through dreams.* Albany, New York: State University of New York Press.

Goerner, S.J. (1994). *Chaos and the evolving ecological universe.* New York: Gordon & Breach.

Goertzel, B. (1993a). *The structure of intelligence.* Springer-Verlag.

—, (1993b). *The evolving mind.* New York: Gordon & Breach.

—, (1994). *Chaotic logic: language, mind and reality, from the perspective of complex systems science.* New York: Plenum.

—, (1995). Chance and consciousness. *PsychoScience,* 2, (1), pp.12–38.

Goldman, D. (1988). *The meditative mind: the varieties of meditative experience.* Los Angeles: Jeremy Tarcher.

Goodwin, B.C. (1994). *How the leopard got its spots: the evolution of complexity.* New York: Charles Scribner's Sons.

Govinda, A.B. (1959). *Foundations of Tibetan mysticism, according the esoteric teachings of the great mantra, Om Mani Padme Hum.* New York.

Greeley, A., & McCready, W. (1975). Are we a nation of mystics? In D. Goleman & R.J. Davidson (Eds.), *Consciousness, brain, states of awareness, and mysticism,* (pp.175–83). New York: Harper & Row.

Green, E., & Green, A. (1977). *Beyond bio-feedback.* Delacorte Press.

Gregory, R. (Ed.), (1987). *The Oxford companion to the mind.* Oxford: Oxford University Press.

Griffin, R. (1989). *Archetypal process: self and divine in Whitehead, Jung and Hillman.* Evanston, Illinois: Northwestern University Press.

Grof, C., & Grof, S. (1990). *The stormy search for the self: a guide to personal growth through transformational crisis.* Los Angeles: Jeremy P. Tarcher.

Grof, S. (1975). *Realms of the human unconscious: observations from LSD research.* New York: Viking Press.

—, (1985). *Beyond the brain: birth, death, and transcendence in psychotherapy.* Albany, New York: State University of New York Press.

—, (1988). *The adventure of self-discovery: dimensions of consciousness and new perspectives in psychotherapy and inner exploration.* Albany, New York: State University of New York Press.

—, & Bennett, H.Z. (1992). *The holotropic mind: the three levels of human consciousness and how they shape our lives.* San Francisco: HarperSan-Francisco.

—, & Halifax, J. (1977). *The human encounter with death.* New York: Dutton.

Gruber & Voneche (Eds.), (1977). *The essential Piaget.* New York: Basic Books.

Guenther, H.V. (1984). *Matrix of mystery: scientific and humanistic aspects of rDzogs-chen thought.* Boulder, Colorado: Shambhala.

—, (1989). *From reductionism to creativity: rDzogs-chen and the new sciences of mind.* Boston: Shambhala.

—, (1992). *Meditation differently: phenomenological-psychological aspects of Tibetan Buddhist (Mahamudra and sNying-thig) practices from original Tibetan sources.* Delhi, India: Motilal Banarsidass.

—, (1993). *The ecstasy of spontaneity: a phenomenological-psychological study of Saraha's* Dohakosa *Trilogy.* Nanzan Institute of Buddhist Studies, University of Nagoya, Japan.

Guilford, J.P. (1979). *Cognitive psychology with a frame of reference.* San Diego: Edits.

Gunter, P.A.Y. (1983). Introduction to the 1983 edition of H. Bergson, *Creative Evolution.* (A. Mitchell, trans.). Lanham, MD: University Press of America.

Hamilton, V. (1988). *In the beginning: creation stories from around the world.* New York: Harcourt Brace Jovanovich.

Happold, F.C. (1963). *Mysticism: a study and an anthology.* New York: Penguin.

Harnad, S.R., Steklis, H.D., & Lankaster, J. (Eds.), (1976). *Origin and evolution of language and speech. Annals of the New York Academy of Science,* 280.

Harner, M. (1980). *The way of the shaman.* New York: Harper & Row.

Head, J. & Cranston, S.L. (1977). *Reincarnation: the phoenix fire mystery.* New York: Julian Press.

Herbert, N. (1987). *Quantum reality.* Garden City, N.Y.: Anchor Books.

Hilgard, E.R. (1977). *Divided consciousness: Multiple controls in human thought and action.* New York: Wiley.

—, (1987) *Psychology in America: a historical survey.* New York: Harcourt Brace Jovanovich.

Hillman, J. (1971). Commentary on Kundalini: The evolutionary energy in man. In G. Krishna, *Kundalini: the evolutionary energy in man.* Berkeley, CA: Shambhala.

Hixon, L. (1978). *Coming home.* Garden City: Anchor.

Hobson, A. (1988). *The dreaming brain.* New York: Basic Books.

Hofstadter, D. R. (1979). *Gödel, Esher, Bach: an eternal golden braid.* New York: Random House.

Huxley, A. (1944). *The perennial philosophy.* New York: Harper & Row.

Huxley, J. (1907/1983). Introduction. In H. Bergson, *Creative evolution.* (A. Mitchell, trans.). Lanham, MD: University Press of America.

Inge, W. R. (1918). *The philosophy of Plotinus.* New York: Longmans, Green & Company.

Iyengar, B.K.S. (1988). *The tree of yoga.* Boston: Shambhala.

Jackendoff, R. *Consciousness and the computational mind.* Cambridge, MA: MIT Press.

James, W. (1890/1981). *The principles of psychology.* Cambridge, Mass: Harvard University Press.

—, (1912). *Essays in radical empiricism.* New York: Longmans, Green.

—, (1902/1929). *The varieties of religious experience.* New York: Modern Library.

Jantsch, E. (1975). *Design for evolution.* New York: George Braziller.

—, (1980). *The self-organizing universe.* New York: Pergamon.

Jaynes, J. (1976). *The origin of consciousness in the breakdown of the bicameral mind.* Boston: Houghton Mifflin.

Jerison, H.J. (1973). *The evolution of the brain and intelligence.* New York: Academic Press.

Judith, A., & Vega, S. (1993). *The sevenfold journey: reclaiming mind, body, and spirit through the chakras.* Freedom, CA: Crossing Press.

Jung, C.G. (1939). *Conscious, unconscious, and individuation.* CW Vol. IX, Pt. I, pp.489–524.

—, (1962). Commentary on 'The Secret of the Golden Flower,' in Wilhelm, R., *The secret of the golden flower,* (C.F. Baynes, trans.), New York: Harcourt, Brace & World.

—, (1965). *Mysterium coniunctionis.* CW, Vol. XIV, Pt. II, Princeton, New Jersey: Princeton University Press.

—, (1973). *Synchronicity: an acausal connecting principle.* CW, Vol. VIII, Princeton, N.J.: Princeton University Press.

Kahler, E. (1956). *Man the measure: a new approach to history.* New York: George Braziller.

Kampis, G. (1991). *Self-modifying systems in biology and cognitive science.* New York: Pergamon.

Kapleau, P. (Ed.), (1965). *The three pillars of Zen: teaching, practice, and enlightenment.* Boston: Beacon Press.

Kauffman, S.A. (1993). *The origins of order: self-organization and selection in evolution.* New York and Oxford: Oxford University Press.

Kellert, S.H. (1993). *In the wake of chaos: unpredictable order in dynamical systems.* Chicago: University of Chicago.

Kellogg, R. (1969). *Analyzing children's art.* Palo Alto, California: National Press Books.

Kelly, S. (1996). Article in *ReVision,* 8 (4).

Kelso. J.A.S. (1995). *Dynamic patterns: self-organization of brain behavior.* Cambridge, MA: MIT Press.

Kernberg, O. (1976). *Object relations theory and clinical psychoanalysis.* New York: Jason Aronson.

Kingsland, K. & Kingsland, V. (trans.; 1977). *Hathapradipika.* Devon, England: Grail Communications.

Koestler, A. (1979). *Janus: a summing up.* New York: Vintage.

Kohlberg, L. (1981). *Essays on moral development* (Vol.1). San Francisco: Harper & Row.

Koplowitz, H. (1983a). *A projection beyond Piaget's formal operations stage: general systems theory and unitary thought.* An unpublished manuscript. A revised version appears in M. Commons and R. Richards (Eds.), (1983b). *Beyond formal operations: Late adolescent and adult development.* New York: Praeger.

Krippner, S. (1990). *Shamanism and 'higher' states of consciousness.* Paper presented at the annual conference of the Lucidity Association, Chicago, Illinois.

Krishna, G. (1970). *Kundalini: the evolutionary energy in man.* Berkeley: Shambhala.

Kuhn, D. (1988). Cognitive development. In M.H. Bornstein & M.E. Lamb (Eds.), *Developmental psychology: an advanced textbook.* (pp.205–61). Hillsdale, New Jersey: Lawrence Erlbaum.

Larkin, J.H., McDermott, J., Simon, D.P., & Simon, H.A. (1980). Models of competence in solving physics problems. *Cognitive Science, 4,* pp.317–45.

Lashley, K. (1956). Cerebral organization and behavior. In H. Solomon, S. Cobb, and W. Penfield (Eds.), *The brain and human behavior.* Baltimore: Williams & Wilkins.

Laszlo, E. (1972). *Introduction to systems philosophy: toward a new paradigm of contemporary thought.* New York: Gordon & Breach.

—, (1987a). *Evolution: the grand synthesis.* Boston: Shambhala.

—, (1987b). The psi-field hypothesis. *IS Journal, 4,* pp.13–28.

—, (1993). *The creative cosmos: a unified science of matter, life, and mind.* Edinburgh: Floris.

—, (1995). *The connected universe.* World Scientific.

—, Csányi, V., Combs, A. L., & Artigiani, R. (in preparation). *The evolution of cognitive maps: new paradigms for the 21st century.* London: Adamantine Press.

Laughlin, Jr., C.D., McManus, J., & d'Aquili, E. (1990). *Brain, symbol and experience: toward a neurophenomenology of human consciousness.* Boston: Shambhala.

Leadbeater, C.W. (1927). Adyar: Theosophical Publishing House.

Levinson, D. (1978). *The seasons of a man's life.* New York: Knopf.

—, (1984). A conception of adult development. *American Psychologist, 41,* pp.3–13.

Lilly, J., & Lilly, A. (1976). *The dyadic cyclone.* New York: Simon & Schuster.

Liu, D. (1986). *T'ai Chi Ch'uan and meditation.* New York: Schocken.

Loftus, E. (1980). *Memory*. Reading, MA: Addison-Wesley.

Lorenz, E. (1963). Deterministic nonperiodic flow. *Journal of the Atmospheric Sciences*, 20, pp.130–41.

Lovejoy, A. (1936). *The great chain of being*. Cambridge, Mass.: Harvard University Press.

Löwenhard, P. (1988). Mind: Mapping and reconstruction of reality. In M. Alonso (Ed.), *Organization and change in complex systems*. (pp. 126–56). New York: Paragon House.

Loye. D. (1983). *The sphinx and the rainbow*. Boulder: Shambhala.

Lu K'uan Yü (Charles Luk). (1972). *The secrets of Chinese meditation*. New York: Samual Weiser.

MacLean, P.D. (1958). Contrasting functions of limbic and neocortical systems of the brain and their relevance to psychophysiological aspects of medicine. *American Journal of Medicine*, 25, pp.611–26.

—, (1970). The triune brain, emotion, and scientific bias. In F.O. Schmitt (Ed.), *The neurosciences: second study program* (pp.336–49). New York: Rockefeller Univ. Press, 1970.

—, (1990). *The triune brain in evolution*. New York: Plenum.

Macy, J. (1991). *Mutual causality in Buddhism and general systems theory: the dharma of natural systems*. Albany, NY: State University of New York Press.

Maharshi, R. (1988). *The spiritual teaching of Ramana Maharshi*. Boston, MA: Shambhala.

Mandelbrot, B.B. (1977). *The fractal geometry of nature*. New York: W.H. Freeman.

Margulis, L. (1987). Early life: The microbes have priority. In W.I. Thompson (Ed.), *Gaia, a way of knowing: political implications of the new biology*. Great Barrington, MA.: Lindisfarne Press.

—, (1988). Speculation on speculation. In J. Brockman (Ed.), *The Reality Club*. (pp. 39–50). New York: Lynx Books.

—, & Sagan, D. (1986). *Microcosmos: four billion years of evolution from our microbial ancestors*. Simon & Schuster.

Marshall, J.C. (1984). Multiple perspectives on modularity. *Cognition*, 17, pp.209–42.

Maslow, A.H. (1962/1968). *Toward a psychology of being*. Princeton, N.J.: Van Nostrand.

Maturana, H. R., & Varela, F. J. (1987). *The tree of knowledge: the biological roots of human understanding*. Boston, MA: Shambhala.

—, —, & Uribe, R. (1974). Autopoiesis: The organization of living systems, its characterization and model. *Biosystems*, 5, pp.187–96.

McDougall, W. (1911). *Body and mind: a history and a defense of animism*. London: Methuen.

Merrell-Wolf, F. (1973) *The philosophy of consciousness without an object*. New York: Julian Press.

Minsky, M., & Papert, S. (1974). *Artificial intelligence*. Eugene, Oregon: Oregon State System of Higher Education.

The Mother (1972). *Questions and answers: 1950–1951.* Pondicherry, India; Sri Aurobindo Ashram Press.

Mountcastle, V.B. (1974). Sleep, wakefulness, and the conscious state: Intrinsic regulatory mechanisms of the brain. In V.B. Mountcastle (Ed.), *Medical physiology* (13th ed., pp.254–81). St. Louis: C.V. Mosley.

Motoyama, H. (1981). *Theories of the chakras: bridge to higher consciousness.* Wheaton, Illinois: Theosophical Publishing House.

Murphey, M., & Donovan, S. (1988). *The physical and psychological effects of meditation: a review of contemporary meditation research with a comprehensive bibliography (1931–1988).* Big Sur, CA: Esalen Institute Study of Exceptional Functioning.

Nagel, T. (1974). What is it like to be a bat? *The Philosophical Review,* 83, pp.435–50.

Nagel, T. (1979). *Mortal questions.* Cambridge, England: Cambridge University Press.

Natsoulas, T. (1978). Consciousness. *American Psychologist,* 33, pp.906–14.

Natsoulas, T. (1983). Addendum to 'Consciousness.' *American Psychologist,* 38, pp.121f.

Neisser, U. (1982). *Memory observed: remembering in natural contexts.* San Francisco: W.H. Freeman.

Newsletter of the International Society for the Study of Subtle Energies and Energy Medicine. (1990). 1, (1). ISSSEEM, 356 Goldco Circle, Golden, CO, 80401.

Neumann, E. (1954/1973). *The origins and history of consciousness.* Princeton: Princeton University Press.

Nikhilananda, Swami (1977). *The gospel of Sri Ramakrishna.* New York: Ramakrishna-Vivekananda Center.

Norman, D.A., Gentner, D.R., & Stevens, A.L. (1976). Comments on learning schemata and memory representations. In D. Klahr (Ed.), *Cognition and instruction.* Hillsdale, New Jersey: Erlbaum.

O'Flaherty, W.D. (1984). *Dreams, illusions, and other realities.* Chicago: University of Chicago Press.

Otto, W.F. (1954). *The homeric gods.* (M. Hadas, trans.). New York: Pantheon.

Ovid (1955). *Metamorphoses.* (R. Humphries, trans.). Bloomington, Indiana: Indiana University Press.

Pagels, E. (1979). *The gnostic gospels.* New York: Random House.

Pagels, H. (1988). *The dreams of reason: the computer and the rise of the sciences of complexity.* New York: Simon & Schuster.

Patterson, C. (1987). Evolution. In R. L. Gregory, *The Oxford companion to the mind.* (pp. 233–44). Oxford: Oxford University Press.

Pearson, C.S. (1989). *The hero within: six archetypes to live by.* New York: Harper & Row.

Penrose, R. (1989). *The emperor's new mind: concerning computers, minds, and the laws of physics.* Oxford: Oxford University Press.

—, (1984). *Shadows of the mind: a search for the missing science of consciousness*. Oxford: Oxford University Press.

Perry, W.G. (1970). *Forms of intellectual and ethical development in the college years: a scheme*. New York: Holt, Rinehart and Winston.

Polanyi, M. (1958). *Personal knowledge: towards a post-critical philosophy*. Chicago: University of Chicago Press.

Plotinus (1930). *The Enneads*. (S. MacKenna, trans.). London: Oxford University Press.

—, (1992). *The Enneads*. (Trans. S. MacKenna, with comparisons to other translations). Burdett, New York: Larson.

Politzer, G. (1928/1974). *Critique of the foundations of psychology*. Paris: Presses Universitaires de France.

Popper, K.R., & Eccles, J.C. (1977). *The self and its brain*. New York: Springer-Verlag.

Pribram, K.H. (1991). *Brain and perception: holonomy and structure in figural processing*. Hillsdale, NJ: Lawrence Erlbaum.

—, (Ed.), (1993). *Proceedings of the first Appalachian conference on behavioral neurodynamics; Rethinking neural networks: quantum fields and biological data*. Hillsdale, NJ: Lawrence Erlbaum.

—, (Ed.), (1995). *Proceedings of the second Appalachian conference on behavioral neurodynamics; Origins: Brain and self-organization*. Hillsdale, NJ: Lawrence Erlbaum.

Prigogine, I., & Stengers, I. (1984). *Order out of chaos: man's new dialogue with nature*. New York: Bantam.

Progoff, I. (1973). *Jung, synchronicity, and human destiny: acausal dimensions of human experience*. New York: Dell.

Putman, J.J. (1988). The search for modern humans. *National Geographic*, 174, (4), pp.439–77.

Radha, S. (1978). *Kundalini: yoga for the West*. Spokane, Washington: Timeless Books.

Ram Dass. (1979). *Miracle of love: stories about Neem Karoli Baba*. New York: E.D. Dutton. *(See also* Alpert, R.)

Rama, S.S. (1971). *Lectures on yoga*. Honesdale, PA: Himalayan Publishers.

—, (1978). *Living with the Himalayan masters*. Honesdale, PA: Himalayan Publishers.

—, (1981). Energy of consciousness in the human personality. In R. S. Valle and R. von Eckartsberg (Eds.), *The metaphors of consciousness* (pp.315–24). New York: Plenum.

—, (1982). *Enlightenment without God* (Mandukya Upanishad). Honesdale. PA: Himalayan Publishers.

—, (1986). *Path of fire and light: advanced practices of yoga*. Honesdale. PA: Himalayan Publishers.

Rapp, P. (1993). Chaos in the neurosciences: cautionary tales from the frontier. *Biologist*, 40, (2), pp.89–94.

Reber, S.A. (1992). The cognitive unconsciousness: An evolutionary perspective. *Consciousness and Cognition,* 1, pp.93–133.

Reps, P. (1961). *Zen flesh, Zen bones: a collection of Zen and pre-Zen writings.* Garden City, New York: Doubleday.

Richards, J.R. (1987). *Darwin and the emergence of evolutionary theories of mind and behavior.* Chicago: University of Chicago Press.

Robertson, R. (1987, unpublished manuscript). *Computer viruses.*

—, & Combs, A. (Eds.), (1994). *A chaos psychology reader.* Lawrence Erlbaum.

Roland, A. (1988). *In search of self in India and Japan: toward a cross-cultural psychology.* Princeton, New Jersey: Princeton University Press.

Rosenthal, D. (1993). State consciousness and transitive consciousness. *Consciousness and Cognition,* 2, pp.355–63.

Rossi, E. (1986). Altered States of Consciousness in Everyday Life: the Ultradian Rhythms. Wolman & Ullman (Eds.), *Handbook of States of Consciousness.* Van Nostrand, pp.97–131.

Rothenberg, A. (1979). *The emerging goddess: the creative process in art, science, and other fields.* Chicago: University of Chicago Press.

Ruelle, D. (1981). Small random perturbations of dynamical systems and the definition of attractors. *Commun. Math. Phy.,* 82, pp.137–51.

Rumi, J. (1988). *This longing: Poetry, teaching stories, and selected letters.* (C.Barks, & J. Moyne, trans.). Putney, Vermont: Threshold Books.

Sacks, O. (1985). *The man who mistook his wife for a hat: and other clinical tales.* New York: Summett.

—, (1985). A new vision of the mind. In J. Cornwell (Ed.), *Nature's imagination: The frontiers of scientific vision.* Oxford: Oxford University Press.

Sannella, L. (1987). *The kundalini experience: psychosis or transcendence.* Lower Lake, CA: Integral Publishing.

Sartre, J.-P. (1957/1966). *Being and nothingness: An essay on phenomenological ontology.* (H. Barnes, trans.). New York: Washington Square.

—, (1957). *Sketch for a theory of emotions.* (P. Mairet, trans.). London.

Satprem (1970/1984). *Sri Aurobindo: the adventure of consciousness.* (L. Venet, trans.). New York: Institute for Evolutionary Research.

—, (1982). *The mind of the cells.* New York: Institute for evolutionary research.

Sayama, M. (1986). *Samadhi: self development in Zen, swordsmanship, and psychotherapy.* Albany, New York: State University of New York Press.

Schumacher, E.F. (1978). *A guide for the perplexed.* New York: Harper and Row.

Schuon, F. (1981). *Esoterism as principle and as way.* (W. Stoddart, trans.). Middlesex, England: Perennial Books.

Schwaller de Lubicz, R.A. (1949/1978). *Symbol and the symbolic: Ancient Egypt, science, and the evolution of consciousness.* (R. Lawlor & D. Lawlor, trans.). Rochester, Vermont: Inner Traditions.

—, (1958). *Le Temple de l'Homme: Apet du Sud à Louqsor.* Paris: Caractères.

Schwartz, G. (1986). Reported by Rupert Sheldrake, in *The presence of the past,* 1988; New York: Random House.

Searle, J.R. (1980). Minds, brains, and programs. *Behavioral and Brain Sciences,* 3, pp.417–24.

—, (1982). The Chinese Room revisited: response to further commentaries on 'Minds, brains, and programs,' *Behavioral and Brain Sciences,* 5, pp.345–48.

—, (1992). *The recovery of mind.* Cambridge, MA: MIT Press.

—, (1993). The problem of consciousness. *Consciousness and cognition,* 2, pp.310–19.

Settegast, M. (1990). *Plato prehistorian.* Hudson, New York: Lindisfarne Press.

Serrano, M. (1966/1968). *Jung and Hess: a record of two friendships.* New York: Schocken; pp.54f.

Shankara (1947). *The crest-jewel of discrimination.* (Swami Prabhavananda & C. Isherwood, trans.). Hollywood, Ca: Vedanta Press.

Shearer, A. & Russell, P. (trans.), (1978). *The Upanishads.* New York: Harper & Row.

Sheldrake, R. (1981). *A new science of life.* London: Blond & Briggs.

—, (1983). Formative causation: the hythothesis supported. *New Scientist,* October 27, pp.279f.

—, (1987). Part I: Mind, memory and archetypes: Morphic resonance and the collective unconscious. *Psychological Perspectives,* 18, (1), pp.9–25.

—, (1988). *The presence of the past.* New York: Random House.

—, (1991). *The rebirth of nature.* New York: Bantam.

—, & Bohm, D. (1982). Morphogenetic fields and the implicate order; a conversation. *ReVision,* 5, (2), pp.41–48.

Silburn, L. (1988). *Kundalini: the energy of the depths.* (J. Gontier, trans.). Albany, New York: State University of New York Press.

Smith, H. (1982). *Beyond the post-modern mind.* Wheaton, Illinois: Theosophical Pub.

Sobel, J., & Sobel, P. (1984). *The hierarchy of minds: the mind levels; a compilation from the works of Sri Aurobindo and The Mother.* Pondicherry, India: Sri Aurobindo Ashram Press.

Sperry, R.W. (1974). Lateral specialization in the surgically separated hemispheres. In F.O. Schmitt & F.G. Worden (Eds.), *The neurosciences: Third study program* (pp.5–20). Cambridge, MA: MIT Press.

—, (1977). Forebrain commissurotomy and conscious awareness. *Journal of Medicine and Philosophy,* 2, pp.101–15.

—, Zaidel, E., & Zaidel, D. (1979). Self-recognition and social awareness in the deconnected minor hemisphere. *Neuropsychologia,* 17, pp.153–66.

—, (1987). The structure and significance of the consciousness revolution. *The Journal of Mind and Behavior,* 8, pp.37–66.

—, (1993). The impact and promise of the cognitive revolution. *American Psychologist,* 48, pp.878–85.

Sprott, J.C. (1993). *Chaotic attractors: creating patterns in chaos.* New York: M&T Books, Henry Holt.

Staniford, P. (1982). Ken Wilber's transpersonal view of evolution. *Phoenix,* 6, pp.163–66.

Stevens, A. (1993). *The million-year-old self.* College Station, TX: Texas A&M University Press.

Stevenson, I. (1974). *Twenty cases suggestive of reincarnation.* Charlottesville, Virginia: University of Virginia Press.

Stone, J.S. (1977). *Meditation for healing!,* Albuquerque, New Mexico: Sun Books.

Storr, A. (Ed.), (1983). *The essential Jung.* Princeton, New Jersey: Princeton University Press.

Suzuki, D.T. (1952). *Essays in Zen Buddhism* (Second Series), Boston, MA: Beacon Press.

Swenson, R. (1989). Emergent attractors and the law of maximum entropy production: Foundations of a theory of general evolution. *Systems Research,* 6, (3), pp.187–97.

Tarnas, R. (1991). *The passion of the Western mind.* New York: Harmony Books.

Tart, C.T. (1975). *States of consciousness.* New York: E.P. Dutton.

Teilhard de Chardin, P. (1959/1961). *The phenomenon of man.* New York, Harper & Row.

Thompson, W.I. (1978). *Darkness and scattered light.* Garden City, New York: Anchor.

—, (1981). *The time falling bodies take to light: mythology, sexuality, and the origins of culture.* New York: St. Martin's Press.

—, (1989). *Imaginary landscapes: making worlds of myth and science.* New York: St. Martin's Press.

Tigunait, R. (1983). *Seven systems of Indian philosophy.* Honesdale. PA: Himalayan Publishers.

Timpanaro, S. (1976). *The Freudian slip: psychoanalysis and textual criticism.* (K. Soper, trans.). London.

Toshihiko, I. (1987) The Ontological Ambivalence of 'Things' in Oriental Philosophy. In J.E. Charon (Ed.), *The real and the imaginary: a new approach to physics* (pp.187–97). New York: Paragon House.

Travis, R. (1976). Foreword to *The selfish gene,* by R. Dawkins. New York: Oxford University Press. Cited in Augros, R. and Stancui, G. (1988). *The new biology: discovering the wisdom in nature.* Boston: Shambhala.

Trungpa, C. (1984). *Shambhala: the sacred path of the warrior.* Boulder, Colorado: Shambhala. *(See also* Fremantle, F.)

Turner, V. (1967). *The forest of symbols.* Ithaca, New York: Cornell University Press.

Underhill, E. (1911/1961). *Mysticism.* New York: E.P. Dutton.

Uttal, W.R. (1978). *The psychobiology of mind.* Hillsdale, New Jersey: Lawrence Erlbaum.

Vandervert, L.R. (1991). A measurable and testable brain-based interactionism: An alternative to Sperry's mentalist emergent interactionism. *Journal of Mind and Behavior,* 12, pp.201–9.

—, (1992). The emergence of brain and mind amid chaos through maximum-power evolution. *World Futures: The Journal of General Evolution*, 33, pp.253–73.

—, (1993). Neurological Positivism's evolution of mathematics. *Journal of Mind and Behavior*, 14, pp.277–88.

—, (forthcoming). Chaos theory and the evolution of consciousness and mind: A thermodynamic-holographic resolution of the mind-body problem. *New Ideas in Psychology*.

Varela, F.J., Thompson, E., & Rosch, E. (1991). *The embodied mind: cognitive science and human experience*. Cambridge, MA: MIT Press.

Vico, G. (1744/1984). *The new science of Giambattista Vico*. (T.G. Bergin and M.H. Fisch, trans.). Ithaca, New York: Cornell University Press.

von Franz, Marie-Louise. (1979). *Alchemical active imagination*. Dallas: Spring.

Walsh, R.N. (1979). Meditation research: An introduction and review. *Journal of Transpersonal Psychology*, 11, (2), pp.161–74.

Waldrop, M.M. (1992). *Complexity: the emerging science at the edge of order and chaos*. New York: Simon & Schuster.

Washburn, M. (1988). *The ego and the dynamic ground*. State University of New York Press.

—, (1990). Two patterns of transcendence. *Journal of Humanistic Psychology*, 30, (3), pp.84–112.

—, (1994). *Transpersonal psychology in psychoanalytic perspective*. Albany, New York: State University of New York Press.

Welwood, J. (1977). Meditation and the unconscious: A new perspective. *Journal of Transpersonal Psychology*, 9, 1, pp.1–26.

Werntz, D., Bickford, R., Bloom, F., and Shannahoff, D. (1982). Alternating cerebral hemisphere activity and lateralization of autonomic nervous function. *Neurobiology*, 4, pp.225–42.

White, J. (1979). *Kunalini: evolution and enlightenment*. Garden City, New York: Anchor/Doubleday.

Whyte, L. (1979). *The unconsciousness before Freud*. London.

Wilber, K. (1977). *The spectrum of consciousness*. Wheaton Ill.: Quest.

—, (1979). *No boundary: Eastern and Western approaches to personal growth*. Boulder, Colorado: Shambhala.

—, (1980). *The Atman project*. Wheaton, Illinois: Theosophical Publishing House.

—, (1981). *Up from Eden: a transpersonal view of human evolution*. Garden City, New York: Anchor/Doubleday.

—, (1983). *Eye to eye*. New York: Doubleday/Anchor.

—, (1986a). The spectrum of pathology. In K. Wilber, J. Engler, and D.P. Brown (Eds.), (1986) pp.107–26.

—, (1986b). The spectrum of development. In K. Wilber, J. Engler, and D.P. Brown (Eds.), (1986) pp.65–106.

—, (1986c). Treatment modalities. In K. Wilber, J. Engler, and D.P. Brown (Eds.), (1986) pp.127–60.

—, (1987). Ken Wilber: An interview by Catherine Ingram. *Yoga Journal,* 76 (September/October), pp.38–49.

—, (1990). Two patterns of transcendence: a reply to Washburn. *Journal of Humanistic Psychology,* 30, (3), pp.113–36.

Wilber, K. (1995). *Sex, ecology, spirituality: the spirit of evolution.* Boston: Shambhala.

—, Engler, J., & Brown, D.P. (1986). *Transformations of consciousness: traditional and contemplative perspectives on development.* Boston: Shambhala.

Wilhelm, R., (1962). *The secret of the golden flower.* (C.F. Baynes, trans.), New York: Harcourt, Brace & World.

Winkelman, M, (1990). The evolution of consciousness: An essay review of *Up from Eden* (Wilber 1981). *Anthropology of Consciousness,* 1, (4), pp.24–31.

Zangwill, L.O. (1974). *Consciousness and the cerebral hemispheres.* In S.J. Dimond and J.G. Beaumont (Eds.), *Hemisphere function in the human brain.* New York: Halsted Press, Wiley.

Zohar, D. (1990). *The quantum self: human nature and consciousness defined by the new physics.* New York: William Morrow.

Index

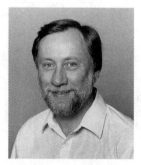